BASH BROTHERS

Other Sports Titles from Potomac Books

The Rocket: Baseball Legend Roger Clemens by Joseph Janczak

Home Run: The Ultimate History of Baseball's Ultimate Weapon by David Vincent

Burying the Black Sox: How Baseball's Cover-up of the 1919 World Series Almost Succeeded by Gene Carney

The Book: Playing the Percentages in Baseball by Tom Tango, Mitchel Lichtman, and Andrew Dolphin

Mickey Mantle: America's Prodigal Son by Tony Castro

BASH BROTHERS

A Legacy Subpoenaed

Dale Tafoya

Potomac Books, Inc.
Washington, D.C.

Library of Congress Cataloging-in-Publication Data
Tafoya, Dale.
  Bash brothers : a legacy subpoenaed / Dale Tafoya. — 1st ed.
    p. cm.
  Includes bibliographical references and index.
  ISBN 978-1-59797-178-2 (hardcover : alk. paper)
  1. McGwire, Mark, 1963– 2. Sosa, Sammy, 1968– 3. Basebal players—United States—Biography. 4. Baseball players—Drug use—United States—History. 5. Doping in sports—United States—History.
I. Title.
  GV865.A1.T34 2008
  796.357092'2—dc22
  [B]

                            2008008982

Printed in the United States of America on acid-free paper that meets the American National Standards Institute Z39-48 Standard.

Potomac Books, Inc.
22841 Quicksilver Drive
Dulles, Virginia 20166

First Edition

10 9 8 7 6 5 4 3 2 1

This book is dedicated to my late, loving father, Daniel Edward Tafoya, who pushed me to complete this once-abandoned project. Thanks for being the best father in the world. I had always anticipated the thrilling moment of one day presenting you the finished product, but fate had other plans. Even in your rest, I hope you're proud, Dad.

CONTENTS

FOREWORD BY FAY VINCENT, FORMER COMMISSIONER OF MAJOR LEAGUE BASEBALL

I came to baseball at about the time two superb players, whose lives are so carefully documented in this book, also burst onto the baseball scene as stars of the Oakland Athletics. Both Mark McGwire and José Canseco were at Candlestick Park in October 1989 when the earthquake hit right before the start of game three of the World Series. They and I were involved in that series and in the next one that the Cincinnati Reds swept in 1990. So, you ask, what are my memories of them and how well did I know them?

To my knowledge, I never met Canseco and McGwire during those years. Perhaps I nodded to them and they to me, but I do not believe we had any kind of conversation. I can recall talking to McGwire only years later at Shea Stadium when I stopped into his clubhouse as I was on my way to chat with Tony La Russa. So what, you say. My point is that they were big stars but not very friendly and perhaps uncertain of how to deal with a commissioner. Others were quite open. I think of Walt Weiss and Carney Lansford especially, as well as Dave Parker and Dave Stewart. In 1989, all of us were waiting to restart the Series, which allowed time for chitchat. It just never happened with Canseco and McGwire.

The book you are about to read is the story of two very different men who played on the same team and whose involvement with performance-enhancing drugs has left them with a confused legacy and an awkward position in the baseball world. Surely they could play and hit. I remember seeing Canseco hit a ball in a play-off game in Toronto that was as hard a hit as anyone there had ever seen. He crushed a ball to left field and then later told the press he had not gotten all of it. Similarly, he and McGwire, with Stewart and Rickey Henderson, led the A's to the sweep in the 1989 Series once we got past the earthquake. The surprise to me is that they only won the World Series once, losing in 1988 and 1990. It was a superb team and they were truly the Bash Brothers. All that and more is here, carefully and even lovingly presented by Dale Tafoya.

As I read this book, I tried to find insights that would explain the many mysteries of these two lives and careers. And there are solid theories and answers here. But the essence of tragedy in the classic Greek dramas is here as well. In those tragedies, the tragic figures, like the two in this drama, struggle against fate, a force they cannot overcome. We watch McGwire and Canseco through the eyes of Tafoya and their teammates as they perform wonderful feats of skill and strength, but we know the outcome. We know the gods win and they will be defeated. But that does not mean this tragedy, like those by the Greeks, is not fascinating. The struggle always is. Especially the most hopeless ones.

As the story told by Tafoya ends, the two protagonists in this drama have themselves been "bashed" by forces they cannot control. I found myself feeling sorry for them in part because I was with them at the peak of their public life and baseball careers, and in part because I believe they never saw the destructive forces coming straight for them. It is their surprise that rings so true and thus enhances the sense of tragedy. Yet, as with all tragedies, there are lessons. And those will continue to play out for these men over the rest of their lives. They are paying a big price for their mistakes. Could they have avoided their fates? I doubt it. But read on, and decide for yourself.

ACKNOWLEDGMENTS

A heart-felt thanks goes out to my Heavenly Father, whose unwavering grace has sustained me. It's been said that if one is obsessed with searching for a particular book, only to discover that none exists, then fate has appointed *that person* to write the book. That's what inspired me. Words can't describe my four-year affair with this once-abandoned project. Rejection discouraged me. When I stumbled into my literary agent, Michael Hamilburg of the Mitchell J. Hamilburg Agency in 2006, he believed in this book and shared his enthusiasm with publishers. Kevin Cuddihy, an acquisitions editor at Potomac Books, Inc., believed in *Bash Brothers*, too. That formula molded and birthed this manuscript into existence. Thank you, Michael, for allowing my subject and writing to overshadow my low profile. Many thanks, Kevin, for your patience and guidance through foreign territory. Thank you, Frank Sanello, for relentless encouragement and injecting your wealth of experience into me.

To the greatest mom and best cook in the world, Vera; God couldn't have chosen a better mother for me. To my grandmother, Connie C. Garcia, who prayed into existence everything I am. To my late grandmother, Primitiva Lafoya, who showered me with unflinching love growing up; words can't describe my appreciation. To my wonderful brothers, Ricky and Robbie, my bash brothers, you're my anchors. To Robbie: you're a great father and I'm so proud of you. To Ricky, I deeply appreciate your wisdom you offered me over the years. The way you can light up a room is truly special. To Tina and Nika, great sister-in-laws, thanks for putting up with my brothers and raising my awesome nephews and nieces. To my cousin Markie, even though we don't talk much, we'll always be best friends. To Keith and Nicole: thanks for your unwavering support. To my aunt and uncle, Christine and Larry

Lopez, God-fearing role models whom I admire: Thanks for your guidance through the recent years. To Larry: Thank you for shouldering my brothers and I through our recent tragedy. We will never forget your refreshing aid during our emotional need. To Armando and Josephine Peraza: Thanks for making my father's final years so fulfilling; and taking us under your wing. To my uncle Dennis: Thanks for always offering sound advice and taking me to A's games when I was a boy. To family and friends I failed to mention, you're not forgotten in my heart.

INTRODUCTION

"They've got a chance to be the best [duo] there ever was. If they stay healthy and if they stay together for 10 or 15 years, I don't see how anybody could be as good as they are."

—Former Oakland A's third base coach Rene Lachemann
October 1988

Nineteen eighty-eight. Mark McGwire had been slamming the weights for over an hour. The weight room, in the bowels of the Oakland-Alameda Coliseum and steps from the A's clubhouse, had been his haven. At six foot five, 220 pounds, and strutting rock-like forearms, McGwire had beefed up the lanky frame he carried during his rookie season in 1987. Stretched across his t-shirt screamed, No Mercy. He stole that phrase from his brother-in-law's bowling team and wore the t-shirt underneath his jersey during each game. Beyond sliding it on, however, he internalized the fearless spirit of the phrase. That attitude intensified his workouts in the weight room and performance on the field.

Moments later, José Canseco strolled into the gym. At six foot four, 230 pounds, he was a twenty-four-year-old oddity. His chiseled face, biceps of steel, and trim waist had once prompted Tigers manager Sparky Anderson to hail him as a "Greek goddess." Observers, though, understood what Anderson meant. In Anderson's four decades of baseball, the sport hadn't seen such an Adonis. Yet Canseco hadn't lifted weights for over two weeks—the hiatus hadn't deflated his strength. He slid on the bench press and lifted "everything in the building," according to former teammate Dave Parker.

McGwire shook his head in disbelief. "You make me sick," he sarcastically barked at his foil.

Seventeen years later, however, the mood wasn't so casual. On

xiii

March 17, 2005, with Americans glued to their televisions and curious congressmen sitting on the dais, glaring down at both and sharpening their inquiries, the muscle-bound duo once dubbed the Bash Brothers marched before the House Government Reform Committee.

Without adoring cheers and a glistening baseball field on which to find shelter, McGwire and Canseco were the subjects of an investigation that questioned the legitimacy of their careers and, ultimately, our National Pastime. Drugs, muscles, accusations, greed, and hypocrisy headlined the agenda. The home run, the celebrated feat that personified their careers, had ironically led them before Congress.

Facing this knee-buckling task, both braced themselves for a different kind of heat. Even voices from their past sensed the silent tension that hovered over the crammed room in the Rayburn House Office Building. "I felt so uncomfortable," remembered Hall of Fame closer Dennis Eckersley, who watched the congressional hearings on television. "It was awful."

"That was the saddest day I had ever spent in sports—without a doubt," admitted Andy Dolich, the marketing force behind the Oakland A's during the 1980s and '90s.

"It bothered me," recalled former A's strength and conditioning coach Dave McKay. "I knew Mark's program, how he took care of himself, and I knew he was uncomfortable there."

"I felt bad for both of them," said George Mitterwald, who managed both when they first teamed professionally in Single-A Modesto in 1984. "It was sad."

"It's a shame it had to come to that point," said Keith Lieppman, who managed them with the Triple-A Tacoma Tigers in 1985–86. "I felt sorry for them."

Some claim that if the Bash Brothers hadn't transformed the game, someone else would have. Unprecedented power, shattered home-run records, and million-dollar lifestyles, generated by slabs of muscle, would have eventually lured any player into the weight room. Other skeptics, hoping to downplay the duo's role, insist that they were nothing more than two burly power hitters who had coincidentally headlined the same lineup for parts of eight seasons. After all, there had been prolific, heavy-hitting duos sprinkled throughout baseball history. In the 1920s, the legendary duo Babe Ruth and Lou Gehrig highlighted the New York Yankees lineup. Three decades later, in the 1950s, Eddie Matthews and Hank Aaron clobbered 863 home runs while teammates for the Milwaukee Braves. The following decade, the 1960s produced heavy-hitting tandems Mickey Mantle and Roger Maris, and Willie Mays and Willie McCovey. One could imagine what those iconic sluggers would have accomplished if they had played in today's supplement-fueled era, which players dub, The Show.

Still, the Bash Brothers, Mark McGwire and José Canseco, ushered a unique brand of player into baseball. After each muscled a tape-measure home run, their ruggedly animated forearm bash at home plate became a swaggering endorsement for strength and testosterone. In Canseco and McGwire, bodybuilding—with all its vanity and supplements—had infected baseball.

"Up until that era, it was considered taboo to lift weights. They were two of the first [sluggers] who proved you can be buff and muscular and still be productive," said Ron Kroichick, who covered the A's for the *Sacramento Bee* from 1990 to 1994. "It was unlike anything the game had seen. Much like Goose Gossage brought intimidation to the mound, they brought it to the plate."

Ripped physiques, mysterious supplements, and personal trainers soon crept into the highly competitive baseball culture. Extensive state-of-the-art weight-training facilities had also emerged in every major league stadium. That muscled-up formula altered the game beginning in the late 1980s.

"They played a big role in the way the game changed," said former teammate Mike Davis. "Prior to Canseco and McGwire, none of the major league teams really had weight rooms. After them, every player started going to weights."

By the late 1980s, Canseco and McGwire merged into one phrase, like Smith & Wesson and Proctor & Gamble. Headlining posters, t-shirts, and magazines, the duo became one of baseball's feature attractions.

"It was like traveling with a rock band with thousands of fans in each city, in the hotel lobby and at the ballpark," former A's public relations director Jay Alves said in a 2004 email. "We set road attendance records. Many times we had to enter hotels through the back entrance." Teammate Greg Cadaret recalled the phenomenon: "It was a cult following. They were a hip and flashy West Coast duo that played in the World Series and attracted a lot of fans."

On the East Coast, players like Mickey Tettleton, a once light-hitting catcher who played for the Oakland A's from 1984-1987, bulked up and bolstered his home-run production with Baltimore and Detroit. Tettleton, who hit only twenty-two home runs during his first four seasons with Oakland, clubbed 224 over his next nine. That power earned him two All-Star Game appearances in 1989 and 1994. "It [weight lifting] helps late in the season," Tettleton told *USA Today* in 1997. "When you feel sluggish, it makes you feel like you have a little left in your gas tank."[1] But it also helped him smash colossal home runs. In 1991, during one week, he crushed two home runs that cleared

Tiger Stadium. Said one former teammate of Tettleton, "I remember when he was getting bigger and I was thinking, 'man, he's getting huge.'"

Five years later, his former teammate in Baltimore, lead-off hitter Brady Anderson, at age thirty two, attributed weight lifting and the over-the-counter nutritional supplement creatine monohydrate to his ripped six-foot-one, 185-pound physique. That combination, he said, also fueled his fifty-home-run season in 1996. In 1997, Thomas Boswell of the *Washington Post* wrote, "A few weeks ago, Yankees shortstop Derek Jeter encountered Anderson near the batting cage. Jeter just started laughing. 'Fifty homers and 110 RBI from a leadoff guy,' was all he said. Then he walked away."[2]

The bodybuilding movement spread. Player by player, team by team, and from weight room to weight room, players added strength and transformed their physiques. While many players camouflaged their steroid use with nutritional supplements, such as creatine, some weren't that naïve. Steroid use "wouldn't surprise me," San Francisco Giants general manager Brian Sabean told *USA Today* in 1997. "If it gives somebody an edge, guys are going to use it. Look how it's affected other sports. We'd really have our head in the sand if we thought it wasn't here in baseball."[3]

Either through steroids or natural means, several mediocre players soared to new heights and a few already talented ones reached stardom by adding muscle and acquiring strength. That left unparalleled greatness reserved for those naturally gifted. That transformation showered them with millions.

Jason Giambi, a slim, sweet-swinging, free-spirited rising star for the Oakland Athletics, pounded the weights. Soon, his sizzling line-drive doubles that pierced the right-center-field alley gained wings and trajectory, soaring over the fence. In 2000, he blasted forty-three home runs, capturing the American League's Most Valuable Player award. After the 2001 season, he signed a seven-year, $117 million contract with the New York Yankees.

Mike Piazza, a sixty-second-round draft pick by the Los Angeles Dodgers in 1988, climbed through the minor leagues and gained freakish strength. As a right-handed slugger, his booming home runs toward right field arched eyebrows and became his trademark. With his powerful wrists, when the ball met his bat there was a unique-sounding explosion. In 1999, he signed a seven-year, $91 million contract with the New York Mets.

Sammy Sosa soon curled dumbbells and caught the wave in 1993. Over the next thirteen seasons, he averaged forty-two home runs. That's a staggering increase compared to the ten he averaged during his first seven seasons in professional baseball beginning in 1986. As Sosa's back widened, so did his wallet. In 1997, Sosa inked a four-year, $42.5 million contract with the Chicago Cubs, becoming the third highest player in baseball at the time.

Barry Bonds added slabs of muscle and morphed into arguably the greatest slugger of all time. Bonds, the son of former All-Star Bobby Bonds, the cousin of Hall of Famer Reggie Jackson, and the godson of the legendary Willie Mays, was groomed for greatness. Before his transformation and rigorous tear-dropping battles with weights in the gym, he had already been destined for Cooperstown. But complementing his polished swing and astute approach was his strength that propelled him past the forefathers of the game. In 2001, he slammed seventy-three home runs, shattering the single season record of seventy, established by Mark McGwire three seasons earlier. After that season, he inked a five-year, $90 million contract with the San Francisco Giants.

Before those players, though, bench-pressed their way through the new millennium and earned millions, the Bash Brothers pioneered the movement during the 1980s. Silencing decades of tradition that insisted weight lifting did more harm than good for a player, both proved muscle *could* elevate them to superstardom. Bill Bathe, a former teammate in the minor leagues and major leagues, christened both as the forefathers of a new era that whirled through every level of baseball. "They had a big impact on baseball," said Bathe. "They had a huge affect on high school and college players who wanted to emulate them during that era."

Their trailblazing fame, however, didn't only compel their peers to the weight room; it also translated on the field. From the time both barged into the major leagues to their retirement in 2001, home-run totals increased by thirty percent. Though one may blame that increase on the juiced balls, expansion teams' watered-down pitching, and hitter-friendly stadiums, the Bash Brothers ignited that era. "They changed baseball," said former A's television broadcaster Greg Papa. "They brought the Incredible Hulk into baseball—that humongous player that thrived. They may have not been the very first [weight lifters] in the sport, but they were the most obviously noticed by the rest of baseball."

Fans took notice, too. They crammed onto the left-field bleachers two hours before game-time to watch them take their ferocious cuts in the batting cage. When Canseco and McGwire strutted into the cage, players stopped stretching, reporters stopped writing.

Everyone watched. "They hit balls during batting practice like it was fucking Little League," said Eckersley. "It was intimidating." One by one, both hammered tape-measure home runs into uncharted territory, drawing standing ovations from fans. Such a spectacle over-shadowed the game itself. Perhaps no other duo commanded such silence.

"Back to back, they hit eleven hundred feet worth of home runs on two pitches in one inning in Detroit," marveled former batting coach Bob Watson. "As a hitting coach, you shake your head and say, 'my goodness.'"

That the San Francisco Bay Area boasted such a celebrated duo seemed appropriate. Across the Bay, San Francisco 49ers quarterback Joe Montana heaved his way into Bay Area hearts. His accomplice, legendary wide receiver Jerry Rice, thrilled millions by slanting and snatching down field. The duo fueled the 49ers to four Super Bowl Championships. But it was the 1980s that ushered in other greats: A tongue-hanging Michael Jordon of the Chicago Bulls electrified auditoriums by demonstrating mind-blowing slam-dunks; the twenty-year-old Iron Mike Tyson invaded boxing rings and ferociously roughed up opponents, becoming the youngest heavyweight champion ever; and hockey icon Wayne Gretzky scored his way to superstardom.

In Oakland, Canseco and McGwire climbed through the minor leagues and entertained players and fans by slamming head-scratching, game-swaying home runs. "You will probably never have two of the more dominating players together coming up like that again," said Dave Wilder, the senior director of player personnel for the Chicago White Sox.

But encountering superstardom, flaunting beefcake physiques, and muscling the Oakland Athletics to three straight World Series appearances, including a championship in 1989, can lead to a colorful lifestyle. Away from the stadium, the spending sprees, fast cars, and provocative woman awaited Canseco and McGwire. At the venue, relentless reporters and adoring fans hounded them.

"They were not very easy guys to deal with," said former baseball commissioner Fay Vincent. "Neither one of them were very friendly to me. I would see them on the field and they were kind of distant. Maybe they were a little concerned, I don't know. They weren't very outgoing. Maybe they were worried; they knew they weren't doing things terribly right."

Yet, despite their fame echoing through stadiums across the country, there couldn't have been a more opposite pair of teammates. Canseco, a Miami-groomed maverick, relished the spotlight, while McGwire, a reserved, all-American athlete, shunned it. Teammates they were; brothers they were not. "They were two different people and hung out with two different crowds," said Dave McKay. "They didn't have a lot in common other than playing on the same team. They certainly weren't workout partners. Absolutely not."

But even contradicting personalities, shocking allegations, and a stomach-turning breakup before Congress couldn't rip their names apart. Their names will forever be traced to an era when power and an obsession for greatness doctored the game. "They revolutionized the game," said FOX Sports International baseball analyst José Tolentino, who played with both in the A's minor league system.

Yet, to some, the Bash Brothers foreshadowed baseball's fate. What Canseco and McGwire provided for the A's in the 1980s and '90s is what performance-enhancing drugs provided for baseball after the 1994 strike that canceled the Fall Classic; they revived sluggish fan-interest and resurrected a frail institution into a thriving empire. "They were the face of our franchise," said Sandy Alderson, the former general manager of the Oakland A's.

Meet the Bash Brothers.

NOTES

[1] Pete Williams, "Lifting the Game," *USA Today*, May 7, 1997.

[2] Thomas Boswell, "Late Bloomer—Brady Anderson Has Gotten Better, Later, Than Anybody in Baseball History," *Washington Post*, March 30, 1997.

[3] Pete Williams, "Lifting the Game," *USA Today*, May 7, 1997.

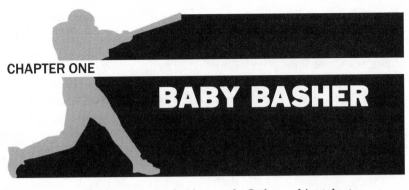

CHAPTER ONE

BABY BASHER

*"Mark was not afraid to work. God gave him talent,
but he worked hard, and that set him apart. God gives
everyone talent. Mark did something with his."*

—Tom Carroll, former Damien High School Baseball Coach
April 2004

If a birth can best foreshadow a legacy, it was Mark David McGwire's.

Ushered into this world and hatched into baseball's grandest nest, the World Series, Mark had no choice. If he had that choice, he might have chosen a birth during The Masters, one of the PGA Tour's most coveted tournaments. But on October 1, 1963, John and Ginger McGwire introduced their second son, Mark, to the world. And on that day, Pomona, California, a suburb scraping the eastern edge of Los Angeles County, became his birthplace.

Eighty years earlier, the city ushered in another phenomena, the citrus-growing industry. Named after the ancient Roman goddess of fruit in the 1870s, the city later blossomed into the worldwide anchor of the citrus market. During that time, shipments of oranges were trucked from Pomona throughout the country, sparking the appetite for California citrus.[1] That oranges once bolstered the economy of Pomona Valley and transformed the community makes the arrival of its freckle-faced redhead even more fitting. On that Tuesday, fate couldn't have picked a more exhilarating time. That week, the hometown heroes, the Los Angeles Dodgers, pummeled their long-time nemesis, the New York Yankees, in a swift four-game sweep to capture the World Series, rousing the Southern California region.

For John and Ginger, however, no celebration matched the joy they felt over their newest son. John, a dentist, and Ginger, a devoted community worker, had met and courted in Seattle during his studies at

1

the University of Washington School of Dentistry. Ginger served as a nurse for two of John's instructors.[2] They later married. Shortly after John graduated in 1963, he planted his practice in the Los Angeles suburb of Claremont. Nestled in a cozy, neighborhood cul-de-sac on Siena Court is where the couple raised their boys: Mike, Mark, Bobby, Dan, and J.J. "They were very invested in their kids," remembered late legendary University of Southern California baseball coach Rod Dedeaux. "We had parent groups and they were very active and unselfish. It wasn't just about [Mark]; every boy on the ball club was one of their boys."

Neighborhood kids felt their warmth, too. Randy Robertson, a childhood friend of Mark's who later competed against him in Little League, played with the boys at the community park in Claremont and enjoyed the hospitality of the couple. "They were very nice and open parents that welcomed anyone into their home," said Robertson. "They were very pleasant and friendly."

One of those neighborhood friends, Scott Larson, remembered climbing up the stairs and playing with Mark in his room. From decorative wallpaper, sheets, and bedspreads to a baseball glove, soccer ball, basketball, and golf clubs, his room was a carnival of sports equipment.

> Mark would be running everywhere in his Adidas sweat suit. He took a lot of pride in the way he looked. We spent a lot of time in his back yard and in the swimming pool. We had a blast. They were way ahead of their time, which was kind of nice because that introduced us all to things we probably would have never done. They were very clean, proper, and well-mannered kids. Those guys had bright red hair. Back then we played a lot of basketball, but Mark couldn't jump.

Robertson, Larson, and Mark mingled around the neighborhood and competed in several sports and activities. With Mark and his brothers befriending other kids, the McGwire's home became a haven and hangout. Seeing friends strolling in the house—without knocking—was not unusual. Once they entered, they watched television, gobbled snacks, and scheduled their entertainment for the day. "Everyone was welcomed," said Robertson. "Having five boys, they had tons of food and soft drinks. We made ourselves at home."

Perhaps that warmth stemmed from John's excruciating childhood. As a boy, he had confronted a fierce challenge. In 1944, in Spokane, Washington, seven-year-old John had been diagnosed with polio, a disease that destroys nerve cells, sometimes causing muscles, mainly legs, to whither and eventually become floppy.[3] Children under five are the most vulnerable to the disease. During the 1940s, the epidemic soared every summer and worried many parents. In 1998, John detailed his battle with polio to *Sports Illustrated's* Rick Reilly for the September issue. "I just collapsed. I was seven years old, walking across the floor of our house, and my legs just gave way."[4]

The disease left John hospitalized and bedridden for several months, eventually forcing him to walk with a limp and wear a brace. Since a polio vaccine had yet to be discovered, John was transferred to another hospital, isolated from other patients. Even his mother couldn't visit him, which forced him to peek through his room window and communicate with her on the sidewalk. John soon battled back and recovered, so much that he later boxed in college and became an avid bicyclist. He also became a dedicated father. "You'd never know he had any kind of disability," said Robertson. "He was always walking and active with his kids. You'd look past the limp. That never seemed to be a deterrent to him."

How John never felt sorry for himself nor allowed his disadvantages to ruin his outlook on life motivated Mark through his darkest moments. In September 1996, Mark expressed his admiration of John to the *Kansas City Star*.

You look at my father, and he didn't have a chance to be an athlete because he was stricken with polio when he was seven years old, mine is really meaningless compared to his life. . . . He has to use a cane. His leg is bowed out, and he has to use a knee brace. But he's dealt with it great. When he was younger, he used to box a lot. But he never had the chance to find out if he could have been a baseball player, a basketball player or football player.[5]

Because his condition prevented him from playing most rigorous sports, John stumbled into golf. He soon gravitated to the sport and injected it into all his boys. Dragging them to the fairways, the boys shared clubs and developed their stroke. Mark quickly became enthralled with the sport, too. Heaving his dad's golf bag over his shoulder, he caddied for him on the course. Once he learned from his dad how to grip a club, he chased his newest passion. "Mark could hit the ball a long way," said Robertson. "The whole family played golf, even Ginger. It was something that the family could do together, unlike baseball or football."

With a putting green strategically placed in his backyard, Mark honed his short game. Besides putting the ball, though, Mark appreciated another component of the game. "The thing I liked about golf was that you were the only one to blame when something went wrong," Mark once said.

Golf dominated the household and became an integral part of their lifestyle. John, however, exposed his boys to an array of athletics, including football, basketball, soccer, and baseball. He also passed along some gifted genes. The boys sprouted and carried their tall, lanky frame into several sports.

Mike, the senior of the bunch, played soccer on the varsity team for Claremont High. He became a psychologist and earned a finance degree. Bobby, John's third son, played golf for Damien High and became a contractor. Dan, the tallest at six foot eight, starred as a quarterback for San Diego State and played for the Seattle Seahawks for four years, while the youngest, J.J., starred on the varsity football team for Claremont High and later pursued competitive bodybuilding. Besides Mark, none of them played baseball.

"I was the only brother who played baseball," said Mark in an interview with the *Minneapolis-St. Paul Star Tribune* in September 1998. "I don't know why—it's just the sport that got to me. I thought football was a waste of time. I liked the idea of having a game every day, watching the Dodgers and the Angels, and not living too far from those two stadiums."[6]

Mark enjoyed life and respected people. His easy-going and cheerful spirit sprung from his positive upbringing. Robertson never witnessed Mark throw a tantrum or become angry with anyone. "He was always laughing and in a good mood," recalled Robertson. "He was a happy-go-lucky kid and loved to hang out with people. He was just having fun. That can be attributed to his dad, John, who was always an easy-going and nice guy."

Larson felt Mark's fun-loving, gentle, and likeable persona attracted a variety of people. "He always had the bigger clique of friends, it seemed," said Larson. "He was a gentle giant with a sense of humor and that stood out amongst the other boys."

John coached Mark in Little League and his dedication was felt by the entire team. After Little League games at College Park field, John would linger in the parking lot until the final child found a ride home. Watching his own boys play sports, though, delighted him the most. After games, the boys scrambled around the diamond, sliding on the infield dirt, staining their uniforms. Mark didn't have much reason to slide, though. On the field, he spent most of his time trotting around the bases.

At age ten, Mark clubbed a home run in his first at-bat for his team, the A's. But since his parents were on vacation, he was forced to wait an entire week before he could tell them. "I started in Little League when I was eight years old. At ten, eleven, and twelve, I played in the major division and ironically, I played on the A's," Mark told *Junior*

BASEBALL Magazine in 1996. "I wore green and gold as a kid and I'm still wearing green and gold as a big-leaguer."[7]

Three years later, he shattered Claremont American Little League's home-run record with thirteen. "I guess that really set the tone for him," said Ginger, who served as the team mom. But behind his home runs in Little League, Mark battled nearsightedness, an eye condition that blurs vision from far distances. The symptoms began pestering his life and play. One game, while pitching on the mound, he struggled with his control and walked several batters. John sadly strolled to the mound and replaced him and moved him to shortstop. When he moved to shortstop, the fuzziness he experienced continued. His inability to see things clearly convinced Ginger to make an appointment for him with an optometrist. Robertson recalled Mark's eyesight struggles. "He had problems and always had to get different prescriptions," said Robertson. "But in high school and college, he began wearing contact lenses."

Years later, while playing with the Oakland Athletics, Mark met Stephen Johnson, a Bay Area-based optometrist, who had treated other players on the team. Mark had problems seeing the spin on the ball, so Johnson explored some treatment options. He finally found one.

He had a lot of nearsightedness combined with an extreme amount of astigmatism. So I designed some custom-made, soft contact lenses that significantly improved his quality of vision. We went through several designs in order to realize the best quality of vision. We tinted the lenses yellow and it helped him pick up the spin on the ball better. His prescription was difficult to say the least.

When Mark was traded and played for the St. Louis Cardinals in 1997, he hopped on a plane and continued treatment at Johnson's San Ramon, California, office. "He was very dedicated and had a very good work ethic. He would come into the office whenever he needed to re-fit," said Johnson.

In 1975, at age twelve, Mark attended La Puerta Middle School. Nestled in an affluent area on Forbes Avenue and across the street from the McGwire home, the intimate school carried 250 students and thirteen teachers. One of the teachers, David Fletcher, taught Mark in a seventh grade biology class. "He was an average student. He earned a C. Even though he was taller than the other students, he was never a bully," said Fletcher, who also had Mark's older brother, Mike, in a science class. "We had a burrito machine in the cafeteria and he would wait patiently for his turn in line. He was shy and never got into trouble."

Mark did create headaches for opponents in sports, though. Fletcher also coached Mark in basketball and flag football during a city league and remembered his relentless desire to win. Capitalizing on his size and nose for the ball, Fletcher planted him as quarterback on the football field and center on the basketball court. Even when Fletcher occasionally caught Mark on television later in his career, he spotted the same competitiveness.

> He didn't like to lose—he had intensity in his eyes. On the court, you can give him the basketball and he could lay it in because he was so tall. The last play of the city championship, we were tied and had a few seconds left on the clock, and I told the players to get it into Mark and let him do the lay-in.

Three years later, Mark barged into Claremont High, the local public school. He played football and basketball with Robertson. "He was a big guy," said Robertson, who was forced to guard him on the court during practice. "Back then, no team really had any six-foot-ten guys, so his size was pretty big." But during his first semester at Claremont, he had some friction with the freshman basketball coach. He couldn't see himself playing for the basketball program and was lured to another school.

The next semester he enrolled at Damien High, a private, all-boys Catholic school five miles from his home. The school happened to be Claremont's archrival. "He transferred to play basketball," said Jack Helber, one of Claremont's teachers who later coached him during American Legion ball. "The freshman coach there [Claremont] was not really a basketball guy and the varsity one was kind of passive, not really a go-to guy."

Impressed by its sports program, he marched on the campus and towered over his classmates. At six foot three, he took his size and leaped back to the basketball court. He also enjoyed the change of scenery. Mark starred for his new team as center and shouldered them to the final four of the Division II Southern Section. "He was one of our big men underneath the basket," said Tom Carroll, former baseball coach at Damien. "He was just a good basketball player and did a great job for us."

Because of Mark's size and dominance, his basketball coach, Mike LeDuc, was convinced that he should concentrate fully on basketball play year-round. Every summer LeDuc tried to persuade Mark to commit to basketball, but he wanted to play both sports, according to Helber.

Starring in every sport didn't always come easy for Mark. His prep career was peppered with injuries. As a freshman, he suffered a back injury that hampered his baseball season. A year later, he injured his chest and arm and was sidelined for part of the season. The next year, as a junior, he hurt his knee. Those perpetual injuries drew whispers as to whether he could stay healthy enough to play *any* sport. During his sophomore year, Mark faced another letdown. After starring in Little League at every level, he couldn't crack the varsity squad. Although that discouraged him, he swallowed his pride and began the season with the junior varsity team. His season was cut short, though, when he pulled a chest muscle and was sidelined. During that period, he grabbed his golf clubs and strolled to the links. The injury confirmed his desire to quit baseball. "I was tired of playing baseball and wanted to take a break," Mark once said.

Those words were music to the ears of Jim Obrien, Damien's golf coach, who also lived in Claremont and attended church with the McGwire family. He watched Mark grow up and not only admired his passion for golf but also his stroke. So Obrien asked for Carroll's permission to use him on the golf team during his hiatus. Carroll gave the go-ahead. Taking a sabbatical from baseball, Mark whittled his handicap down to four and fueled Damien's golf team to a league title in 1979. Mark's success on the links wasn't surprising to Carroll. If Mark couldn't find a career in the majors, Carroll figured that, besides his stroke, he exuded the perfect temperament for golf. Despite his success on the fairways, Mark felt compelled to return to baseball. In an interview with Ken Burns of *USA WEEKEND* magazine in 1999, Mark explained:

> I didn't play baseball for a whole year and I really missed it. And I heard it through the grapevine there was some people who wanted to know why I didn't play my sophomore year. They thought I had the talent to play major league baseball, and at the time I never even thought about it. And then all of a sudden I started missing the game. And I said I was going to start playing it again because there is a possibility that I can start playing this professionally and that was the day I started working hard.

He returned to baseball in 1980 and finally made the varsity team as a junior. But this time he made the most of his opportunity. Although he always displayed spurts of power growing up, he focused on pitching. He pitched and anchored Damien's pitching staff, showing glimpses of his potential and hurling them to a league title. "I hit, but I didn't care about hitting," Mark once said. "I cared about pitching. That's all I wanted to do."

Mark stepped up his game during his senior year in 1981. On the pitcher's mound, he overpowered. At the plate, he displayed explosive power. That combination lured a trove of professional scouts to the games where he played. Dominating on the mound and at the plate, he transformed into double threat. Scott Larson witnessed firsthand Mark's eye-opening power. "We were in awe of some of the balls he'd hit," marveled Larson. "There was never any doubt that he was going to hammer the ball."

Besides blasting the ball, Mark was one of the hardest workers on the team. Through his strenuous work ethic, he led by example, though he was perceived as quiet and reserved. After practice, he took extra swings in the batting cage and honed his pitching mechanics on the side. The added practice was attributed to his high demands of himself. Those demands impressed Carroll. "Mark was not afraid to work," said Carroll. "God gave him talent, but he worked hard, and that set him apart. God gives everyone talent. Mark did something with his."

The extra work paid off for Mark, especially on the mound. His pitching abilities overshadowed his powerful swing. He developed faster as a pitcher than hitter. As a pitcher, he embraced the adrenaline rush of controlling the pace of the game. As scouts flocked to the games, they pulled out radar guns and marveled. If he had a chance to land in the major leagues, it appeared pitching would be his ticket. "What impressed me was his composure and how good of a control pitcher he was," said Carroll.

Those qualities molded him into a promising pitching prospect. However, scout Dick Wiencek, who was sniffing for talent for the Detroit Tigers in 1980 and lived only four blocks from the McGwire family, wasn't so convinced. "I saw him in high school, but I didn't like him as a pitcher," said Wiencek. "He was about a fifth-rounder. His talent was to hit—not pitch."

Mark's ideal pitching frame, along with a commanding fastball, intrigued other scouts. Yet his fierce competitiveness and intimidating delivery frightened opposing batters. Carroll said Mark's extreme high kick on the mound and exaggerated stride toward the plate created the illusion that he was nearly hovering over the plate as he released the ball. That scared hitters. Word of his pitching abilities began to spread. One night Mark pitched at Ralph Welch Park in Pomona. With several scouts sprinkled throughout the stands, he unleashed his fastball and shocked scouts. "He's throwing the damn ball over 90 mph tonight," one stunned scout yelled at Carroll.

His talent didn't stop on the mound, however. When Mark wasn't pitching, he hammered breathtaking home runs. His bat began powering Damien to victory and forced Carroll to play him everyday.

Carroll soon inserted him as a designated hitter when he wasn't pitching. Carroll wondered why he didn't recognize his dangerous bat earlier. "We just didn't want him to get hurt because he was the mainstay of our staff," Carroll admitted.

Shortly thereafter, Mark mentioned to Carroll he could play first base, too. Carroll inserted him there when he wasn't pitching. The extra at-bats helped him. Mark was maturing as a hitter and still learning the strike zone. He didn't take many pitches and ripped away. Still, his sizzling bat generated a buzz and attracted major interest. During his junior year, Mark was invited to play for the Claremont Cardinals, an American Legion summer club. "We recruited him as a first baseman and hitter," said Jack Helber, who managed the team. "His pitching was the third part of the package. We knew we were getting a guy who could pitch, but we wanted him as a hitter."

And Mark obliged. For two summers, he traveled around surrounding states and blistered home runs in tournaments, luring scouts to the games. His talent to smoke a baseball impressed Helber far more than his mediocre heater. "He was one of our regular starters in the rotation, and I guess, with his size, I might have expected an outstanding fastball. He was imposing on the hill, but I still feel he was developing," Helber said.

According to childhood friend and teammate, Randy Robertson, during a game, he blasted a home run into another county. The ball traveled out of the McKenna College ballpark, over the Cypress trees, passed Claremont Boulevard in Los Angeles County, and bounced onto a nearby street that entered San Bernardino County. "At our field, there's a prevailing wind blowing out to left field about 3:00 everyday, so his high, booming home runs got a lot of help," chuckled Helber.

Helber also remembers spearheading a road trip to Ogden, Utah, where the team was scheduled to play in a round-robin tournament. As the team bus passed through Baker, California, near the Blood Baker Grade, an area noted for its staggering head-on collisions, the brakes gave out. With the team scheduled to play its first game the following night, Helber used the emergency brake and nursed the bus to a nearby twenty-four-hour Shell station at midnight. But after the mechanic checked the bus, Helber received some grim news. "We were going to have to leave it there for three days for repair," said Helber.

Draped with uncertainty, the team slept overnight at a Holiday Inn, while Helber pondered his options. He found one in Claremont. When John and Ginger heard the news from their home, they offered their own van to transport the team the rest of the way. Mark's brother, Mike, then scurried the van to the team and flew back the following day. Gathering a few more cars, the team crammed in and again departed for Ogden. "Because Mark and I were the older guys on the team, we helped drive the team all night," said Robertson.

When the team finally arrived, however, they had missed the first game and barely made the second one. The team rushed onto the parking lot, dressed into their uniforms, and hopped on the field, but it was too late. Tournament officials forced them to forfeit the game. His club lost their second game, too. That meant the team would have little room for error the remainder of the week-long tournament. One more loss could send them home, a sour ending to an exhausting road trip. Mark wouldn't let that happen, though. Batting against Ogden, the team that hosted the tournament and had them forfeit its first game, Mark clubbed a game-winning home run to win the tournament. "I thought that was just desserts," chuckled Helber. "We didn't lose another game and won the tournament."

But it was at the Pomona Elks Tournament that spring where Mark sparked the interest of Art Mazmanian, the legendary head baseball coach at Mount San Antonio Junior College in Walnut, California. Since Damien was one of the twenty-four high schools in his district, Mazmanian went to the tournament and hoped to scope local talent. He found it that night. "He pitched and I was very impressed," remembered Mazmanian, who coached at Mt. SAC for thirty-one years. "But I knew we weren't going to get him because he could play for a Division I school."

That didn't calm his enthusiasm. Mazmanian was so stirred about Mark's pitching future, he approached John and Ginger after the game. He assured them he would alert the University of Southern California. Later that evening, he phoned one of his best friends, Marcel Lachemann, the University of Southern California pitching coach who lived around the corner from him. As a high schooler, Lachemann had pitched for Mazmanian and both remained close. "I told him, 'You have to see this boy, McGwire,' and they called him and eventually recruited him," said Mazmanian. "That was the only time I had ever seen the kid pitch in high school."

The same year Carroll bumped into Lachemann at Anaheim Stadium. Lachemann approached Carroll about promising talent on his squad. Carroll uttered one name: McGwire. After Carroll told Lachemann McGwire was a six-foot-five pitching prospect, he immediately pulled out his notebook and jotted down his name, phone number, and schedule. Lachemann made the trek to see Mark pitch and wasn't disappointed. Mark not only shone on the mound, but he blasted two home runs during the game. "I thought he was definitely a pitching prospect," Lachemann said in 1998. "And, obviously, he could swing the bat, too. He was big then for a high school senior, but obviously, not as big as today."[8] His performance sold Lachemann and by the third inning he popped his head into Damien's dugout and told Carroll, "I've seen enough. I'm going to make arrangements to bring the 'Old man' down."

That man was Rod Dedeaux, the head baseball coach at USC, and the most iconic name in college baseball. Under his tutelage, USC polished, produced, and packaged a trove of big leaguers, including Dave Kingman, Tom Seaver, and Fred Lynn. Playing in the Pacific-10 Conference, one of the most talent-laden in the country, Dedeaux captured eleven national titles and twenty-eight conference championships. USC wasn't the only college that showed interest, though. Another Pac-10 powerhouse, Arizona State University, was mulling over Mark. Dick Hines, an assistant coach for ASU, spotted Mark pitching for the Claremont Cardinals during the summer and expressed his interest.

In Rob Rains's book, *Mark McGwire: Home Run Hero*, Mark offered his perspective:

> Hines said he'd like to fly me to Tempe to visit the campus and promised to contact me with the details. After a week or so, I still hadn't heard from him, so my dad called ASU and the trip was arranged. I went to Tempe, enjoyed myself, and was told they were still interested in me and would give me a call soon.

That call never arrived. Shortly thereafter, with the season winding down, USC offered him a scholarship to pitch for its legendary program. "The second-to-the-last week of the season [USC] gave me a call," McGwire told the *Daily Trojan* in 1984. "The next thing I knew I was sitting at Dodger Stadium with Rod Dedeaux."

In a stellar senior year, Mark batted .359 with five home runs and amassed a gaudy fifty-three RBIs. When he wasn't taking his cuts, he hurled a 5–3 record with a stingy ERA of 1.90 on the mound. After brooding over his decision with his family, Mark tentatively accepted the offer from USC. Mark also had a professional option. In June, during Major League Baseball's amateur draft, the Montreal Expos selected him as a pitcher in the eighth round. That year, during a strike-shortened season, the Expos captured the National League Eastern Division title and advanced to the championship series. Even with its success on the field, however, the organization remained active in stocking its farm system, especially with pitching. Courted by scout Jack Papke, the Expos dangled a $8,500 signing bonus before him. If he signed, he would report to Calgary, Alberta, its Rookie League affiliate.

Mark had to make a choice: the thrill of playing professional ball or accepting a free education and play for a Division I powerhouse. With the Expos offer on the table, Mark weighed those figures against the value of the scholarship. In the end, he decided that the value of the scholarship at USC outweighed the Expos' lackluster offer. So he stuck with USC. "I really wanted to sign, but the money had to be as much as the scholarship and it wasn't," Mark said in 1984. "I'm glad I'm here. I now realize I was not ready at seventeen for the minor leagues."[9]

Things, though, took a scary turn. Shortly thereafter, while Mark prepared to play another summer with the Claremont Cardinals, he complained of relentless stomach pains and scurried to the hospital. During the visit, the doctor diagnosed him with appendicitis and mononucleosis.[10] That setback forced him out of action for several weeks. "It was frustrating for him," said Robertson. "His energy was zapped. And when he did come back, he was still kind of weak." Though Helber missed Mark's potent bat in the lineup, he eagerly awaited his return. "He missed the first twenty games," said Helber. "We were concerned if he would even be able to go on the road with us, but he managed to get healthy enough to play the rest of the summer."

When Mark fully recovered, he powered the Cardinals to the state playoffs during his final summer with the team. He batted .426 and launched thirteen homers, shattering his team's previous record. Mark's next stop was to one of the nation's most notorious college baseball programs, where his talent would be showcased. For Mark, no more cozy cul-de-sac on Siena Court and no more private schooling. A baseball diamond nestled on the field of a celebrated university awaited him. Even he couldn't predict where this next ride would take him.

NOTES

[1]   Kathy Weiser, "Legends of America," January 2006, http://www.legendsofamerica.com/CA-inlandEmpire3.html.

[2]   Rob Rains, *Mark McGwire: Home Run King* (New York: St. Martins, 1990), 17.

[3]   "The Disease and the Virus," http://www.polioeradication.org/disease.asp.

[4]   Rick Reilly, "The Good Father," *Sports Illustrated*, September 7, 1998.

[5]   Dick Kaegel, "His Eyes Are On the Prize," *Kansas City Star*, September 9, 1996.

[6]   Jim Souhan, "First, McGwire Sees It," *Minneapolis-St. Paul Star Tribune*, September 9, 1998.

[7]   "An interview with Mark McGwire," *Junior Baseball Magazine*. http://www.juniorbaseball.com/wheniwasakid/mcgwire.shtml.

[8]   Jim McConnell, "Mac's Start Came in Southland," *Daily News of Los Angeles*, September 9, 1998.

[9]   Valerie Mendoza, "Chasing Home Run Records Nothing New For Big Mac," *Daily Trojan*, September 10, 1998.

[10] Rob Rains, *Mark McGwire: Home Run King* (New York: St. Martins, 1990), 27.

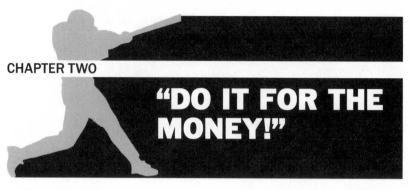

CHAPTER TWO

"DO IT FOR THE MONEY!"

"I told him, 'Jose, don't do it for me; don't do it for the team; do it for yourself; do it for the money; you have tools; you might be able to sign and make a lot of money."

—Luis Brande, former Coral Park High baseball coach
May 2007

Nineteen fifty-nine. José Canseco, Sr., wanted out. He recognized Fidel Castro's communist movement overwhelming his country, Cuba, and figured it was only a matter of time before the Marxist regime completely suffocated his earnings. Under the Batista regime he lived comfortably, but Castro claimed power and overhauled the government, altering its economic parity. By 1960, after the United States refused to refine a shipment of Soviet crude oil, Castro nationalized all major U.S. petroleum companies, including Texaco and Esso. He also seized all American-owned properties and companies. Those changes trickled down to the professional class, including José, Sr. He had already lost his job as an executive for Esso Standard Oil and had been forced to support his family by teaching English. He soon lost his house and car. In the film *Fidel Castro*, directed by Adriana Bosch, Professor Jorge Domínguez described Castro's strategy.

> At some point in February, March, 1959, Fidel Castro had come to the decision that there could not be a revolution in Cuba, that he could not build the Cuba that he wanted, unless he extirpated the United States from Cuba. And at that point, there was very little the U.S. government could do to shake that conviction.[1]

The revolutionaries had also ripped out the spirit of the island nation, banning professional sports, including baseball, a phenomenon sweeping through the country. At one time or another, American players like Ty Cobb, Babe Ruth, Jackie Robinson, and Christy Mathewson had all graced the ball fields of Cuba. In 1959, however, during a Triple-A game between the Rochester Red Wings and the Havana Sugar Kings, Castro supporters interrupted and fired aimless gunshots in Gran Stadium at midnight.[2] After two players suffered flesh wounds, Red Wings manager Cot Deal pulled his team off the field and scurried to a hotel in downtown Cuba. Baseball commissioner Ford Frick soon intervened and moved the Sugar Kings to New Jersey in 1960. Castro, meanwhile, nationalized the sport by creating an amateur league. By 1962, many Cuban players saw the writing on the wall and moved to the United States, where they hoped again to play baseball. That sadly marked the end of professional baseball for Cuba.

"Castro began nationalizing, confiscating, and appropriating American properties, the big corporations," said Amaury Pi-Gonzales, who serves as a Spanish broadcaster for the Anaheim Angels and also left Cuba when he was seventeen in 1961. "There was a lot of panic in Cuba. And with the missile crisis, there were rumors that there was going to be a world war. Those question marks made it very uncomfortable. Then it came down to the upper-middle class."

Those troubling signs saddened José, Sr., who had worked too hard to watch his livelihood crumble. Providing for his wife, Barbara, and nine-year-old daughter, Teresa, pushed him to find a way out. He pleaded with the government to exit the country, but his application was denied. His skills and education were invaluable and made it difficult for the revamped government to allow such expertise to leave the country.[3] So he endured the tumultuous times.

Shortly thereafter, the size of his family increased. On July 2, 1964, while living in Regla, a suburb of Havana, José, Sr., and Barbara gave birth to twins, Osvaldo and José Canseco y Capas, Jr. In 1986, José, Sr., explained to a reporter how he distinguished his identical twins.

> I think José is maybe an inch taller and he has a birthmark behind a knuckle on his right hand. When the boys were little, I identified them that way. Now they have the same long necks and broad shoulders. Sometimes I have to look at them twice. And they have the same personality; they're both very nice guys. They take after me.

His babies weren't the only good news. Months later, he learned of a Castro-sanctioned plane bound for Florida. During that time, Castro had approved Cuban nationals to immigrate to the United States. The prospect of leaving Cuba was bittersweet, though. While the economic advantages of relocating to America had been tempting, José, Sr., recognized that leaving Cuba would mean abandoning his family and friends. But he pondered the welfare of his family and ultimately decided the risk of relocating was worth taking. In December 1965, the thirty-six-year-old father packed his family into a tiny plane, and they flew across the Florida Strait. In an interview with Bruce Jenkins of the *San Francisco Chronicle* in March 1986, José, Sr., explained his dramatic exile from Cuba.

> When Castro took over, in 1959, I was in the prime of my life. I worked for an American company [Standard Oil], a good job. Suddenly, it was as if the roof collapsed on our heads. I did not side with the system, and I had to get out. Everything I had worked for, my plans for my family, they were all shattered, like a piece of glass. I told my wife, "This is it for us here. There is no future."[4]

The risk proved worthwhile. Landing in South Florida, they settled in the city of Hialeah. José, Sr., soon secured a job as a territory manager for Amoco Oil, while Barbara cared for the children. Aside from his job at the oil company, he also worked as a security guard. He took nothing for granted, though. He had labored hard for this opportunity and guarded his family from complacency. He challenged his children to pursue excellence. While José, Sr., was the disciplinarian, Barbara played the role of nurturer and provided balance. Anna McCarter, a friend of the family who later became José's girlfriend, described Barbara and her family.

> Everything was for her boys. They were a very close family. They did a lot of vacationing and cruises. I can remember us coming home from school at lunchtime and she always had awesome meals for us. She would tell me, "I can't believe you can eat as much as my boys." José, Sr., was like a father to me. When he worked at Amoco and he saw that my tires were bad, he told me to come by the station and get some new tires. His dad was strict, but being twin boys, they got away with murder.

Barbara also wrestled with nagging health problems. While giving birth to José and Ozzie, she received a desperately needed blood transfusion. The family, however, soon discovered the blood had been infected with hepatitis.[5] Because she was already a diabetic, her condition worsened. She didn't, however, allow her sickness to sap her love for her children. She adored them. She always felt her boys were destined for greatness. After Barbara made an abrupt visit to a psychic, their auspicious future became clearer. "She didn't go to a fortune-teller or anyone like that," José, Sr., told *Sports Illustrated* in 1986. "No, the woman she saw was more serious than that, a real psychic. And she told my wife that both of our boys would become popular in sports, but that one of them would get there first and would become very famous."

In 1975, the family moved to the Miami suburb of Westchester. Groomed in a bilingual community, the boys spoke English and Spanish. Little Havana, blocks from their neighborhood, had been the hub of the Cuban exile community. The twenty-five-block ethnic enclave was soaked with small shops, restaurants, cigar factories, car dealerships, and everything Cuban. With the rich smell of Cuban coffee whirling through the vibrant strip, elderly Cuban men gathered around tables, smoked cigars, played dominoes, and chatted about great Cuban ball players like Tony Pérez, Tony Oliva, Luis Tiant, Jr., and Minnie Minoso. "Cubans are in love with baseball, especially back then," said Jorge Díaz, who roomed with José while playing in the minor leagues at Madison, Wisconsin, in 1983. "Those old men would go to the high school games and argue about everything from Cuba to baseball and his dad was like that. It was just part of their tradition."

José, Sr., followed that lore and taught his boys baseball. When he had spare time, he drove them to a nearby school and pitched to them. While he never played competitive baseball, he followed the sport when he lived in Cuba. Val Lopez, who played sports with the Canseco boys in Miami, remembers José, Sr.'s dedication to the family. "He was a hard worker," said Lopez. "He was always very helpful around practices and games. He loved his kids."

Luis Brande coached those boys at Miami's Coral Park High in 1981. As a coach, Brande eschewed becoming too close to his players' parents. Because tough decisions, such as trimming the roster and benching players, are a necessary evil that some emotionally driven parents can't comprehend, he cautiously kept himself at a distance. Even then, Brande admired José, Sr.'s commitment. "I saw him act like an excellent father. He attended every practice and every game," remembered Brande. "He was very dedicated and was an integral part of their lives. Whatever they accomplished in baseball, they owe a lot of it to their dad."

On the baseball field, however, they battled an element more daunting than a sweeping curveball: The criticisms heaved by their father. From the stands, José, Sr., barked at them and ridiculed their play. His badgering made them squirm in the dugout. Even when José and Ozzie dazzled on the field, he demanded improvement. For the boys, nothing satisfied him. "He was there at all the games, screaming at us the same way he had been doing ever since we were little boys," José admits in his book, *Juiced*. "If you did something wrong, you always knew you would hear from him."[6]

The hard-nosed father had paid a price for his family's comfortable lifestyle in America and hoped to sway them from mediocrity. He expressed that conviction through pushing them to improve. "He was very strict," said AmauryPi-Gonzales, who covered José with the Oakland Athletics beginning in 1985. "That's the way Cuban fathers are. They come to a country with millions of people, so much money and temptations, so he looked hard after them. He protected them."

In 1978, at age fourteen, José and Ozzie played for Carol City Optimist Little League at Risco Park in Miami Gardens. During that time, the area embraced baseball and boasted several up and coming stars, including Danny Tartabull and Rafael Palmeiro. Another player, Charles McCool, who currently works as a Virginia-based travel consultant, remembers the talent-laden area, as well as the Canseco boys. "It was a phenomenal place to play baseball," wrote McCool in an email in 2007. "Their team, the Yankees, had bright yellow uniforms. They were tall, skinny boys and pitched. One funny memory was when they pitched with a runner on first base, they would look through their legs at the runner—instead of turning their head over the shoulder."

Val Lopez, who currently operates an accounting firm in Coral Gables, Florida, remembers the overflowing talent saturating the region. "The talent level was tremendous," said Lopez. "Back then, there was so much talent, but not as many schools as today, so that made it difficult to make the teams."

A year later, José and Ozzie attended Miami's Coral Park High. Gifted and athletic enough to play most sports, both focused on baseball. Ozzie, however, garnered the most attention. Nicknamed Obbie growing up, Ozzie was an overpowering pitcher. Lopez, who cruised his rusty, four-door Toyota down Coral Way and picked them up at their home on 102nd Avenue before the games, praised his abilities. "I always felt Ozzie had more potential and talent than José," said Lopez, who shared and headlined the starting rotation with him on the junior varsity team in 1980. "He had a tremendous arm."

There was one part of José's game, though, that was electrifying: when he grabbed a bat, his lightening bat speed and power mesmerized observers. In the fall of 1981, Brande implemented a weight-training program during the off-season. With the *Rocky* theme song, "Gonna Fly Now," echoing throughout the gym, his players paired off and rotated from station to station every three minutes. At each station, they focused on specific muscle groups. Brande also set up a hitting tube station just outside the gym. He made rag balls out of elastic tape for his players to hit against the side of the building. As Brande browsed through the stations and evaluated his players, José, a sixteen-year-old, unleashed his swing. To this day, Brande reminisces on his explosive swing.

The first thing I noticed was his swing. His hand speed and strength was unbelievable. The barrel of the bat use to crash against a thick, rubber hitting tube and he hit it so hard, it almost bent. His lightening quick hands and power he generated was impressive. Back then, he had a closed batting stance and had a very long, swooping swing. He was extremely powerful. You could tell he was uniquely gifted.

José also enjoyed gliding through the other stations and lifting weights. He soon began witnessing the benefits. "Weight training was working for him," said Brande. "One day, after he hit, he came up and told me, 'hey, coach, check out my abs.' He felt he was getting stronger and I was very happy about that. I thought he was going to be awesome."

In the batter's box, when José connected, the ball traveled over Coral Park's twenty-foot-high fence in left-center field, bounced on Twelfth Street and over nearby duplexes. Lopez remembers pitching to him during an intersquad game. He hurled an inside fastball, and José smashed the ball to the houses on Twelfth Street. "You could tell the amount of power he generated," marveled Lopez.

He peppered that street with majestic blasts. The school couldn't contain him. Seven years later, in 1988, Miami-Dade County commissioners renamed Southwest 12th Street from the Palmetto Expressway to Southwest 107th, Jose Canseco Boulevard. Coral Park High officials also considered renaming their baseball field "Jose Canseco Field." Lopez said José carried a tall and lanky frame in high school and he had not yet fully developed into the slugger he later became. Lopez attributed José's astonishing power to his quick hands and bat speed. "He wasn't a bulky kid, but he had tremendous bat speed," said Lopez.

José flaunted another weapon in his arsenal. When he wasn't clobbering baseballs into nearby duplexes, he unleashed a cannon from the outfield. Brande remembered his low, steaming, skidding, one-hop throws to home plate from deep right field. "He had a rocket for an arm," said Brande. "He wanted to play third base, but at that time, I couldn't see him as a third baseman, so I moved him to right field, but he didn't like that; he wanted to play the infield."

Before the 1981 season, Brande had envisioned José and Ozzie headlining his varsity squad. They both were juniors and displayed the talent to help his team. Since several of his players from the previous season had graduated, he had several openings on the roster. Brande, who had coached at Mississippi State and sat under the guidance of legendary coach Ron Polk, ran a structured practice. He earned the reputation as a strict coach with little tolerance. For him, baseball was a microcosm of life and he injected that philosophy into his practices. "He was the type of coach who didn't put up with anything," recalled Jorge Díaz.

During his practices, however, José loafed. That saddened Brande, who had always instilled hustle into his workouts and felt it showed desire, determination, and passion. "It was a tragedy to see a player with great gifts like he had, not hustle," admitted Brande. "He went through the drills, but didn't do them with the intensity that I would have liked." Brande cut José and demoted him to junior varsity. Because Ozzie hustled and shined on the mound, he made Brande's varsity squad. "Obbie hustled and did the right things all the time. But José had a different personality. He was a little more reserved and aloof," said Brande.

While Lopez admitted José rarely gave 100 percent during practices, he did notice him hustling during games. Brande eventually replaced José on the team with a short, scrappy player named Santialonso. Though being half the size of José, Santialonso hustled. He sprinted on the base paths and chased every ball in the outfield. He bunted and stole bases. He arrived early for practice and departed late. Aside from talent, he had been everything José wasn't during practice. "At that juncture, for me, it's a no-brainer: You keep that kid and send José down to J.V. and hopefully he'll get it, but I'm not sure he got it."

For Brande, José's lackadaisical work ethic didn't convince him he wanted to play. His patience soon dwindled. After José loafed around the bases during a running drill, an angry Brande pulled him behind the first base dugout and raised his voice: "I told him, 'José, don't do it for me; don't do it for the team; do it for yourself; do it for the money; you have tools; you might be able to sign and make a lot of money.'" Brande's decision to demote him was backed by his players. Before the season, he polled his team, asking them to rank the players. After the poll, Brande learned his team's perception coincided with his decision. "They had the same impressions as I did. We had a point system and he didn't receive enough votes to make varsity," said Brande. "It's too bad because he definitely had the talent." Still, Brande blamed José's nonchalant attitude on his immaturity and makeup. He never disrespected him, questioned his authority, or disrupted the team.

Away from the field, José and Ozzie roamed the campus and played pick-up basketball games with Lopez. "He was well liked. He was charismatic and great with the ladies—that was never a flaw," said Lopez. "He carried himself well and as he grew into his high school years he became more confident and cocky."

It wasn't José's charisma, however, that enticed Anna McCarter, who shared a homeroom class with him. Besides being sophomores, they shared other interests. While José played baseball, Anna, five foot eight with an athletic build and extravagant looks, played left field for Coral Park's softball team. After exchanging flirtatious glances in class, José abruptly showed up to one of Anna's practices. A girlfriend of hers eventually told her of José's interest. José and Anna's relationship soon blossomed into more than classmates. Now a firefighter for Miami-Dade County, McCarter recalled the courtship. "He finally got up the nerve to come to one of my practices," chuckled McCarter, who said both met when they were sixteen. "After that, we pretty much started dating and hanging out. That lasted off and on for twelve years. He was always very quiet and shy. He was not a ladies man in high school. That's for sure. He was always a nice guy and would do anything to help anyone."

Others noticed José's tender side, too. Comprised mostly of Cubans at the time, Coral Park high school carried two levels with portables running along the left side. On the upper level, Cynthia Hart shared an English class with him. "He was very nice and polite," said Hart. "But if he saw a guy mistreating a girl, he would become somewhat of a hot head."

His interest in women, fast cars, and baseball were some of the distractions that affected his grades. If he had ambitions of attending a prestigious university after graduation his enthusiasm for academics wouldn't be his ticket. He maintained a C average. "As you get more into sports, you know, unless you study really hard, your grades will go down," José told the *Miami Herald* in 1986. "We'd go out and practice, and, by the time we got home, we'd just want to go to sleep."[7]

The following year, in 1982, José finally made the varsity team. Brande, though, had left coaching and pursued the pharmaceutical industry. During his senior year, José batted .400 and powered the lineup. Because of his explosive power, he was later named to the first team All-Greater Miami Athletic Conference. "He was lackadaisical, getting by on his natural talent," Coral Park's varsity head baseball coach Sal Pirrotta told the *Miami Herald* in April 1986. "He'd field a ball, examine the label, take his time and still throw the guy out. That's the way he played the game back then."[8]

His bat, though, crowned him the team's Most Valuable Player. José's power also sparked the interest of Camilo Pascual, a Cuban-born scout for the Oakland A's. A year earlier, long-time baseball scout Dick Wiencek, who became the vice president of scouting shortly after Walter A. Haas purchased the team from Charlie O. Finely in 1980, had hired Pascual. With the late Billy Martin briefly becoming the general manager and on-field manager, the organization planned on rebuilding the franchise by stocking the farm system with fresh talent.

The franchise began this strategy by hiring scouts. Pascual had been one of those scouts hired to scope the Florida region. "I hired him right away because of his influence with the Venezuelan and Cuban kids," said Wiencek, who met Pascual while he scouted for the Washington Senators in the 1950s.

In the 1960s, Pascual pitched for the Minnesota Twins, boasted a tantalizing curveball and led the American League in strikeouts from 1961 to 1963. His son, Bert, had also played for Coral Park the previous season. During the season, Pascual periodically threw batting practice to the team and marveled at José's strength. "He was a great hitter with a lot of power," said Pascual, who currently serves as a scout for the Los Angeles Dodgers. "He made a scout out of me."

Not many scouts shared his enthusiasm, however. José's name, in fact, didn't appear on the Major League Scouting Bureau, a centralized list of the top prospects in the country eligible for the draft. His defensives lapses at third base cautioned many scouts. That didn't sway Pascual. When the 1982 Amateur draft rolled around in June, several A's scouts flew to Oakland and mulled over prospects with Walt Jocketty, the A's director of minor league operations at the time. During a preliminary meeting at the Oakland-Alameda Coliseum, Pascual marched in and told the gathering, "I want to draft José Canseco."

Wiencek, who hadn't heard of José or ever seen him play, asked, "How good is the kid?"

"I like him so much, I'll give him my own money," insisted Pascual.

Pascual, who always carried wads of cash, reached into his pocket and dumped several thousands on the table. After brooding over what section of the draft to select José, Pascual suggested selecting him in the middle part of the draft because, "I don't think any other teams like him." His strategy paid off. After several rounds had passed, no teams had shown interest in him. So the Oakland A's selected its wildcard, José, in the fifteenth round, the three-hundred-and-ninety-first overall pick. "I don't know why he was overlooked by the other scouts," said Pascual. "He was always a powerful hitter. He just had some problems with breaking balls." Pascual negotiated with the family and handed him a $10,000 signing bonus. "The dad really wanted his kids to play professional baseball," recalled Pascual.

Despite scouts' lack of interest in José, Anna wasn't shocked that he had signed a professional baseball contract. She figured Pascual spotted him launching enormous shots onto nearby streets. "He probably was at one of his high school games and saw José hitting balls on roofs of houses. If someone sees somebody hit like that, they're like, 'Wow!'"

José packed his bags, grabbed his bat and strolled into professional baseball. Bound for the Pioneer League in Idaho Falls, Idaho, he embarked on endless bus rides through the Rocky Mountains and the first step to the big leagues. Leaving Miami behind, but not its lore, he plunged into baseball's sifting process—the minor leagues, a system that had both shaped and shattered the dreams of many aspiring players. "I wasn't disappointed in being drafted in the fifteenth round," Canseco said in 1986. "I only played one year of varsity high school baseball. I was glad to be drafted at all."

NOTES

1   Jorge Domínguez, *American Experience: Fidel Castro,* by Adriana Bosch, PBS, 2005.

2   Cesar Lopez, "Professional Exodus: Timeline 1959 to 1983," *Cubanball.com,* http://cubanball.com/Images/History/Timeline/Time1959/time1959.html/.

3   José Canseco, *Juiced* (New York: HarperCollins, 2005), 17.

4   Bruce Jenkins, "A Canseco Hears America Singing," *San Francisco Chronicle,* March 18, 1986.

5   José Canseco, *Juiced,* 40.

6   José Canseco, *Juiced,* 30.

7   Joel Achenbach, "From Out of Left Field," *Miami Herald,* September 21, 1986.

8   Bob Rubin, "If Canseco Calls, It's a Homer," *Miami Herald,* April 25, 1986.

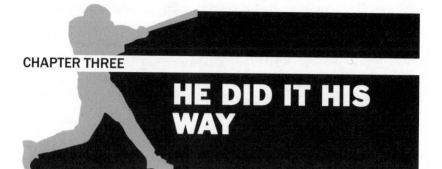

CHAPTER THREE

HE DID IT HIS WAY

"He was the most incredible hitter I've ever seen in my life. With or without [Steroids], Jose Canseco would have been the best player God has ever created. He was unbelievable."

—Former minor league teammate and FOX Sports baseball analyst José Tolentino
June 2007

Nineteen eighty-two. Leon Baham scratched his head. The seventeen-year-old José Canseco had just dribbled a two-hopper to shortstop and darted passed the first base bag. He was safe. "No, he didn't?" Baham asked himself. The next day mesmerized Baham even more: while manning the outfield, Canseco backpedaled near the warning track in right field, snatched a line drive, whirled, and fired a bullet to home plate, beating the runner tagging from third. Out. By the next day, Baham had enough. The tall and gangly teenager strolled into the batting cage and smashed a baseball out of Idaho Falls's McDermott Field, traveling some five hundred feet.

Canseco was an oddity in the Oakland Athletics organization, but not just for his talent. Prized by A's scout Camilo Pascual, he was one of the few high schoolers drafted by the organization. He had just received his high school diploma, reported to the Pioneer League in Idaho, and strolled into a locker room filled with men. One of those men, Leon Baham, quickly recognized that Canseco wasn't your average player. He brought with him from Miami a cluster of tools that electrified the field and awed his teammates. "I knew he was special right away," said Baham, who had just been drafted that year by the A's as a shortstop from Brigham Young University in the eighteenth round. "He was six foot three, 170 pounds, who could hit, run, and throw like that? That was scary. He didn't do anything over a long period of time, but he did just enough where you'd ask, 'This kid is seventeen?' He had a ton of talent."

Those gifts were showcased during Canseco's first workout in Idaho. His explosive, raw abilities became a phenomenon on the field. In bursts, he showed off his rifle of an arm, freakish speed, and how far he could smash a home run. His displays of power lured several coaches to linger around the batting cage to watch him hit. Some couldn't comprehend a middle-round, seventeen-year-old having so much power.

The A's director of player development, Keith Lieppman, was Canseco's first manager in professional baseball in Idaho Falls. Lieppman remembered when he showed up for the two-and-a-half-month league and impressed, especially during his moments inside the batting cage. What Canseco brought to the organization was rare and Lieppman hoped to steer his talent in the right direction. A former player himself, Lieppman spent nine seasons in the A's minor league system, but never broke into the major leagues. He then decided to take a shot at coaching and landed his first job in 1981 as a manager for the Modesto A's, the organization's Single-A affiliate before managing in Idaho. For Lieppman, Canseco was a caliber of player the organization hadn't seen. "You just saw that tremendous bat speed and great arm," said Lieppman. "During that time, we didn't get many tool guys like that often, where you'd say, 'this guy has a chance to be something special.' We had something to work with."

A friend of Canseco's on the team, Dave Wilder, remembered watching him blast tape-measure home runs. He knew Canseco possessed the weapons to become a star. He projected that Canseco just needed time to develop, learn the game, and hone his approach. His talent was crude, inconsistent, and immature, and desperately needed direction. "He was hitting the ball 500 feet, even back then," remembered Wilder. "He hit balls as far back then as he did in the big leagues. He just didn't do it as consistently. You'd see him hit balls and you'd say to yourself, 'oh shit!' Even at eighteen, he was dominant. It just took him a couple of years to figure things out."

Still, most felt Canseco had a long way to go. Though Baham admitted he was taken by his bursts of talent, he recognized Canseco needed refining and polishing. "He was six foot three and didn't know what the hell he was doing," chuckled Baham. That Idaho Falls' McDermott Field was a mausoleum for power hitters made Canseco's power even more unearthly. The pitcher-friendly ballpark helped pitchers like Dave Weatherman, who starred for California State-Fullerton and was drafted in the thirteenth round by the A's in 1981. Weatherman remembered how even the deep dimensions in center field couldn't contain Canseco. "That place was a canyon," said Weatherman. "But he was smashing them way out of there."

Canseco, however, wasn't a smash hit in the clubhouse. He was a teenager. His maturity hadn't caught up with his athleticism. His communication skills couldn't match his arm strength. His drive fell short of his foot speed. His confidence couldn't keep up with his bat. While his body appeared groomed for professional baseball, at the time, his mind wasn't. That immaturity exposed him and aggravated coaches and teammates. "He was a kid amongst a bunch of college guys," said Wilder. "He was very immature and goofy and a lot of guys took it negatively. He was inexperienced and didn't have confidence. He grew up in professional baseball. Coming from Miami to Idaho Falls was a big adjustment for him, but he handled it."

Other players didn't think so. In the locker room, players participated in kangaroo court, a light-hearted, fun tradition where they jotted down the transgressions of a teammate and tossed it in a box. An assigned player, who played the presiding judge, reached into the box, read the complaints to the team and decided on sanctions. "José made the box every time," said Lieppman. "There was always a big fuss over him refusing to wear shower sandals in the shower. Back then, locker rooms weren't as quite as nice as they are today, and it was a policy to wear them, but for some reason, he never seemed to want to do that."

Since Canseco was the youngest on the team, his antics weren't detrimental to the team, but were aggravating enough to bother players and coaches. "One coach called him a 'Dog,'" according to a teammate. The badgering soon began taking its toll on him, so Canseco started barking back. "After a while, he didn't take it well," said Lieppman. "The older guys picked on him a lot, but he fought back as best he could. He took a lot of heat from players. There were issues."

Wilder felt sorry for Canseco. Because Canseco was raised in the flair and diversity of Miami, Wilder noticed that he was having a difficult time adjusting to a different culture in Idaho Falls. Signing a professional baseball contract was a culture shock of its own. That combination overwhelmed him. While Wilder admitted teammates ragged Canseco, he also believed they looked after him. "He never did anything that was bad or prompted us to view him as a bad teammate or that he was going to become one," said Wilder. "He was always at the game early and worked hard."

Wilder admitted some players, including coaches, overlooked his challenges and weren't as tolerant. "He was dogged a lot in his early minor league years," said Wilder. "But some of the people that took advantage of him when he was younger, weren't able to take advantage of him later in his career. Nothing was handed to him."

Things didn't get any smoother in the community. One night,

Baham and Canseco picked up a cab from a restaurant, but didn't have enough money to pay for their entire fare home. Halfway to their apartment, they hopped out of the cab and started walking the rest of the way. As they rounded a corner, though, the Idaho Falls police pulled alongside them. After a hostile interrogation, the officers released them. Baham, an African American, remembered the culture shock.

> They wanted to know where we were going. It was really difficult. We're in part of the country where people like José and I weren't seen all over the place. We had a lot of problems with the local people and police. We didn't drive anywhere because no one had a damn car. At that time, we were only making $600 a month. So we took cabs and walked everywhere. But we dealt with it.

Several players purchased twenty-five-dollar bicycles and perused the town. The club, however, enjoyed most of its time on the road. Passing through Calgary, Medicine Hat, Lethbridge, and Great Falls, the team more than made up for their hometown's boredom. "He was fun to hang out with. We had some good times—some crazy times," remembered Baham. "We'd go on the road and he'd always get laid. Were they always the best looking women? No. But he did okay."

On and off the field, though, Canseco wrestled with the demands of professional baseball. His raw abilities landed him in the minor leagues, but taming himself was his fiercest challenge. Receiving a salary for playing baseball meant accountability. The daily grind conflicted with his sub-par work ethic. His strong-willed personality clashed with authority. The change of scenery revealed his vulnerability. Canseco was forced to grow up.

"It just seemed like a game to him," said Baham. "He almost seemed like a deer staring into headlights when he first got there. He was kind of like, 'what the hell am I doing here?' He was quiet and didn't say much. He was always hard on himself and thought he should get four hits every night. He didn't have those skills as an adult to communicate with people."

Adding to his restlessness was some coaches' opinion that Canseco lacked drive. His lethargic body language and disinterest during practice, for example, angered coach Grady Fuson, a fiery twenty-four-year-old hired by Dick Wiencek to help scout and develop the minor league system in 1981. Though functioning in different roles, he and Canseco together climbed through the organization. Yet, from the start, Canseco and Fuson never clicked. Currently serving as the vice president of scouting and development for the San Diego Padres, Fuson reflected on his run-ins with him.

I was probably one of the naysayers [of Canseco] at the time because I'd been with him so much and questioned his makeup. There was no doubt [about] the upside skill he had as far as strength and arm strength. There was also speed there. He was very raw in 1982 and he started becoming a little bit of a baseball player by 1984. He was a very difficult person. Once the game started, he gave you everything he could, but wasn't much of a practice player. . . .You didn't know where his work ethic would take him, or if he had the passion and interest in the game to really make the most out of his abilities.

That was evident when he played defense. Once Canseco was drafted as a third baseman, the organization quickly realized he lacked the reflexes and soft hands to patrol the hot corner. With Canseco's size and strong arm, some teammates figured that he would be out of his element and it would be a waste to put him at third. Since he had played the position at Coral Park, they gave him a shot. He botched grounders and looked clumsy, which concerned coaches. "We hit him 15 groundballs, and he hadn't picked one up yet," remembered Dick Wiencek. "I said, 'what the hell? I just paid this kid $10,000' . . . we were concerned, and I told the manager, 'We better try this kid at first base or the outfield.'"

Playing in Idaho Falls was an adjustment period for Canseco. His first experience in rookie ball challenged him physically and mentally. By the end of the season, he batted .263 with only two home runs. Despite those statistics, the A's drooled over his potential and felt that by smoothing his rough edges they could mold him into a superstar. The next season, in 1983, the A's sent him to Madison, Wisconsin, to play for its Single-A affiliate, the Madison Muskies. Playing in the Midwest League, Canseco would face a higher caliber of pitching, which the A's hoped would accelerate his development.

Nineteen eighty-three. Hall of Famer Eddie Matthews leaned against the batting cage and barked. "Hit the fucking ball hard, José! That's all you gotta do!"

The fifty-two-year-old Matthews was a hitting coach for the Madison Muskies. A legendary bomber himself, Matthews hammered 512 homers during his seventeen-year career. When he first laid eyes on Canseco's titanic blasts out of Madison's Warner Park, he smirked and applauded such strength. That's why he loved Canseco, in a bruiser-to-bruiser kind of way. He pulled the eighteen-year-old aside and injected him with his own experience. He mentored Canseco. After games, Matthews dragged him to a local pub and analyzed the art of hitting over a beer. Matthews saw himself in Canseco and carefully guarded him from coaches trying to soften his game. For example, during batting practice, one coach instructed Canseco to bunt. Matthews flipped out. "You don't tell that guy to bunt," he yelled to the coach. "What the fuck's wrong with you? Look at his size!" Matthews then steered his focus back on the eighteen-year-old. "Just swing for the fences, José," he shouted.

Canseco's power—not his hustle—dubbed him a prospect. He understood his value to the organization. That year the Oakland A's finished fourth in the American League West and the sinking team desperately needed a franchise player. Canseco had all the tools to become one. To make him comfortable, the Muskies roomed him with Jorge Díaz, a catcher and fellow Cuban who had also graduated from Miami's Coral Park High in 1979. Growing up, Díaz lived blocks from Canseco and played baseball in the area. Díaz was three years older than Canseco, and the organization hoped his maturity would rub off on the crude prospect. They became friends and explored Madison. Díaz, who played catcher for the University of Florida, remembered Canseco as an aloof teenager who could hit like a man.

> Mentally, he was a goofy and immature kid. But his talent was obvious. He was head and shoulders above most players you run into in professional baseball. He could run, throw, and his bat [speed] was unquestionably the fastest I'd seen. We would laugh, because the way the ball left his bat and traveled, was not common for a eighteen-year-old. He was a goofy kid with all kinds of tools.

Canseco sharpened those tools in the weight room. He loved lifting weights. He religiously lifted before each game in Madison. His passion for weight lifting overshadowed his intensity for the game. He felt the benefits of strength training provided a psychological edge that fueled his confidence, something he lacked growing up. Díaz claimed that Canseco refused to go to the ballpark unless he worked out. Lifting made him feel strong before a game.

> In the weight room, he worked as hard as anyone. His passion was for weight lifting, not baseball. The only place he really worked hard was in the weight room. Even when he wasn't doing that well early in his career, he lifted. But it was difficult for a skinny kid like that to put on any weight. At eighteen and nineteen, it was very difficult for him to acquire muscle mass that the other older guys had. His body wasn't mature enough.

Neither was his knowledge of the sport. Canseco didn't appreciate the history of the game and its forefathers. He'd rather discuss his other interests: blondes, hot rods, and weight lifting. To Canseco, researching the history of the game couldn't help him hit a curveball. Everyone recognized he was playing professional baseball because of his explosive talent and not his love for the sport. "Back then, he probably couldn't name you twenty big leaguers," chuckled Díaz. "His talent got him there not his work ethic. I really don't think his dream was to become a big leaguer. He didn't care that much about the game. He wasn't a student of the game like some players coming in."

Díaz actually felt Canseco's disregard toward the game championed his approach in the batter's box. He was oblivious to the reputation of other prospects. Whether he faced a first-round pitcher everyone feared or a sixty-third-round afterthought, he didn't care who he faced at the plate. "Some players would be awed by it, but he didn't give a shit," said Díaz. "They would still have to throw the ball over the plate and he still had to hit it. He was indifferent about it because they all put pants on the same way."

Canseco's stay in Madison was short. He struggled. In thirty-four games, he batted .159 with only three home runs. The curveball and slider were pitches that troubled him the most. The A's demoted him to Medford, Oregon, to play in the Northwest League, a short season Class-A league, where most collegiate players first report after signing. The A's hoped the change of scenery would improve his play.

Canseco had just purchased his first hot rod, a Trans Am, and refused to leave the car in Madison. Instead of flying, he wanted to drive to Oregon. The A's reluctantly handed him the cash designated for the flight to use for gas and instructed him to immediately report to Medford. Canseco, though, relaxed in Madison for three more days. As the season started, Medford coaches wondered of Canseco's whereabouts. They phoned Díaz. "I told them he left a few days ago and I didn't know where he was," admitted Díaz, who later joined Canseco in Medford that year. "But he wrecked somewhere on the way, so it took him about a week and a half to get there. But when you're a prospect, you can get away with it."

Canseco's girlfriend at the time, Anna McCarter, received a call from his mother, Barbara. "He was either falling asleep or it was so foggy he couldn't see to pull over on the road," recalled McCarter. Canseco finally arrived in Medford two days late and nursing a dent on his Trans Am. Because he missed the mandatory preseason workouts, he wasn't in good graces with the organization. When Canseco strolled into the locker room, Medford manager Dennis Rogers immediately ordered him to cut off his long, wavy, shoulder-length, black hair to a "respectable length." By doing this, Canseco, voluntarily or not, would present himself as a young professional athlete, according to the organization's standards. They also hoped his fresh image would alter his attitude. Canseco resisted, however, and argued with coaches over the length. "It took him almost two days to get it right," said Dennis Rogers.

By that time, Canseco had sapped the A's patience. Scouts felt his behavior and play in Medford would decide his fate in the organization. "If you can't do anything with him, he's done," an A's scout told Rogers. But Rogers, who always granted new players a clean slate, decided to make his own evaluation of him. Even though Canseco was a gifted prospect and tapped to play most games, Rogers warned him that if he loafed during drills and games, he would eliminate his playing time. Rogers schooled him on hustle. "If you can hustle, no matter what transpires—even if you roll an 0 for 4 with four strike outs, I'm going to play you. We're here to help progress your career, but you have to give back to the game," Rogers told Canseco.

Hustling didn't translate into immediate success for Canseco. As in Madison, he struggled and his strikeouts piled up. His failures drained him and crushed his spirits, which weighed on his play. He wore his slumps on his sleeve, and some questioned if he had the fortitude to battle through the anguish of a full season. Even Rogers spotted his discontent but encouraged him to keep battling. "Before professional baseball, no one gave him a framework on how to deal with adversity," said Rogers. "Or when you fail, it doesn't make you less of a person and if you don't get a hit, life won't end. I don't think anyone addressed those issues with him before he left Miami."

Roger's loyalty to Canseco was put to the test, however. During a game at Spokane's Avista Stadium, Canseco hit a sky-scraping pop-up that floated endlessly in the air. All four infielders, including the catcher, trying to gauge its trajectory, swerved around the infield before converging near the mound. Untouched, the ball finally dropped on the mound. "He hit it so high, he probably could have run around the bases," said Rogers. After the play, Rogers figured Canseco would be standing on third base. When he turned around, though, he discovered Canseco had stopped at first. After the inning, the steaming Rogers pulled him aside. "Grab a seat," Rogers told Canseco, who had already grabbed his glove and prepared to sprint to left field. Rogers benched him for three games. "That was the first part of our deal that he didn't live up to," said Rogers, who's currently the head baseball coach for Riverside Community College in Riverside, California. "I really have no desire to fine players, so I'd rather hand them the worst penalty: taking away the opportunity to play."

During his time on the bench, Canseco apologized to Rogers and assured him he wouldn't loaf during games. Rogers inserted him back in the lineup. Rogers claimed Canseco exploded during the second half of the season. He played as if he belonged on the field. He also fueled the lineup and carried the team. "He took off from there," said Rogers. "He finally looked like he enjoyed coming to the ballpark and settled in with the club. He became a big catalyst to the success of our team."

The incident soon forged a bond between Rogers and Canseco. Before one game, Canseco had just received his paycheck but encountered an emergency and needed additional funds. He walked into Roger's office and explained his crisis. "I loaned him one hundred dollars," remembered Rogers. During the conversation, Rogers spoke prophetically to Canseco and predicted he would one day enjoy a prosperous baseball career. "You're a millionaire—you just haven't collected," he told Canseco.

Those words inspired Canseco and he began hitting with more confidence. Even though he was a headache for coaches, they looked past his antics when he stepped into the batting cage. They lusted over his power. "José had a spat with a few coaches, but he knew his talent," said Díaz. "We would see a bunch of coaches surround the batting cage just to see him hit. Even as a skinny kid, he would stand straight up in the batters box and hit balls that we hadn't seen. We had to laugh. That was an eighteen-year-old hitting the ball 500 feet?"

First baseman José Tolentino also admired Canseco's quick bat. He was the cleanup hitter and batted behind Canseco in the lineup. From the on-deck circle, he watched Canseco and was convinced he would soon star in the major leagues. "He was the most incredible player I've ever seen in my life," said Tolentino, who starred for the University of Texas at Austin and currently serves as a FOX Sports International baseball analyst. "He was unbelievable."

Tolentino's compliments reached new heights after watching Canseco crack his bat while slamming a home run. When Canseco trotted across home plate and discovered it was cracked, he walked to a nearby tool shed on the baseball complex and nailed it back together. During his next plate appearance, he crushed another home run using the same bat. "I remember picking up the bat and thinking, 'they just sent this kid down from where I want to go play,'" remembered Tolentino. "But a few games later, I realized he just didn't know how to play the game yet."

Canseco began digesting his talent and how it grabbed the organization. He clearly had leverage other players didn't. He also attracted observers off the field—the Medford Police. After one game, he cruised his Trans Am down one of the main streets of Medford and pulled alongside Tolentino's Porsche. At a stoplight, Canseco revved his engine and taunted Tolentino, challenging him to a race. Tolentino indulged him. "I'm thinking, 'I'm going to blow him away,'" said

Tolentino. "So we're going 80 on a 45 mph zone, and he blew me away. But we both ended up getting tickets. That was something strange for me, but an everyday thing for him."

So was amusing his teammates. Despite his run-ins with coaches, Canseco meshed with players in Medford. During long bus rides through the Pacific Northwest, he joked with them and wasn't afraid to be the center of laughter. "He was liked by most," said Díaz. "He was a likeable guy and everyone wanted to be around him. He was a good clubhouse guy and didn't make any waves. On the bus, the guys would say, 'Look at José' and we'd look at him and his tick would go wild. He could laugh at himself."

Playing in Oregon proved to be a perfect fit for Canseco. He blasted several home runs out of Medford's Miles Field. For the first time in professional baseball, he began translating his bat speed into games. He also honed his defense in the outfield. Dennis Rogers spent endless hours hitting him fly balls from all angles of the field. Canseco learned how to read the ball off a bat, take appropriate routes, and cover the outfield. He soon developed into a bona fide outfielder. "We worked with him for three or four days a week on fundamentals and getting breaks on balls," said Rogers. "We worked him in center field, which allowed him to move left to right. We stayed on his butt about getting reads on balls during batting practice. We gave him a game plan everyday . . . because he had no foundation set with him when he left Miami."

Canseco played so well in Medford, the A's toyed with the idea of promoting him to Modesto, California, to play in the California League, the elite level of Single-A baseball. Although they phoned Canseco to prepare him, he refused, according to Díaz. "I'm not going anywhere," Canseco told the A's. "You just moved me from Madison. . . . I'm doing well here . . . so if you want to trade me, trade me." Canseco said he enjoyed playing in Medford and was already exhausted from traveling cross-country. His wreck on the way to Medford also sapped his energy. He was finally playing well and couldn't understand why the A's wanted to send him to California. "He was hot," said former teammate Brian Guinn. "He didn't want to go to Modesto. He had come from Madison to Medford and he was doing well."

Canseco remained in Medford for the duration of the season. In fifty-nine games, he batted .269 with eleven home runs, fifteen doubles, and forty RBIs. Those statistics crowned him the Northwest League's top professional prospect, according to managers. "They [the A's] couldn't get rid of him," said Díaz. "He understood they couldn't do anything to him. . . . He knew that if they got rid of him, every other team would be lining up to get him."

After the season, the A's sent Canseco to Instructional League in Scottsdale, Arizona. Designed for the top prospects in the organization, the instruction began in the middle of September and concluded at the end of October. With the league held at Scottsdale Community College, players worked on targeted areas of their game and received individualized attention from several coaches, which is impossible during the high-paced regular season. By this time, Canseco had earned the reputation among coaches as a moody, hardheaded pouter. Those concerns welcomed Karl Kuehl, who became the A's farm director during the 1983 Instructional League. Kuehl had established himself as a hard-nosed instructor with a proven nose for talent. He sported a wide range of experience spanning three decades. He managed, coached, and scouted in the major leagues. He also brought an awareness of the game's mental side and how it helped performance. With such affluent credentials, the A's felt Kuehl could tame Canseco.

"Even before I saw him, people told me, 'this guy has a really quick bat, but we know you're going to change him . . . he's got to be changed,'" remembered Kuehl. "And I saw some of that, but a lot of it was just immaturity. He was alright."

Kuehl decided to evaluate Canseco for himself. After watching him blister balls to every part of the field during a game, Kuehl was so impressed that he told the instructors he had no plans on overhauling Canseco. "I'm going to leave that guy alone," Kuehl told the A's instructors. "I don't want anyone changing him. He just has to come up with a solid plan and learn to execute [it], but you can't teach that kind of bat speed."

While Kuehl admired Canseco's dangerous swing, he recognized that he lacked strategy, direction, and consistency at the plate. When he connected, though, the ball jumped off his bat. By teaching him a plan at the plate, Kuehl felt Canseco could become more seasoned there. But whether or not Canseco remained in Arizona loomed larger. On a Saturday afternoon, during workouts, Canseco botched a baserunning drill and engaged in a heated confrontation with coordinator Fred Stanley. That evening, an upset Stanley informed Kuehl of the incident and recommended a three-game suspension for Canseco. On top of that, Stanley assigned him as the team's batboy during his suspension. Since Kuehl was on the road performing scouting duties, he backed Stanley and upheld the discipline. Later that evening, Stanley notified Canseco of the suspension, which happened to land during the same week Oakland A's manager Steve Boros was scheduled to visit Scottsdale and evaluate the minor league prospects. Fuming, Canseco wanted out. He marched back to the hotel, phoned his mother, Barbara, packed his bags, and prepared to catch a flight back to Miami.

"He came to my hotel room with his bags packed and wanted a ride to the airport," said Dennis Rogers, who monitored the players at the hotel during Instructional League.

Rogers soon phoned Kuehl, hoping he would urge Canseco to stay. But Kuehl refused. "I'm not going to talk him out of it," Kuehl told Rogers. "The only thing you can tell him is that if he decides to go home, I'm going to let his father know why he's coming home. . . . Don't try to talk him out of it. This guy has a chance to be something special and he's going to find out he has to be a part of the team and adhere to the team rules. The sooner the better."

Rogers still felt he could persuade Canseco. "He was headed home, so we drove him around," said Rogers. "But on my part, there was never any indication that he was ever going home." During the drive to the airport, Rogers and pitching coach, Howard Ashlock, delayed enough time to convince Canseco to swallow his pride and apologize to Stanley. Canseco adhered to Roger's advice and stayed. He figured that missing three games couldn't compare to the prospects of a baseball career, according to Rogers. So the next morning, he reported to the ballpark and fetched bats after his teammates. Nothing, however, prepared him for the mockery he faced. In his book, *Juiced*, Canseco recalled the humility of being the batboy: "I was the first one they had ever tried to ridicule like that, making me run around to pick up after them. They all taunted me the whole time, like I was some kind of animal."

Instructional League coach Dave McKay remembered, "He acted as if he enjoyed doing it, so they let him do it the next day and the next day." Kuehl remembered a heated Canseco enduring the embarrassment. "You could see the smoke coming out of his ears. He was hot and had veins sticking out of his neck."

When Canseco finished serving his suspension, Boros had already left town. Some wondered how Canseco would perform after his tumultuous week, when he returned to the lineup. In his first game back, facing the Cubs at Mesa's HoHoKam Park, Canseco channeled his anger during his first at-bats and clobbered a home run that cleared the center-field light tower, estimated at 475 feet. His next at-bat, he drilled a line drive that crashed off the left-center-field light tower. That Canseco emotionally rebounded from a taxing week impressed Kuehl more than his majestic long balls. "That was incredible power," said Kuehl. "I turned to the instructors next to me and said, 'we thought this guy was going to be something special, but he is something special.' When you can get angry and emotional and be at your best, I felt this guy was going to be awesome."

Those mammoth home runs in Mesa skyrocketed his value to the organization and generated a buzz throughout professional baseball. Baseball publications began heralding him as one of the top minor league prospects. Concerns, however, over whether his antics would overshadow his talent loomed into the off-season. With a turbulent year-and-a-half worth of professional baseball under his belt, Canseco left his mark on the organization detrimentally and beneficially. Waving his powerful bat in the batter's box and instigating fits for coaches on the field, Canseco made it clear that, if he were to make it to the major leagues, he would do it his way.

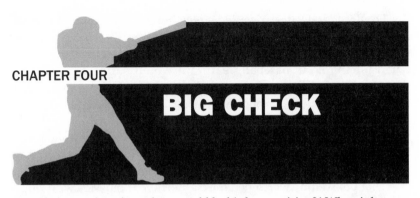

CHAPTER FOUR

BIG CHECK

"I had always thought, 'where would be his best position?' When it became apparent that he wanted to focus on hitting exclusively rather than pitching, it was sooner than I felt, so we certainly discussed that along the way. But I was just thinking about what's best for the kid himself. There was zero doubt that keeping the options open was the only intelligent way to go about it."

—The late legendary USC coach Rod Dedeaux
June 2004

Rod Dedeaux shrugged his shoulders every time. After hearing several professional scouts bark at him for inserting freshman Mark McGwire at first base during a game, he took it in stride and weathered the barrage. "What are you doing having McGwire at first base?" screamed a pitching-minded Boston Red Sox scout, who feared an injury would cut short McGwire's future on the mound. "He's a damn pitching prospect!" Dedeaux, however, eyed his players through a broader lens and kept a deeper purpose in mind.

During his forty-plus years of coaching, Dedeaux had successfully tackled such projects before. Perhaps no other collegiate coach possessed the instincts and patience to masterfully groom prospects. In 1969, flame-throwing pitcher Dave Kingman marched into the lore of the University of Southern California and transformed into the nation's most feared collegiate power hitter. A few years later, in 1971, pitcher and football player Fred Lynn played for the storied university and fell under the spell of Dedeaux and departed a sought-after slugger, too. Both played in the major leagues and smashed their way to distinguished offensive careers. "For some reason, he had that knack for being able to figure out certain things," marveled former University of California baseball coach Bob Milano, who faced USC in the Pacific-10 Conference. "He was very good at putting the pieces together."

For decades, Dedeaux could be most recognized for his gentle direction with players. He didn't limit or corner their potential; he allowed and released it. In fact, Dedeaux strongly opposed the designated hitter role in baseball, fearing it would suffocate a player's development. For his own players, though, his influence transcended teaching and mentoring. They viewed him as their "grandpa." He nurtured each player's spirit and molded and steered his team. "My whole philosophy was anytime you can do two things well, leave both avenues open," said Dedeaux. "Because you never know which way you will lean and become better. So keep all options open."

That philosophy welcomed the eighteen-year-old McGwire when he arrived on campus in 1982. Even with glimpses of explosive power he displayed during his senior year at Damien, he eyed a brilliant career on the mound, beginning with the Trojans, or so he planned. He embodied the ingredients of a touted pitcher, and observers always reminded him of it. "I went to USC to learn how to pitch," McGwire once said.

The university had witnessed this before. Over the years, its legendary baseball program had spit out many major league prospects. As the team captured victories and stacked championships, it also blazed an acclaimed past. Playing its first game in 1889, the baseball program competed intermittently for the next three decades, until finally regrouping in the 1920s. That decade, Sam Crawford spearheaded the program and helped develop the California Intercollegiate Baseball Association in 1927. The 1930s belonged to Sam Barry, who steered the team to dominance, snatching five CIBA titles.[1]

The following decade, after Barry joined the Navy in 1942, Rod Dedeaux grabbed the mantle and guided the Trojans to uncanny heights, capturing eleven national championships and twenty-eight conference titles over the next forty-five seasons. His leadership and success prompted the university to build a stadium on campus and name it after him. On March 30, 1974, Dedeaux Field opened its gates and hosted the nation's elite collegiate stars and fiercest rivalries. Because USC developed future big leaguers, such as Tom Seaver, Rich Dauer, Ron Fairly, Roy Smalley, Fred Lynn, Dave Kingman, and Steve Kemp, its legend permeated throughout the university. Former USC pitcher Phil Smith described the lore of the revered collegiate stadium.

> Even if you played for unbelievable high school programs, I don't think anyone's really equipped to walk onto Dedeaux Field. Mentally and physically you may think you're ready to go out there and play with the top players. But when you see the stadium and all the plaques on the wall, you're taken aback. You don't realize the mystique until you get there and the pieces of the puzzle come together.

After capturing a national championship in 1978, though, the base-ball program uncharacteristically sputtered. Engulfed in a post-season drought spanning three straight seasons, there were whispers that Dedeaux had coached too long and the game had passed him by. His off-the-field business endeavors had flourished and afforded him the financial freedom to voluntarily earn a salary of one dollar per year to coach. Because of Dedeaux's multi-million dollar trucking firm, DART (Dedeaux Auto Repair and Transit), booming and demanding most of his time, some felt he couldn't offer the necessary focus to operate a successful college program. "Some felt he had lost it by then and should have retired after his championship in 1978," said USC historian and author Steven Travers. "By the time McGwire and [Randy] Johnson got there, the program was in dire straights. They had talent, but had a couple of really bad years."

The team's pitching had also faltered toward the end of the season. McGwire entered the program and hoped to rekindle its winning tradition. He marched on the mound and fired an impressive fastball with good command. But besides his lively arm, he had a strategy on the mound. Adding a change-up and a biting curveball to his pitching repertoire, McGwire was developing into a promising, well-rounded hurler. "He wasn't just a thrower, but he was a pitcher," remembered Dedeaux. "During his freshman year, he was really showing he could pitch and began getting recognized. He was definitely a major-league pitching prospect."

Teammate and starting pitcher Phil Smith also admired his pitch-ing mechanics, but recognized he needed more polishing to strut into the big leagues as a pitcher. "He threw pretty hard but his fastball was a little straight," said Smith. "He had a decent off-speed pitch with good control, but he would have had to work to make it as a pitcher."

Steven Bast, who currently serves as a sports medicine doctor in South-ern California, also teamed with McGwire at USC. Bast remembered McGwire more as a control pitcher than a flamethrower. He hurled an above-average fastball but relied on location to stifle hitters. "He wasn't 'Roger Clemens-overpowering,' but he threw hard and kept the ball down," Bast told the *St. Louis Post-Dispatch* in 1998.

However, with an established starting rotation, McGwire didn't pitch in many Pacific-10 Conference games, which usually fell on week-ends and highlighted the team's top three starters. Besides an occasional start, he appeared in relief during non-conference games during the week. He observed and learned about life and competition in one of the most elite conferences in the country. "We played [USC] six times that year, but he didn't pitch at all," recalled Milano. "He only came in and played first base late in one game."

The complexity surrounding McGwire was that he hit too well. With the overflowing talent on the squad, even highly recruited freshman players rarely barged into the starting lineup. That year was no different. With starter and senior first baseman Dave Smith, a left-handed hitter, looming, McGwire had to wait for his chance to play. After Smith pulled a hamstring while running the bases during a game that season, McGwire replaced him at first base for three weeks. "That was a big concern because he was replacing a four-year starter who played great defense and hit well," said Phil Smith. "With a jet stream toward right field, that ballpark was made for a left-handed hitter. So he stepped in as a right-handed hitter where it's much more difficult to get the ball out of that part of the park."

McGwire appreciated his opportunity. In twenty-nine games, he clubbed three homers and drove in eleven runs. Even with a fledgling batting average of .200, he impressed the coaches and team enough to generate promise for the following season. When he did struggle at the plate, it was later attributed to problems with his contact lenses. "He didn't miss a beat," said Smith. "His performance set the tone for the next year. When the program recruited for the next season, it didn't have to worry about first base. He pretty much locked it up in a little less than a month assignment."

He also developed and showed poise on the mound. He pitched in twenty games and compiled a record of 4–4 with a 3.04 earned run average. He also saved two games and struck out thirty-two hitters in 47 1/3 innings. For Dedeaux, those statistics proved he could survive at the college level. He also expected to insert McGwire into his starting rotation the next season.

Playing baseball was only one feature of McGwire's life at USC. Being away from his family for the first time, albeit fifty miles away, McGwire stayed in a two-bedroom apartment on Ellendale Place, minutes from USC. Rooming with teammate and childhood friend Randy Roberston, they hosted several teammates on Thursday nights. "We use to drop by and watch television shows like *Cheers*, *Night Court*, and *Hill Street Blues*," said Smith.

After the gathering, they poised themselves for Fraternity Row, a carouse where students and alumni streamed onto Twenty-eighth Street on Thursday nights. The affair oftentimes spilled into the weekend. With student housing and bars running alongside the street, students tailgated before home football games, partied, and reveled in the university's distinguished tradition. While McGwire enjoyed rubbing shoulders with friends, he also valued time alone. "We had a blast," said Smith. "But sometimes he stood back. He wasn't much of a partier. It was all about playing ball for him."

While some financially challenged teammates clawed their way through the perils of college life, McGwire lived comfortably. That advantage allowed him to focus on baseball. Smith said McGwire eluded financial challenges other players faced. "He came from a well-to-do family," said Smith. "There were some players that didn't know how they were going to make it. They didn't have a monthly stipend check attached to a scholarship and their parents weren't well off."

Classmate and friend Steven Travers met McGwire in 1982 at a USC fraternity gathering. While Travers had pitched in the Minor Leagues with the Oakland Athletics that summer, he was released and enrolled at the university. During that time, Travers mingled with the players and lived in the same apartment complex as McGwire. "He was as neat a person as you'd ever see," said Travers, who remembered when McGwire returned to his apartment and unpacked after touring with Team USA in 1984. "Every single piece of clothing was perfectly folded and creased. He was a very ordered individual."

McGwire couldn't control his encounter with love, though. During the season, Dedeaux hosted a team party at his surfside home on Seal Beach. Dedeaux not only invited his players to the barbeque but also his batgirls, who were students, too. During games, both groups didn't mingle much. While the players stretched and practiced, the girls showed up minutes before game-time. Occupied with their responsibilities, the girls fetched bats after hitters and brought jackets for pitchers after they completed an inning. "During the season, we never really had a chance to interact with them," said Smith, who drove his 1968 Volkswagen and picked up McGwire before the gathering. "From the dugout, we'd say, 'hey, she's pretty,' but when the game started, we were focused."

That intensity lifted at Dedeaux's house. For the first time, the girls and players, loosened by food and drinks, socialized. During the party, McGwire eyed Kathy Hughes, one of Dedeaux's favorites. "I used to call her my 'Queen B,'" recalled Dedeaux. "She was my head batgirl." McGwire and Kathy instantly connected and became inseparable—flirting and joking with each other for the remainder of the evening. By the end of the night, they planned a second date. As people filed out of the home, Mark told Smith to drop him off at her place. "He was smitten with her—no doubt," said Smith. "That was the first time he had ever shown interest in a girl that I ever saw. He was such a quiet and shy guy and to my knowledge, he never had a girlfriend. He was pretty excited during the drive back."

His crush lingered. They dated for the rest of their stay at USC. "She was a very nice girl," said Robertson. "There were always a good couple. She was very supportive of him." McGwire also earned admiration from his peers. Besides showcasing his talent, his humil- ity and hard work earned their respect. While some teammates jeered at opposing players from the dugout, trying to rattle them, he astutely studied the game and allowed his bat to do the taunting. "He wasn't the high-fiving, cheerleading, jump up and down type," said Smith. "He wasn't cocky or arrogant. He was respectful and a great team player. If you came off the street and didn't know him, you'd see his physical stature and the kind of player he was, you might be in awe. But he was always one to stick out his hand and say, 'hi.'"

Dedeaux admired his attitude and remembered how respected he was among teammates. "He was an All-American Boy. He was re- served, but not shy. He was a natural leader by example. He was very popular and well liked. He liked to play the game and knew how to play it. I think that marked his career." Former baseball publicist for the USC sports information office Nancy Mazmanian doesn't remem- ber McGwire carrying the flair and swagger that usually accompanied a highly touted player. "I didn't get a sense that Mark was a star," Mazmanian told the *St. Louis Post-Dispatch* in 1998. "He didn't have that sense about him."

Stardom, however, pulled him after his freshman year. McGwire was one of four players on the team selected to play for the Anchorage Glacier Pilots of the Alaskan Summer League. The invite-only league had been the playground for elite college players every summer. Scouts arrived in clusters to scope top-shelf talent. USC third base coach Ron Vaughn and San Diego State head coach Jim Dietz compiled the roster and tapped McGwire to pitch in the land of the midnight sun. "He was going up there as a pitcher," recalled Vaughn. "He had potential as a pitcher and with work, he could have pitched in the big leagues."

As the summer approached, Dietz mulled over the roster and dis- covered that all three of the first basemen scheduled to play for the Glacier Pilots wouldn't arrive by opening night. During that time, the Major League Baseball June amateur draft passed by and snatched two of those first basemen and both signed professional contracts. The other player battled grade problems. With no first baseman, Dietz scratched his head and phoned Vaughn. "We just need a power-hit- ting first baseman," Dietz told Vaughn.

Vaughn recommended McGwire. "I told him, 'we already have one. Why don't we just pitch him every fifth day, and when he's not pitching, let him play first base. He's got power and with some adjust- ments, he'll hit,'" remembered Vaughn. Dietz agreed, and by opening night, McGwire manned first base. But even though McGwire dem- onstrated power at the plate, his batting approach and long swing concerned Vaughn. "He was really long with his swing and gangly," said Vaughn. "In his first move, his lower half flew open. So we did a lot of soft-toss right away."

Vaughn tinkered with McGwire's swing all summer. He convinced him to visualize a volleyball jammed between his knees when he batted. That drill kept his knees balanced and prevented him from pulling off pitches. If the ball dropped from between his knees during his swing, he again practiced the drill. "But he took it a step further and discovered it was easier to keep his knees together if he became pigeon-toed in the batters box," said Vaughn. "Then with the upper half, we shortened his swing and got more extension up front. He was outstanding at going to right center and centerfield."

Vaughn's suggestions paid off for McGwire. By lowering his hands, revamping his stance, and compacting his swing, McGwire transformed into the most dominant slugger in the Alaskan League. Dick Lobdell, the former radio play-by-play broadcaster for the Glacier Pilots, remembered his offensive explosion to start the season. "He immediately started hitting. He had a good swing and made contact. With the aluminum bat and with him being a big, strong guy, he got a lot of base hits. When he extended, he could hit the ball a long way. He also played a very good first base."

The original plan for McGwire to tune-up his pitching mechanics throughout the summer was short-lived. He pitched in one game and couldn't survive an inning. He allowed two hits, two walks, and four earned runs. To this day, McGwire holds the highest earned run average in the history of the Glacier Pilots, infinity. He patrolled first base for the remainder of the summer. "He was hitting so well, we just left him at first base," said Vaughn.

Off the field, he also charmed his way into the hearts of the Alaskan natives. Lobdell remembered the team traveling to Fairbanks to play the Goldpanners. During the trip, McGwire came down with an eye infection. That setback forced him to miss one game. Instead of playing, McGwire strolled up to the broadcaster's booth and assisted Lobdell with color commentary. "I found him very engaging. He seemed to be very well grounded," said Lobdell.

Lobdell also recalled the most stomach-turning game in Anchorage history. On July 7, the Glacier Pilots and Anchorage Bucs were locked in a 0-0 pitcher's duel heading into the bottom of the ninth at Mulcahy Stadium. With McGwire looming in the on-deck circle, Bucs manager Dennis Mattingly warned pitcher Don August, who was throwing a no-hitter, not to leave McGwire a pitch over the plate. He also offered August the option of walking him. "I told him, 'If you walked him, it won't be a big deal because the guy couldn't steal a base at midnight,'" Mattingly said. August decided to challenge

McGwire. He centered a fastball over the plate, and McGwire blasted a mammoth, game-winning, walk-off home run to capture the victory. Watching McGwire's swing was enough for August. When he saw the ball collide with McGwire's bat, he immediately looked down and moped toward the dugout. "He hit that ball so far it was a little dot leaving in the dark," Mattingly told the *Anchorage Daily News* in August 1998. "That ball had stewardesses, movies, the whole thing. It was just smoked. That was one of the furthest balls I had ever seen hit in this park."

McGwire, though, marveled at the significance of the home run more than the distance. "I'm dreaming," McGwire said after the game. "To break up a no-hitter, too. How often do you see that?" But for McGwire, his stay in Alaska wasn't entirely packed with excitement. Away from the field, he missed his family and battled long bouts of homesickness. For the first time, the nineteen-year-old was separated from his family and Kathy for a lengthy period. "I was away from home for the first time in my life with a group of people I didn't know," McGwire told the *Daily Trojan*. "I didn't have the support of my family and friends and I went through a very bad period of homesickness."[3]

Not many visiting players conquer Alaska, however, because of the chilly climate and rickety fields. By April, the fields are oftentimes draped with snow, which makes its year-round upkeep impossible. Being far away from home also saps the spirit of players, who are expected to work side jobs to support themselves. The league recruits local families to host players, hoping to provide stability and a family environment. Dennis Mattingly, a staple in Alaskan baseball for decades, described the daunting elements that sometimes overwhelm visiting players.

"Some players don't have a problem adjusting. But others can't seem to make the adjustment. The weather up here is not conducive to what they've been use to. Coming from California and Texas, where it's hot and muggy, they play on beautiful ballparks, but that's not what Alaska has. I tell the kids, 'if you wanted to come and see beaches and girls, you came to the wrong place.'"

McGwire stayed with Glacier Pilots general manager Ron Okerlund. At Okerlund's home, he spent most of his time on the phone with Kathy. "He was homesick," Okerlund told the *Anchorage Daily News* in 1998. "It was his first time away from home. He was on the phone all the time." With his heart back home in Southern California, his potent bat terrorized pitchers in Alaska. In forty-four games, McGwire batted .404 with ten home runs and forty-four RBIs. His electrifying performance during the summer steered his focus toward hitting and becoming an everyday player. "Somewhere along the line up there in Alaska, it hit me, 'You know, I'd rather play every day than every fifth day.' Then I started getting some hits," said McGwire. "Ron Vaughn, who's one of my biggest mentors as a hitter, pretty much started me and taught me everything I needed to know."

But convincing Dedeaux back at USC about his decision to narrow his focus on hitting was another hurdle. Dedeaux valued pitching, and with the season a few months away, he felt McGwire could help solidify his rotation. Apart from the team's needs, though, Dedeaux still perceived McGwire as having the makeup and tools to be a major league pitcher. McGwire soon flew back home and talked with Dedeaux. "I remember hearing that Dedeaux was not happy that Mark had played in Alaska and was used primarily as a hitter," said roommate Randy Robertson. "He really wanted to use him as a pitcher and a hitter."

Dedeaux felt it was premature to insert him at first base everyday. With McGwire still physically developing and learning how to pitch, Dedeaux didn't want to abandon McGwire's arm just yet. And with highly recruited freshman, flame-throwing left-hander Randy Johnson from Livermore, California, making his debut, USC seemed poised for a string of success. Dedeaux planned on including McGwire in the pitching rotation. Before the season, USC's 1983 media guide screamed, "Pitching will be back to USC's standard of Excellence. One of the main reasons . . . is the return of sophomore starter McGwire." By mid-season, McGwire shattered those plans and showed where his future in the game would be—smashing home runs in the heart of the lineup. "Even Rod [Dedeaux] didn't want me to play everyday because I was pitching well," McGwire told the *Minneapolis-St. Paul Star Tribune* in 1998. "Until he saw those three-run homers. He liked those three-run homers."[4]

Even after McGwire pitched effectively in seven starts during the season, his explosive bat finally convinced Dedeaux. He believed McGwire had a major league arm, but soon bowed to his Hall of Fame swing. Dedeaux backed off and admired.

> I had always thought, "where would be his best position?" When it became apparent that he wanted to focus on hitting exclusively rather than pitching, it was sooner than I felt, so we certainly discussed that along the way. But I was just thinking about what's best for the kid himself. There was zero doubt that keeping the options open was the only intelligent way to go about it.

McGwire rewarded Dedeaux with monstrous, game-swaying home runs. With each at-bat, he gained more confidence. During clutch moments in the crucial games, he came through with momentum-changing hits. His ability to handle pressure championed his lethal bat. Smith remarked:

> He had such an explosive, unbelievable swing. As teammates, our biggest concern was how he would be able to adjust to the off-speed pitches. And what's he going to do when, after seeing an 85-86 mph change-up, he faces a 93-95 mph fastball. As he developed and got better, it was amazing how he kept adjusting. We found out he had great bat-speed.

McGwire also instilled fear into opposing coaches. Bob Milano guided the University of California Golden Bears for twenty-two years and amassed the most wins in the program's history (688). Earning Pacific-10 Conference "Coach of the Year" honors in 1980 and 1992, he witnessed a trove of touted prospects whirl through the conference. During his second series against USC in 1983, Milano spotted another. "I said to myself, 'this kid is going to be dangerous,'" said Milano. "He had unbelievable power. If you made a mistake, he would put it in play with some authority."

From Arizona to Washington, McGwire arched eyebrows. During his sophomore year, he batted .319 and clobbered nineteen home runs. He also drove in fifty-nine runs in only fifty-three games. With his pitching days behind him, McGwire generated glowing anticipation for his junior year. His raw power impressed his biggest fan and friend Randy Robertson.

> I didn't think he had that power to be consistently hitting home runs. Growing up, he wasn't as disciplined a hitter. He would swing at balls from his head to toes. So you could get him out by not throwing him good pitches. He would get himself out. When he came back from Anchorage, he learned that he didn't have to swing at every pitch. He became a more disciplined hitter. That's the change I saw in him.

By 1984, most teammates believed McGwire would land in the big leagues. They had already witnessed several prospects burn through the conference and don a major league uniform. That assured them McGwire would be next. He dominated top-shelf collegiate pitching and held his own at first base. During an exhibition game against the Los Angeles Dodgers in the spring, however, he found out for himself. Facing former Cy Young–award winner Fernando Valenzuela, McGwire smacked a game-winning, two-run single to beat the Dodgers 2-1. "It was the peak of Fernando-mania when he was dominating the big leagues," said Smith. "McGwire was battling up there with those guys."

During his junior year, McGwire elevated his work ethic. Smelling a career in professional baseball, he refused to let complacency lower his spot in the draft and slash his payday. If that meant curtailing his social life, he welcomed the challenge. On one occasion, when Robertson invited him to join a group of teammates for a night on the town, he declined and stayed in his apartment and curled dumbbells. "His work ethic was unbelievable," said Robertson. "He worked the hardest way that I've ever seen anyone work." Minimizing distractions allowed him to concentrate on his game. And his game soon reached historic heights. The twenty-year-old blistered tape-measure home runs and attracted head scouts across the country. Major league teams assigned scouts in pairs to observe him and report on his progress. Oakland A's scout Grady Fuson relished his size and stroke. "For a big man, you could tell he had a lot of athleticism. He was very tall, slender with rounded shoulders and there really wasn't any bulk or strength to his body. But he certainly took the country by storm that year and we felt he'd be an impact player."

On May 13, McGwire clubbed his thirty-first home run against cross-town rivals, UCLA. By the end of the season, he hammered thirty-two home runs and shattered the Pac-10 Conference single season record of twenty-nine, established by UCLA's Jim Auten in 1979.

He launched a homer every 7.75 at-bats. He also batted .387 and drove in eighty runs. His power propelled him to become the most cherished collegiate slugger in America. "He had some fabulous days," Dedeaux told the *Montreal Gazette* in 1998. "He was hitting the ball over our center-field fence, which is a forty-foot-high screen 400 feet away. I called it light-tower because when he got hold of one with an aluminum bat, it wound up on top of the light tower."

With his home runs rippling throughout the country and his popularity reaching its peak, McGwire decided to enter the June amateur draft. "Over the last two weeks, the top scouts have been watching," McGwire told the *New York Times* in 1984. "I've heard reports that they think I have major league power." During his three-year stay at USC, he batted .302 with 54 homers and amassed 150 RBIs.

His dominance and startling home run pace amazed teammates but also spoiled them. "It was unbelievable. I've never seen anything like it. He hit for high average and turned into an awesome hitter. Every time he came to the plate, you would know he's going to hit a home run," said Robertson. "Each big game or whenever we needed something, his big bat came up and we were like, 'oh yeah, he's gonna go deep.' And sure enough, he did."

Milano still shakes his head over a two-run homer McGwire smashed at Evans Diamond in Berkeley, California. The ball traveled over the left-center-field fence, crashed into a recreational sports facility and landed near a ladder connecting three levels. "I assumed it traveled 480 feet," marveled Milano, who reminded his pitchers not to let McGwire beat them. "As soon as he hit it, it was gone. Those were the only two runs they scored all day."

Phil Smith remembered a prodigious McGwire blast at Arizona State's Packard Stadium. "It's still circling the planet," bragged Smith. "It went up into the night and never came down."

Those blasts became McGwire's trademark. Though he had reached amateur stardom, he never flaunted it. Since his teammates figured he was in store for a hefty payday when the amateur draft rolled around, they began teasing him and calling him "Big Check." He shunned such accolades, though. They reminded him about his success in the attempt to pry out any ounce of emotion. "He was embarrassed," said Smith. "He was shy and humble, so we tried to engage him in a conversation to talk about it. That's just the way he was."

Dedeaux flagged down his friend, Oakland A's scouting director Dick Wiencek, who held the tenth pick in the draft that year. "He told me, 'you better get down here and see this kid,'" recalled Wiencek. "So I spent a lot of time at USC that year. Then I made sure every one of my scouts would also see him. The hardest thing to get in a baseball draft is a power hitter who can drive in runs and there's usually only about five of them in the draft every year. So I made up my mind that I wanted to take him first pick."

Drafting and grooming college players had been a strategy for Oakland. The rebuilding franchise pursued players who could swiftly contribute to the parent club, and dipping into the college pool accelerated the process. The organization felt it could improve faster by drafting established collegiate players than seventeen-year-old high schoolers. "If you work for the Yankees or Braves, teams that win every year, you can afford to take some high school players," explained Wiencek. "But if you work for a team that's in the cellar, you can't afford it."

That made McGwire even more appealing for Wiencek. He cherished McGwire and felt he was only three years away from the major leagues. But with nine teams ahead of him, he doubted his chances. "We didn't think we'd have a chance to get him and never thought he'd be around for the tenth pick," admitted Wiencek.

Neither did the New York Mets, who were selecting first in the draft. During the week of the draft, Mets scouts and executives scoped the crop of top prospects and decided on McGwire. Mets scouting director Joe McIlvaine was so intrigued, he jotted on his scouting report that one day McGwire would probably be the most productive home-run hitter in the major leagues. McGwire sensed the Mets' interest, too. The night before the draft, he called Nancy Mazmanian. "Nance, this is Mark. . . . I just wanted to let you know my dad is meeting with a scout from the Mets right now. I might be the number one pick in the country tomorrow. Is there somebody I should call to talk about this?"

During that same night, McIlvaine phoned John McGwire, hoping to gauge their interest.

> We talked for forty-five minutes and all I was looking for was some assurance that his son would consider signing with us. We hadn't even discussed a dollar amount. But he deferred and said, "well, we'll have to think about it." So I just kept pecking away. After talking on the phone with his father that long, it was very clear to me he wasn't interested in signing with us. I think he was very interested in trying to find a way to keep his son on the West Coast. It wasn't a matter of money, but interest.

Meanwhile, McIlvaine saw the writing on the wall and selected high school outfielder Shawn Abner from Mechanicsburg, Pennsylvania. After that, Billy Swift, Drew Hall, Cory Snyder, Pat Pacillo, Erik Pappas, Mike Dunne, Jay Bell, and Alan Cockrell were all snatched, leaving McGwire roasted and stuffed on a platter for the A's. "I jumped out of my chair and yelled, 'he's still there . . . he's still there,'" Wiencek said. "I was relieved because my friend Jack Mckeon, who was the general manager for the Padres at the time, had the eleventh pick and told me he was going to pick him next." The Oakland A's pounced on the chance and selected Mark McGwire as its tenth pick. "We were very lucky to get him," said Wiencek.

Even though the A's lusted after McGwire's bat, they hadn't decided on a position for him. They had already drafted a touted, power-hitting first baseman, Rob Nelson, from Mt. San Antonio College in Walnut, California, in the first round the year before, in 1983. That was one of the challenges for Wiencek to sell McGwire to the A's front office. He explored moving McGwire to third base or the outfield. Either way, the A's felt McGwire could soon become a threat in its lineup.

"At the time of the draft, we considered Oddibe Mcdowell, Shane Mack, and McGwire, and we picked McGwire because of his power potential," said former A's general manager Sandy Alderson, who also traveled to USC and scouted him. Wiencek, who lived only four blocks from McGwire in Claremont, negotiated with the family and signed him at the Beverly Hills Hilton in August 1984. McGwire received a signing bonus of $145,000.

The adrenaline rush of signing a professional contract was only the tip of the iceberg. That season, Dedeaux also tapped McGwire to represent the United States and play baseball in the 1984 Olympics in Los Angeles. Highlighting Team USA, collegiate standouts such as Will Clark, Cory Snyder, Oddibe Mcdowell, B. J. Surhoff, Barry Larkin, and Billy Swift also teamed with McGwire. Hailed as one of the most talented amateur baseball squads ever assembled, undefeated Team USA bulldozed through competition in the round-robin section of the tournament. The team's momentum was quenched, however, when they ran into a sizzling Japan team, who edged them 6-3 in the championship game at Dodger Stadium, shocking the world and grabbing the gold medal.

To McGwire, however, the frustration of playing on a heavily favored team that underachieved couldn't haunt him too long. Professional baseball called his name. Shortly thereafter, he cleared out his apartment, packed his bags, and traveled north to the slower paced region of the Central Valley. In Modesto, California, home of the Oakland A's Single-A affiliate, and a springboard for other greats such as Reggie Jackson, Rickey Henderson, and Rollie Fingers, McGwire eyed a similar fate.

Author's note: Rod Dedeaux passed away on January 5, 2006, but graciously granted an interview to the author for this book in 2004.

NOTES

1 Jim Gigliotti, "Trojan Memories," *Trojan Family Magazine*, Spring 1999, http://www.usc.edu/dept/pubrel/trojan_family/spring99/baseball/ baseball4.html.

2 Neil Miller, "The Summer of '98," *Trojan Family Magazine*, Spring 1999, http://www.usc.edu/dept/pubrel/trojan_family/spring99/baseball/ baseball1.html.

3 Jim Souhan, "McGwire: Record-setting Slugger Resisted," *Minneapolis-St. Paul Star Tribune*, September 9, 1998.

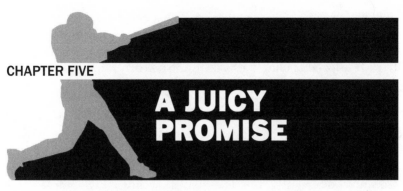

CHAPTER FIVE

A JUICY PROMISE

"I remember having conversations with him about it [steroids]. He was lifting but not to the point where he was making huge gains. We'd talk about the dangers of steroids. He'd tell me, 'I'm going to come back massive, bro, that your eyes will explode. You won't even recognize me.' He was hungry to get bigger and get to the next level, especially after closure to his mom. Back then, there were people who were saying there was nothing wrong with it, and those were the guys that were talking with him at the gyms in Miami. But it seemed like his mind was made up to get bigger."

—Former teammate and Modesto A's centerfielder Rocky Coyle
June 2007

Nineteen eighty-three. Canseco finally returned to Miami. After driving through unfamiliar spots across the country and becoming accustomed to the less-than-glamorous demands of professional baseball, he was exhausted. When he returned to Westchester, friends and family bombarded him with inquiries about his brief minor league career. He also checked in with Ozzie, who after briefly pitching for Miami-Dade Community College was drafted by the New York Yankees in January 1983. Ozzie had just returned from North Carolina where he pitched for the Greensboro Hornets, the Yankees Single-A affiliate. The brothers spent the off-season lifting weights at Miami Court Club and a twenty-four-hour gym. Canseco also enjoyed Miami's colorful nightlife. "He was heavy into weight lifting and always talked about going home to sculpt his body," said former minor league roommate Brian Guinn. "He and his brother always talked about the night life in Miami and weight lifting—typical twenty-year-olds."

Canseco enjoyed his life away from baseball. Because he was reluctant in accepting baseball as a year-round passion, he distanced himself from the sport, especially during the winter. Spending time with his family and girlfriend, Anna, demanded most of his time. That reflected in his off-season regimen. "He wouldn't pick up a baseball bat until he got to spring training, which used to amaze me," said Jorge Díaz. "He loved playing softball. During his early minor league years, that's how he trained. He would hit the ball a million feet. Then he got to spring training and was just, you know, José."

That March, Canseco flew to California to meet with his friend Brian Guinn, whom he played with in Medford. Since Guinn lived in the Bay Area, he and Canseco caravanned from there to Arizona for spring training, reporting to the Athletics' minor league camp. Guinn, who currently runs a baseball academy in El Sobrante, California, remembered meeting Canseco when they played together in Medford. "He was young, rambunctious, loved weight lifting, driving fast and one of the nicest guys you'll ever meet," said Guinn. "Right away we hit it off." After arriving in Scottsdale, Arizona, Canseco pounded the weights and hit mammoth home runs. One of his admirers was Jackie Moore, an A's coach and confidant of Billy Martin.

Moore remembered during one spring training an argument that ensued between Canseco and A's player Rickey Henderson and pitcher Mike Norris. They argued over which player was the fastest in camp. The fuss led to an impromptu fifty-yard dash in the outfield. Henderson blazed and secured a comfortable lead entering the final ten yards. But Canseco, exploding with deceptively long strides, burned past Henderson and won the race. "He outran the whole group," said Moore, who was also Canseco's first major league manager in Oakland. "That's just how fast he was. He could do it all. He was the perfect specimen for a major league player."

During the final weeks of spring training, the A's decided to send Canseco and Guinn to their Single-A affiliate in Modesto, California. Farm director Karl Kuehl told Modesto A's manager George Mitterwald that Canseco would be playing for him all summer. Kuehl also warned him of Canseco's aloof reputation. That didn't bother Mitterwald, who played catcher for the Minnesota Twins and Chicago Cubs in the 1970s. He welcomed the challenge. "They told me, 'If he gets a hang nail, he doesn't want to play and he doesn't run balls out,'" remembered Mitterwald. "But I told them he was going to play everyday for me. Even if I chew his ass out, I'm not going to sit him on the bench—he's going to play."

Concerns over Canseco's staggering strikeout totals had also reached Mitterwald. The previous season, in 1983, he whiffed 114 times in 285 at-bats. He tried to pull every pitch and hadn't figured out the strike zone. By playing him every day, Mitterwald hoped to help curb those totals and offer him enough at-bats to be consistent at the plate. Even with the raw tools Canseco displayed during spring training, though, Mitterwald felt he had the talent to one day be a superstar. "You can't teach a guy to hit a baseball over 500 feet," said Mitterwald. "He had a great arm and could run. He had tremendous ability."

But Mitterwald's fascination with Canseco clashed with Modesto coach Grady Fuson, who grew frustrated with his half-hearted effort. Fuson acknowledged his skills but felt he lacked the hustle required to thrust him into the majors. "Grady and I were buddies, but I told him, 'you may not like his attitude or certain things about him, but he's got the talent to make it big in the major leagues.'"

Canseco showed up to Modesto and roomed with Guinn. Canseco didn't connect with many teammates, but he felt comfortable enough with Guinn to ask him to be his roommate. Guinn attributed Canseco's standoffish nature to his perception that coaches and players had mistreated him since he signed with Oakland in 1982. He rarely allowed people in his inner circle. "He didn't trust anyone," said Guinn. "If he didn't trust you, he wouldn't come around you. He was on-guard all the time. They did so many things to him in the minor leagues and that didn't sit too well with him." Girlfriend Anna McCarter also spotted his frustration. "Sometimes he would get upset when a lot of politics were involved or he felt that because he was Latin, he wasn't getting what he should be getting. He didn't believe he got the same respect that other players got." One player he did click with was Rocky Coyle, a scrappy outfielder who signed with the A's after terrorizing an Independent League in New York. "He was a good teammate and always kind to my family. I always have good memories of him."

Mike Cobleigh, who served as a groundskeeper at the ballpark, claimed Canseco didn't mesh with too many teammates. "He didn't seem to have the same openness and relationship that other players had with each other." Cobleigh also recalled a much leaner player than what he later became. "He was a lot thinner. He bulked up quite a bit over the next few years. He was slender." Dan Kiser, the general manager of the club at the time, had heard scouts rave about Canseco and looked forward to watching him play. "He was flamboyant on the field, but he seemed kind of reserved off the field," said Kiser.

Away from the park, Canseco and Guinn rented an apartment off Interstate 99, minutes from John Thurman Field. It didn't take long for Guinn to discover that Canseco's expertise rested on the field—not shuffling utility bills and maintaining the upkeep of their apartment. "I took care of everything," said Guinn. "I was older than him, so he just gave me the money and I paid the rent and took care of all the bills while he just played baseball." Both clicked. Since Guinn's off-season home was only sixty miles from Modesto, in Richmond, after home games they sometimes hopped on Interstate 120 and drove to his place, ate dinner, and slept overnight.

Grady Fuson admitted he never had the best relationship with Canseco. In Modesto, Fuson established a money-based reward program geared toward compensating players when they excelled, but fining them when they failed during situational hitting or missed curfew. He fired off several fines at Canseco during the season. Fuson hoped his tough love would ignite his work ethic.

> He had such tremendous skills that people continued to kiss his ass and let him get away with things; I guess I was the bad guy because I wouldn't let him get away with anything. He always owed money and never paid. It got so bad that when we would get on the bus for a road trip I would tell the trainer, before he passed out the meal money, "give me Canseco's [money]" and I would take out what he owed in fines.

Nothing crushed Canseco, however, more than an unexpected tragedy he faced at the start of the season.

One night, he received a call from his sister, Teresa. She informed him that his mother, Barbara, was gravely ill and he should fly back to Miami. Nothing prepared him for that disheartening moment, which made baseball seem meaningless to him. Even battling health conditions, Barbara had showered her children with love and glued the family together. The news shocked Canseco. "He told me she was in a coma," Guinn recalled. "He was quiet—it hit him pretty hard. He didn't really elaborate too much."

Canseco immediately flew back to Miami and scampered to see Barbara at Miami's Cancer Research Center. By that time, she had suffered a brain aneurysm and was on life support. Since her brain had expired, the family prepared for the inevitable and had to decide how long to rely on technology to preserve her body. Her condition shattered Canseco. McCarter remembered:

"We didn't know she was sick. She was fine but all of a sudden she had the aneurysm. I remember being frantic and trying to get him home before she passed. When he came home, the family decided to take her off the respirator. The doctors had already announced that there was no brainwave activity. He had always looked forward for his mom to see him play in the major leagues and that never got to happen, which was very sad. He wasn't even able to share any of his wealth he had with her. . . . He never got to wine and dine his mom like he always talked about. She was so proud of her boys."

With her condition beyond his control, he made a promise to her he could control. As Barbara lay on her hospital bed connected to machines, Canseco promised he would transform himself into the greatest athlete in the world, no matter the price.

Canseco remained in Miami for the funeral services and spent a month away from baseball. In *Juiced*, Canseco expressed his sadness over his mother's death:

> I went into shock and cried for hours. I just couldn't believe that my mom was dead. Out of nowhere, overnight, she was suddenly taken from me, and I would never be able to talk to her again. She had protected me and my brother all those years, and gave us so much love and support and encouragement—but she would never see me play professional baseball. I was a wreck. I was just devastated, and all my family members knew it.[1]

Roommate Brian Guinn recalled how her death crushed him. "His mother was his heart," recalled Guinn. "He had a lot of deep-seeded anger." Teammate Rocky Coyle remembered how much Barbara meant to him and also noticed how her sudden death weighed on him. "I know how much he loved his mother and it was a real troubling time for a nineteen-year-old," said Coyle.

During his time of grieving, Canseco honored his mother and, for the first time, decided to pour his life into baseball. That meant his drive would catch up with his talent. Back in California, however, his extended absence concerned A's management. Wondering if he would return to Modesto, teammates heard whispers that the organization might release him. When teammate José Tolentino strolled out of the clubhouse and onto the field before a game, he noticed manager George Mitterwald engaging in an animated discussion with someone on the phone. "I asked him what happened and he said, 'you're not going to believe this, but the A's wanted to release Canseco,'" recollected Tolentino. "But he told them if they do, they're going to be releasing the next Mickey Mantle."

Rocky Coyle also heard the rumors. "They were like, 'Where is he?' I actually overheard some management in the clubhouse that didn't know I was in the training room, say, 'If he didn't show up, they were thinking about releasing him.' He really hadn't proven himself at that point," remembered Coyle. "They were getting tired of it." A's farm director Karl Kuehl, however, claimed he never planned on releasing Canseco and, in fact, graciously offered him as much time as he needed to recover from the loss. Kuehl vehemently denied those clubhouse rumors.

He was very close to his mother and we put absolutely no pressure on him to come back right away. The Yankees had put a considerable amount of pressure on his brother. The day after the funeral, they called his brother and badgered him about coming back and for that reason, I wanted to leave him alone. That was really important to him because if we brought him back while he was still going through the trauma, he wouldn't have been the player he was during the second half of the season. He returned a better player than before her death.

When Canseco returned to Modesto in June, he pushed himself and focused on his promise. That created a larger wedge between him and his teammates. He told Guinn he wanted to become the greatest player that ever lived. He also became a loner, according to Guinn. "He was in his own world, so I just left him alone," said Guinn. Coyle also noticed a more tight-lipped and bottled-up Canseco upon his return. "He was very quiet and more reserved," said Coyle. "He was going through a grieving process with no one to grieve with and still trying to be a ball player."

Darlene Westley, a long-time fan in Modesto who hosted barbeques for players, reflected: "He liked to be by himself." A's instructor Ted Polakowski believed those sad moments to be a turning point for him. "It was traumatic to the point where it was first a negative and then became a positive. He began to grow up," said Polakowski. Canseco soon dropped his outside interests, intensified his time in the weight room and sharpened his skills on the field. He applied himself, for the first time. Tolentino connected his transformation and rejuvenated work ethic to his mother's death. "He went from being a great 'maybe' to becoming the player he became," explained Tolentino. "When she died, he turned the page from being a punk and getting tickets to becoming a superstar."

George Mitterwald also recognized Canseco's newfound enthusiasm for the game. Mitterwald said he clobbered a home run to left-center field that he estimated traveled 530 feet during a championship series against Bakersfield. "He came back and played hard," remembered Mitterwald. "It was amazing." Canseco smashed fifteen home runs and drove in seventy-three runs for Modesto. Batting a career high of .276, he also lowered his strikeouts. He improved in every offensive category and even swiped ten bases. His bat also helped Modesto capture the California League championship in 1984.

Those totals weren't enough, however. Canseco eyed a legendary career and wondered how his obsession with weight lifting could fuel that dream. During his stay in Modesto, he became intrigued with anabolic steroids, a synthetic male hormone that increased muscle size at an accelerated rate. The controversial drug had revolutionized competitive athletics in the 1960s and '70s, including bodybuilding, football, and track and field. When athletes used steroids, it ignited their natural abilities and offered them greater chances to champion competitions. Since the International Olympic Committee had figured steroids provided an unfair advantage for its athletes during competitions, they banned the drugs in 1976. Other sports entities such as the National Football League and Major League Baseball had yet to establish a policy on the drugs. Guinn recalled Canseco's curiosity with steroids in 1984. "We talked about steroids before he got on them," said Guinn. "He imagined how far his home runs would travel if he were on steroids. He wanted to be a certain type of player, to see how much weight he could lift and how far he could hit the ball."

Coyle recalled that steroids became a thought-provoking discussion with a handful of players in Modesto. "I remember having conversations with him about it," said Coyle, who was one of the several weight lifters on the team. "He was lifting but not to the point where he was making huge gains. There was nobody really saying it was bad except for a couple guys that knew. We'd talk about the dangers of steroids. We would always go back and forth on that. Back then, there were people who were saying there was nothing wrong with it, and those were the guys that were talking with him at the gyms in Miami. He seemed his mind was made up to get bigger."

While several players lifted weights, some were curious. Others feared the drug's rumored health dangers. Still, some plunged into the steroid culture and Canseco wasn't the first, according to teammates. Before Canseco carried his fascination back to Miami, he bumped into some teammates and predicted an improved physique He flew back to Miami and found a source. He learned how to inject the chemicals and watched how steroids intensified his workouts in the gym. By January, he looked into the mirror and noticed his increased muscle. The results pleased Canseco; after pounding the weights for two years, he never witnessed such results. In four months, Canseco swelled his physique and couldn't wait to see how his newly acquired muscle would electrify his game. "I started with light stuff that off-season before the 1985 season, your basic testosterone, liquid form, combined with some Deca Derbol. I lifted weights seriously all the way through spring training the next February," Canseco wrote in his book, *Juiced*. Tolentino reflected, "He had seen other players doing it, but he wanted to do it better."

Nineteen eighty-five. Canseco strutted into Scottsdale and reported to spring training carrying twenty-five pounds of extra muscle. Whispers of his steroid use permeated the camp. The once gangly Canseco had noticeably filled out. Leon Baham, who played rookie ball with the then-skinny seven-year-old in Idaho Falls in 1982, was one of the first to spot his new physique. "Back then, he was six-foot-three, 170 pounds, but when I saw him two years later, he weighed 220, so right away I knew something bad had happened," chuckled Baham. "You had to be from Mars to not know what he was doing."

Catcher Bill Bathe had played in the organization for four years and had observed Canseco climb through the minor leagues, playing with him during several instructional leagues and intrasquad games. He, too, noticed his rapid muscle gains and even probed him about it. "He told me he had been lifting weights for eight hours a day, which I didn't think any human being could do," said Bathe. "He looked like Charles Atlas with muscles coming out everywhere. It was night and day from when he left and came back."

Rocky Coyle, who teamed with Canseco in Modesto, cruised into the minor league complex in Scottsdale, and saw him sliding out of his car. He donned a sleeveless cut-off shirt. "I was like, 'Holy Cow! You're huge,' I told him. He said he had been lifting. Then I smiled and remembered our conversations in Modesto. I really believe he was the catalyst for steroids in baseball."

Canseco casually discussed his steroid use with a handful of teammates that spring. "He was never discreet about it [steroid use]," confirmed former A's pitcher Steve Ontiveros. "The guy leaves 180 pounds and comes in 250. Come on, we weren't stupid." Canseco encouraged Tolentino to work out with him during the off-season. "He invited me to Miami to perfect my body," said Tolentino, who declined the offer. "But I didn't think I needed it. He wasn't peddling it, but he was a friend lending some advice. He even told me, 'José, I'll buy it for you.'" Since Canseco had already admitted to his steroid use in *Juiced*, Tolentino felt comfortable enough to describe his interactions with him during that time. Canseco boasted about how steroids fueled his confidence and quickened his swing. "I just want to take the whole bat rack and go hit," Canseco told Tolentino. "It gives you confidence and makes you quicker. It's crazy." Former roommate Jorge Díaz, who worked out with Canseco in Medford, Oregon, in 1983, watched him struggle to pack on weight. That all changed in 1985. "Steroids made him a monster in six months," said Diaz. "Every player knew what he was doing."

One of those players, Greg Cadaret, spotted acne on Canseco's back and figured he used steroids. "We all knew what happened. He showed up to spring training that year and people talked about his acne and how much he blew up. He blew up so quickly. When we left at the end of the 1984 season, I was bigger than him. When he comes to spring training, I looked like his little brother. That was the first expo-sure for most guys to steroids."

Anna McCarter said Canseco never shared his steroid use with her. Because he was obsessed with getting bigger and spent so much time in the gym, she thought his increased size was the result of hard work. "He really kept that part from me," said McCarter. "I never knew he was on steroids. I still don't and to this day, he's never admitted that to me. That was one thing he always kept to himself." To this day, McCarter flips through her photo albums and reminisces on his dra-matic transformation. "He went from a scrawny little toothpick to Conan," she admitted.

Minor league pitching coach Gary Lance, too, figured Canseco attained his swelled physique through hard work in the gym, a daily regimen of his since he arrived to spring training. One night, approach-ing midnight, Lance cruised the A's van back to his hotel when he spotted Canseco strolling along the sidewalk. Canseco had already been disciplined several times for a few minor incidents, including missing curfew, so Lance flagged him down and prepared another lecture for him. As Lance pulled over, though, he noticed something strange about Canseco: he was dripping with sweat. Puzzled, Lance probed him. Canseco told him he had been having trouble falling asleep and assured him that he had been lifting weights at a twenty-four-hour Nautilus gym and was headed back to his room. Relieved, Lance appreciated Canseco's dedication but also encouraged him to work out before his curfew.

"That was the first time I'd run across twenty-four-hour gyms," said Lance. "He was soaking wet and I could tell he had been lifting weights. He worked his butt off. He lifted weights hard. His body did get much bigger, and that's because of his hard work. Everyone else was prob-ably sound asleep or watching television, but he was lifting weights."

Canseco grabbed his bat and strolled into the batting cage and ripped home runs that traveled even farther than before. He began luring opposing players to stop stretching and admire his hitting ses-sions. After each ball exploded off his bat, admirers followed the trajectory and speed at which it left the ballpark. He peppered the street that ran alongside the left-field fence, East Van Buren, with mam-moth blasts that interrupted traffic. "Numerous times during batting practice and games, he'd hit balls and you would hear tires screeching and balls crashing onto cars on the street," said former A's manager Jackie Moore. "It was almost a dangerous situation, because, hell, no one could ever hit a ball that far. Everyone would stop what they were doing and gaze and be awed by it all. That was something we had never witnessed before."

Canseco flexed his muscle during games, too. He dominated, and by the end of spring training, he felt he should have made the big league roster. Since Canseco was only twenty years old, though, Karl Kuehl figured it wouldn't hurt to polish him in the minor leagues for another year. The organization was also grooming a herd of sparkling prospects, such as Terry Steinbach, Rob Nelson, Todd Burns, Stan Javier, Luis Polonia, Dave Wilder, José Tolentino, Darrel Akerfelds, and Mark McGwire. So Kuehl hoped to keep that nucleus playing together and felt, with time, they would trickle into Oakland and contribute.

Kuehl informed Canseco he would spend the entire season with the Huntsville Stars, the A's new Double-A affiliate in Alabama. "I was adamant and told everyone, including José, it doesn't matter what kind of year he has, he's going to play the whole year in Double-A," remembers Kuehl. "I always felt that it was important for players to have a good year and put up some numbers, so they knew what it took to finish off a season."

Canseco then left Arizona and hoped to take the Southern League by storm. With the phrase "Stars" stretched across his jersey, he hoped its aura would follow him throughout his career.

NOTES

[1]   Jose Canseco, *Juiced* (New York: HarperCollins, 2005), 41.

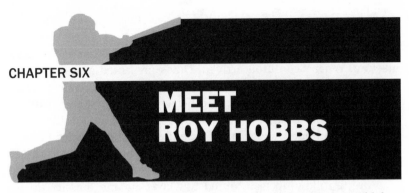

CHAPTER SIX

MEET ROY HOBBS

"That was the first time I'd ever seen a guy that looked like he could do whatever he wanted. He was in that kind of zone. If we needed a home run in the eighth or ninth inning, he'd hit one. If we're down by three runs in the ninth with two out and two strikes, he hits one over the light tower. He was hitting balls out to all fields. He could never do that and suddenly he's hitting sliders out to right, fastballs out of center, and changeups out to left. That was incredible stuff."

—Former Huntsville Stars teammate and Oakland A's reliever
Greg Cadaret
August 2007

Nineteen eighty-five. Equipped with a recently constructed state-of-the-art baseball venue, Joe W. Davis Municipal Stadium, and considerable fan interest, Huntsville Stars general manager Don Mincher hoped to field prospects whose play could match the hype before its inaugural season. The pressure to pack the 10,000-seat stadium, later dubbed the Crown Jewel of the Southern League, and compete among the league's heavy-hitting minor league affiliates also weighed on Mincher's mind. Failure on both fronts could sap fan interest and lend credence to why professional baseball had never lasted in Huntsville, Alabama.

Though Huntsville had briefly hosted the Huntsville Professionals, the city's first professional baseball team, of the Georgia-Alabama Class-D League in 1930, it folded after that summer. "The club found it hard to compete for fans against the then-popular local cotton baseball teams," *Huntsville Times* columnist John Pruett said in a February 2008 email. But Mayor Joe W. Davis wanted professional baseball in his city. In 1984, he tried to convince local officials as well as minor league franchise mogul Larry Schmittou, who had owned the Double-A Nashville Sounds of the Southern League and had recently purchased the Evansville Triplets of the American Association, that his city could support a minor league team.

When Davis heard that Schmittou moved his Triplets to Nashville and became the Triple-A affiliate of the Detroit Tigers, leaving his Double-A franchise without a home, he called Schmittou and set up a meeting. When Schmittou arrived, Davis presented a stadium proposal before city officials. Because he refused to endorse an alcohol-free stadium, however, reluctant city officials initially voted against the proposal. Davis, though, didn't give up. "The stadium wouldn't have been built without Mayor Davis," admitted Schmittou, who had the option of selling or moving the franchise elsewhere. "I didn't want to give up the franchise and wanted to remain in the Southern League."

After a follow-up visit, urged by Davis, he and the city finally forged an agreement that required him to designate one alcohol-free section in the stadium for fans and guarantee additional seats if demands increased. "Needless to say, we sold two tickets for that section," recalled Schmittou, who also served as the vice president of the Texas Rangers, at the time. "That's how we wound up going to Huntsville and they [the city] built us a nice stadium." Schmittou soon reached an agreement with the Oakland A's, whose agreement with their previous Double-A affiliate in Albany, New York, had expired, to become their new affiliate. The prospect of professional baseball returning to Huntsville left the city drenched with enthusiasm. "We never had minor league baseball before [besides 1930] and we were excited about Oakland coming into our stadium," remembered Mincher, a long-time Huntsville resident.

Marketing a player who could thrill the fans and carry his team seemed like a perfect start to Mincher. Rob Nelson appeared to be that player. At six foot four, the left-handed first baseman sported a long but powerful swing. Nelson was drafted in 1983 as the seventh player in the country from Mount San Antonio College in Walnut, California. The A's cherished its first-round investment. With an entire season of Class-A baseball under his belt, Nelson had blasted nineteen home runs for the Madison Muskies in 1984. He embodied all the characteristics of a touted prospect. For scouts, Nelson was a can't-miss major leaguer whom the A's could build its franchise around. With those credentials, Mincher couldn't wait to see him. "The big player that we were hyped up about was Rob Nelson," remembered Mincher, who currently serves as the president of the Southern League.

Nelson also played adequate defense at first base. Those skills intrigued the A's, which hadn't produced a power-hitting first baseman through its farm system since its arrival in Oakland in 1968. In 1981, the A's hoped Kelvin Moore, who feasted on Pacific Coast League pitching in Triple-A with Tacoma that year, would be that player; he fizzled out, though, in the big leagues. They felt Nelson, however, could patrol the position and power the lineup in the future. "Rob was supposed to be the answer," recalled Gary Lance, the Huntsville Stars' former pitching coach. "The big, tall, left-handed powerful swinger . . . they felt he was the main cog in the machine."

Meanwhile, back in Scottsdale, Arizona, Canseco and Nelson, along with several minor leaguers assigned to play for Double-A Huntsville, boarded a plane bound for Alabama. Prospects Terry Steinbach, Luis Polonia, Tim Belcher, Stan Javier, Darrel Akerfelds, and Eric Plunk were also among those players on the flight. As the plane glided into Huntsville International Airport, Canseco gazed over the city and elbowed teammate Rocky Coyle. "What is this God-forsaken place we flew into?" Canseco asked him.

After players filed out of the plane and marched onto the runway, a cluster of fans and media welcomed them as they passed through the lobby. Some players had never expected this type of interest and figured they wouldn't encounter such attention until they landed in the major leagues. But with the city overjoyed at the prospect of hosting professional baseball, players appreciated the warmth. "We had reporters and people crammed into the airport," recalled Coyle. "They treated us like celebrities around town. That place was electric. It was a magical time." Rick Davis, the Stars former radio play-by-play announcer, was also at the airport and spotted Canseco. "He looked like a Greek god stepping out of that airplane," said Davis.

Once the Stars prepared themselves for their first workout of the season, they were informed that the groundskeepers were still grooming the field at the stadium. The delay forced them to practice on a nearby field, Huntsville Park. Fans still flocked to watch them practice. During the workout, Canseco took his cuts and clobbered enormous shots, drawing "oohs" and "aahs" from the fans. That display mesmerized fans and set the tone for a heart-felt bond between him and the city. "His flash made him such a fan favorite here," said former Stars batboy David Sharp. "Fans are drawn to that kind of player. He had superstar written all over him. Everyone knew he was going to make it to the big leagues."

For Sharp, though, to land a job as batboy came as a surprise. Before the season, the fourteen-year-old student had coincidently combed through the *Huntsville Times* and spotted an advertisement. The clip informed readers that anyone interested in serving as batboy should come to the stadium and fill out an application. Sharp jumped on the opportunity and leaped to the ballpark. His enthusiasm paid off. "I was one of the lucky ones they chose," said Sharp, who earned four dollars a day for his duties. "The Stars were the biggest thing going in town and that was the time of my life." During the season, Sharp idolized

Canseco and how he demolished a baseball. Besides being a player with immense talent, Canseco carried the swagger of a celebrity and attracted a slough of attention. For Sharp, he embodied all the traits of a superstar, and he hoped to one day emulate him. "It was amazing— the raw strength he had," remembered Sharp, who currently serves as a high school teacher for Huntsville City Schools. "It just seemed like he hit everything solid. He was my hero."

More impressive, however, was Canseco's generosity. Before games and during rain delays, players frequently sent Sharp to the concession stands to buy them food. When he returned to the clubhouse, he sorted through the orders and disbursed the food. "He always tipped better than anyone else," said Sharp.

The Stars opened the season and played an eight-game road trip in Birmingham, Alabama, and Columbus, Georgia. After dominating the road trip, the Stars returned home and an overflow crowd of 11,000 fans stuffed the stadium. That was good news for Stars manager Brad Fischer, who recognized his team carried the talent to dominate the league. "Boy, this city had better get ready because we really have a great team," he told reporters before the game. But it was Canseco who snatched the spotlight. Wearing number 44 in honor of childhood hero, Reggie Jackson, he clobbered game-swaying, thunderous home runs throughout the home stand. "He hit a number of home runs during the home stand to either tie or win the game," said former teammate Darrel Akerfelds, who pitched on the starting rotation for the Stars. "It was incredible stuff."

Bob Mayes covered the Stars for the *Huntsville Times* in 1985. Before the season, his editor told him to sniff out stories on Akerfelds, who, besides pitching, had played linebacker for legendary football coach Lou Holtz at the University of Arkansas in 1983; Tim Belcher, whom the Oakland A's had just plucked from the New York Yankees in a controversial compensation pick in 1984; and Stan Javier, son of former major league infielder Julián Javier. Rob Nelson was also an intriguing story to cover. No one focused on Canseco. "We had seen that he showed a lot of promise during the spring, but he still wasn't a guy that we were all that excited about," said Mayes, who ironically wrote the first nationally published story on Canseco for the *Sporting News* in 1985. "He was below the radar."

Not for long. The twenty-year-old thrilled fans by blasting monstrous home runs that cleared the fence and practically rolled onto Memorial Parkway, the street running alongside the left-field fence. He bombarded the area with so many blasts, fans began calling him José Parkway. "They called him that because he hit balls that seemingly reached the parkway. That, however, was impossible, because the road was a good 600 feet or more from the fence," Mayes wrote in a January 2008 email.

He also launched balls over a scoreboard on a berm behind the center-field fence. Canseco's freakish power soon became the main attraction in Huntsville. Besides Canseco's home runs, Mincher said fans marveled at the distance. "He came here and just blew us away," Mincher remarked. "It was unbelievable because we really hadn't heard much about this guy. But once we laid eyes on him and saw what he could do, he was so impressive. No one expected this kid to hit balls like he did. We hadn't seen anything like that before. He brought an excitement and it was a delightful surprise."

So was his muscle-bound physique. When Mayes flipped through the Stars' media guide before the season, it listed Canseco at six-foot-three, 180 pounds. Yet, when he saw the two-hundred-and-twenty-five pounder strut out of the dugout and onto the field before a spring training workout, he remembered the reactions of the players and coaches in the A's organization. "When I got to spring training, he came to camp and the players were shaking their heads," said Mayes. "Even [manager] Brad [Fischer] told me, 'this just doesn't seem like the same kid that was in the organization last year; he looks totally different.'"

Pitching coach Gary Lance didn't have to face the batting cage to recognize Canseco was taking hacks. While Lance worked with pitchers in the bullpen before games, he heard the distinct sound of a ball exploding off a bat behind him. He immediately traced it to Canseco. "You could really tell when he was in the batters box," recalled Lance, who also threw to him at times during batting practice. "It was actually scary the way the ball shot off his bat with such velocity. He had such bat speed and good hand-eye coordination. "

Though steroids and weight lifting fueled Canseco's strength and confidence, which powered his bat, he also became a student of hitting. Instead of hacking carelessly at most pitches as he did previously, he developed a studious approach at the plate. He began expecting specific pitches during certain counts. When he finally realized he could launch home runs to every part of the field, he became even more difficult to pitch. He crushed pitches on the outside corner of the plate over the right-center-field fence. The combination of steroids and his development as a hitter morphed him into the most electrifying player in the Southern League. Steroids invaded Huntsville. "There were a small handful of us that knew what he was doing, but others chose not to ask questions," said Rocky Coyle. "Some figured he was a kid that finally developed. Back then, some people didn't know about the weight lifting culture."

Huntsville Times' John Pruett wrote a column on February 13, 2005, and assembled facts and time-frames pointing to Canseco's steroid use in Huntsville in 1985: "With the understanding that the conversation was off the record, the now-deceased former owner of a local gym once acknowledged that Canseco used to regularly buy steroids at his gym during those three months with the Stars," Prutte wrote.

Away from the gym, he developed even more when former major league slugger Bob Watson came to Huntsville and tutored him. After a sparkling nineteen-year playing career, accumulating a .295 batting average with 184 home runs, Watson was lured by Karl Kuehl to become the A's minor league hitting instructor. Kuehl and Watson had crossed paths before. In 1965, while Kuehl scouted for the Houston Astros, he signed the nineteen-year-old Watson to his first professional contract. Now, twenty years later, they reunited with Oakland. One of Watson's assignments was to mentor the up-and-coming prospects; Canseco was on top of his list.

"I was assigned to make sure he had the basics," said Watson, who spent parts of the season in Huntsville. "He was a good student and listened well. I wanted him to hit the ball to straightaway or right field. Once he figured out that he didn't have to pull the ball to hit a home run, he was lethal."

Over time, Kuehl noticed that Watson's influence had helped Canseco's approach in situational hitting. What Canseco lacked as an eighteen-year-old free-swinger in Idaho Falls, he acquired three years later in Huntsville. Canseco not only impressed observers with sky-scraping home runs, but he also absorbed the nuances of hitting, which elevated his game. Hiring Watson had paid dividends for the organization. "Bob did an outstanding job with him," said Kuehl. "He helped him develop a plan at the plate so he wasn't going up there without a strategy. After awhile, he knew what he was doing and Bob was instrumental in getting his approach started."

His head-turning home runs, though, garnered him the most attention. Play-by-play radio announcer Rick Davis claimed Canseco crushed a ball that scraped a gold ball atop the seventy-foot-high left-field flagpole. "He didn't just hit home runs, but he hit bombs," said Davis. "I don't remember any of his home runs that barely cleared the fence. Some of the outfielders didn't even give their pitchers a courtesy jog. He hit rockets. He hit balls so hard they knuckled out there."

By May 10, Canseco led the Southern League with fifteen home runs, ten RBIs, and a .352 batting average. For those gaudy statistics, he earned a spot on the Southern League all-star team, which was scheduled to play an exhibition game against the Houston Astros at Birmingham's Rickwood Field in June. Garnering the most votes of any player in the league, Canseco became the unanimous choice of the field managers and reporters covering the teams. "It was almost like the prophecy to his mother had come true," said Coyle. "He became an icon in Double-A and no one becomes an icon at that level. He was packing out the stadium. He was something you'd never seen before. Word quickly spread around town about this Cuban kid hitting balls near Memorial Parkway."

Canseco took his show on the road, too. Facing the Orlando Twins at Tinker Field, Coyle took his lead off second base when Canseco lifted a ball to center field. Once the ball was struck, Coyle figured one of the outfielders would casually coast back and catch it, so he scrambled back to the bag to tag up. But the ball kept traveling and soared over the fence, 420 feet from home plate, crashing off the Citrus Bowl's rafters, which loomed behind the fence. "He would break bats and hit balls over the fence," said former teammate David Wilder. "He would smash 400-foot home runs and claim he didn't get it all and he probably didn't. At the time, Cecil Fielder was also in the Southern League, but he couldn't match what Canseco was doing."

Back in Huntsville, Canseco blasted a home run that disappeared into the night. When the ball exploded off his bat, it darted so high that a security guard, standing on the berm behind the left-center-field fence, looked up and tried to follow its trajectory. But the ball had disappeared. "It was like you were seeing something like you had never seen before," marveled Coyle. "That berm was so far out there and the security guard was looking straight up, but the ball kept rising." Local businesses also embraced Canseco. After a home run, workers at Huntsville Lumber, a company located on Memorial Parkway, showed their appreciation by flashing the building's lights on and off, lighting up the sky over the stadium. Tales of Canseco's power spread throughout the country.

Jealousy, though, spread in the Stars' locker room. Canseco commanded attention on and off the field. He headlined local newspapers and became the most sought-after interview in Huntsville. Even in spite of the Stars' dominance in the standings and how manager Brad Fischer injected team play into his players, everyone wanted to talk about Canseco. That rubbed teammates the wrong way. After a game, beat writer Bob Mayes strolled into the locker room, hoping to elicit comments from utility infielder Chip Conklin, who had smashed a game-winning, two-run home run.

"Why don't you ask José?" Conklin barked at Mayes. "I have no comment."

"Players were jealous of the coverage he received," said Mayes. "He became somewhat of a prima donna in Huntsville." Off the field,

Canseco blazed his car throughout the city, and where he showed up became the buzz around town. That he lured a throng of beautiful women away from the field also irked teammates. "That didn't sit too well with some of the guys—a Cuban born with all the girls—and that sparked some of the jealousy from some of the players, especially from Huntsville, Alabama," said Wilder. "He had everything in the palm of his hand. A lot of players ended up becoming resentful and didn't like that at all."

Before a game, Canseco clashed with Brad Fischer. During the week, Canseco had been fined for missing curfew, and Fischer had established a rule that if a player didn't pay his fine on payday, he wouldn't play in the game. Canseco had a reputation for not paying his fines, so when he strolled into the clubhouse and didn't see his name in the lineup, he marched into Fischer's office. "What's going on? I'm not in the lineup card," Canseco asked Fischer.

"Well, you know the rule, if you don't pay your fine then you don't play," said Fischer.

'You can't do that to me—I'm the best player in this league . . . I'm tearing this league apart!" Canseco shouted.

Fischer grabbed the line-up card again and showed it to him, hoping he would finally convince Canseco that the rules still applied to him. Fuming, Canseco barged back into the locker room, took a collection from his teammates, and paid his fine.

"He was always in and out of trouble with the organization," said former teammate Steve Ontiveros. "And we'd get wind of it as minor leaguers, and say, 'Oh José did this and he did that!' We were like, 'Why was he doing that?'"

An injury, however, paused Canseco's flair for the dramatics. During a game in Greenville, South Carolina, Canseco was hit on the hand by a Duane Ward pitch and suffered a broken finger, which forced him to the disabled list. The A's called up outfielder Wilder from Single-A Modesto of the California League to replace him on the roster. After Wilder's arrival, he and Canseco became friends and roommates. After a few days, though, Wilder learned that Canseco's fascination with weight lifting and sculpting his body absorbed his life. He habitually arose early in the morning and interrupted Wilder's sleep by convincing him to train with him at a nearby gym. "He was a work out freak," said Wilder. "We'd go to the gym in the morning and he'd slide on two 45-pound plates to start his workout. He had energy and never stopped. He ate great food and his work out regimen was better than any athlete I'd seen. He knew what he was doing."

The injury sidelined Canseco for three weeks. When he returned to the lineup, however, he didn't miss a beat. On June 25, the Stars

opened the second half of the season on the road against the Birmingham Barons, and Canseco blasted three home runs and collected nine
RBIs, capped by a sixth inning grand slam. When he warmed up in the
on-deck circle and prepared for his final at-bat, opposing fans hoped
to see him smash his fourth home run of the game. With two out,
though, hitter Stan Javier would have to get on base. The Birmingham
pitcher managed to get Javier out, which elicited boos from the fans.
Girlfriend Anna McCarter watched Canseco dazzle on the field and
joked with José, Sr., when they visited Huntsville.

> We had this joke going. Because the cotton candy lines were always so
> long, I used [to] bet his dad that José was going to hit a home run. But
> his dad told me, "no, he just hit one last game." Then I said, "I don't
> care; he's going to hit another one. If I win you're going to have to buy
> me cotton candy." He had to wait in a lot of cotton candy lines, that's
> for sure.

His five-hit game was impressive enough to convince Kuehl, who
was in the stands, to phone A's general manager Sandy Alderson. "This
kid is ready to play in the big leagues right now," Kuehl told Alderson.
What convinced Kuehl of Canseco's progress wasn't just his monstrous home runs and the way he awed crowds, but how he
transformed into the toughest out in the Southern League. "It was his
day-in and day-out consistency," remembered Kuehl. "He was just
not giving at-bats away. He was locked in and was a tough out every
time he walked to the plate." By July 1, Kuehl was convinced that
Canseco had nothing else to prove in Double-A. The A's promoted
Canseco to its Triple-A affiliate in Tacoma, Washington, where he
would play in the Pacific Coast League, the final step before the major
leagues. But before the season, Kuehl had guaranteed Mincher that
Canseco would play the entire season in Huntsville. Canseco's play
forced him to break his promise. "Before the season, I remember Karl
Kuehl, the Oakland A's farm director, told me Canseco would be with
us the entire season," said Mincher. "but later he came up to me at the
All-Star break and said, 'Don, I'm sorry, I lied to you, we have to take
this kid.'"
After learning of Canseco's abrupt departure for Tacoma, Mayes
remembered the sadness hovering over Huntsville. While fans
wouldn't dare stop rooting for the Stars, Canseco had been the figure
that represented the city's romance with baseball. For fans, his departure left a void. "He kept saying he didn't want to leave and enjoyed
Huntsville," said Mayes. "He was the darling of the fans and they
were very unhappy when he left. It wasn't quite the same."

Canseco did leave behind a trail filled with memories. Canseco belted twenty-five home runs and drove in eighty runs in fifty-eight games. Complementing those statistics were his batting average of .318 and slugging percentage of .739, which later crowned him the Southern League's most valuable player, despite playing only half a season. "He always had bat speed, but it was confidence that, more than anything, made him the player he became," said Wilder. "The strength gave him the confidence that he didn't have as a kid."

Before his final game in Huntsville, Canseco had one more fan to entertain. He pulled batboy Sharp aside. "Since it's my last night here, I want you to go throw with me," Canseco told Sharp. Numb, Sharp appreciated Canseco's gesture, and both played catch near the left-field line during warm ups. While the news had spread throughout the city that Canseco was headed for Tacoma, fans leaned over the rail and begged for his autograph. "All the fans wanted his autograph, but he was throwing with me," recalled Sharp. "He had a nasty knuckleball and when he threw it, I could hardly catch it. I could never forget that night."

Meanwhile, trumpeted reports of Canseco's feats and how he dominated the Southern League had reached the Pacific Northwest. Players who had watched Canseco play in Huntsville and during spring training bragged about him to others on the team. Some players were intrigued and looked forward to seeing him, but others felt the higher caliber of pitching in Triple-A would bring him down to earth. "When the A's were about to call him up to Tacoma, I told the guys, 'You haven't seen anything like this,'" said Tacoma catcher Mike Ashman. "But we had some former major leaguers on the team, and they were skeptical; they've heard it before."

José Tolentino, who had played with Canseco in Modesto the previous season in 1984 and in other minor league stops, also warned his teammates. "Everyone was talking about him," remembered Tolentino. "Some players began saying, 'he's not going to be that good—wait until he gets up here and starts seeing some good breaking balls on the outside corner,' but I told them this guy is the real deal. He can wait until the ball is practically on top of the plate to make a decision and put a powerful swing on it. I told them they had never seen anyone like this."

Back in Alabama, Canseco hopped on a plane to Tacoma on his birthday, July 2. During the batting session before his first game, he clubbed a home run over Cheney Stadium's thirty-two-foot high center-field fence, 425 feet away from home plate.

In a game or practice, no player had ever cleared those spacious grounds and hit a ball over the center-field fence in its twenty-six-year history. On only one pitch, Canseco had left his mark on Tacoma. "They became believers after about a day," chuckled Ashman, who played with Barry Bonds in Triple-A with the Pittsburgh Pirates organization the following year. A few nights later when Canseco took his cuts in the cage, he not only drove the ball over a fence 370 feet away, but over a 120-foot light tower as well.

"He hit the ball as hard as anyone I had ever seen hit a baseball," said Bob Christofferson, the head groundskeeper for Cheney Stadium at the time. "He hit some long balls in batting practice. We had a place called tightwad hill in right field. People would stand on the [hill] to watch him hit. At the time, I thought he was a can't-miss Hall-of-Famer."

Not many players conquered Cheney Stadium. Over the years, its heavy, damp, dead air and deep dimensions had victimized many elite sluggers and knocked down the fiercest of drives. That element helped Tacoma's pitching staff post one of the stingiest earned run averages in the league each year. In fact, many scouts felt that if one can success-fully hit in Tacoma, one could hit in the major leagues. But even the pitcher-friendly confines of the stadium couldn't contain Canseco, who even drew comparisons with past great sluggers. "Everybody you talk to says he has [Mickey] Mantle's power and [Willie] Mays' speed," Tacoma Tigers' general manager Stan Naccarato told reporters in 1985. "I've been here twenty-six years working with the club and we've never had this before. People are coming up to me and asking, 'How's the club doing?' and 'How's Canseco doing?' There's electricity in the air."

Canseco launched so many balls out of Cheney Stadium during batting practice that Naccarato hired kids to shag balls in the parking lot. In exchange for the balls, he offered them tickets to the game. He soon barred fans from coming into the stadium during batting practice and even pondered the strategy of finding a company to advertise its name on the ball to help negate the cost for new ones. "He's busting us in batting practice," a budget-conscious Naccarato told Dave Newhouse of the *Oakland Tribune* in September 1985. "Those balls cost us $2.50 a rattle, and we have to have people standing outside the park when he's hitting. One night, he took seven pitches and hit seven out."

Tacoma Tigers assistant general manager Ron Zolo cringed when the Albuquerque Dukes rolled into town. The Dukes, the Los Angeles Dodgers' Triple-A affiliate, not only lured an array of pestering sports-writers, but also carried a cloud of arrogance. That aura paraded into town in 1981, touting their newest diamond, Mike Marshall. At six foot five, 220 pounds, the twenty-one-year-old prospect was matched by none—for good reason. Sporting a cannon for an arm and drilling baseballs to all fields, Marshall resembled a machine built for base-ball. Pounding 34 homers and driving in 137 runs, while batting a scorching .373 that year, Marshall captured the Pacific Coast League's first Triple Crown, stirring glowing anticipation in Los Angeles. "They basically anointed him to the Hall-of-Fame," remembered Zolo, who had witnessed hordes of talented prospects rocket through Tacoma.

For Zolo, though, even Marshall's glimpses of greatness, which he displayed when he roared through the Pacific Coast League, couldn't match Canseco's exploits four years later. "Marshall wasn't close to Canseco," recalled Zolo. "He was physically the best specimen I had ever seen as an athlete. If I've ever seen a can't-miss-looking player it was he. He was head and shoulders better than anybody I had ever seen come through Tacoma." On July 6, Canseco blasted his first home run for Tacoma, a three-run shot to power the Tigers over Portland in ten innings. He immediately silenced critics who believed he couldn't maintain his torrid pace facing Triple-A pitching. The following week, he hit three home runs in three games.

Ashman overheard a conversation between Canseco and pitching coach Chuck Estrada in the dugout in Vancouver, British Columbia. Canseco asked Estrada for his advice on the pitches he'd see during his next at-bat. "He's going to try to throw you a slider at your back ankle," Estrada told him. Canseco marched out of the dugout, stepped in the batter's box, and slightly backed off the plate, gearing for a slider. "The pitch was a slider down and in and he hit the ball 450 feet," confirmed Ashman. "There was a four-lane road above the stadium and the ball landed on the other side of the road. One time, he hit the back of a truck. It was phenomenal."

Tales of Canseco's legend spread, and he was soon likened to Roy Hobbs, the fictional character played by actor Robert Redford in the Oscar-award winning movie *The Natural* which had been released the year before. After the death of his father, Roy Hobbs crafts a bat out of a tree struck by lightning and morphs into the greatest player in the world, leaving onlookers mesmerized. Canseco shared those attributes. "He was the only player that I had ever seen where teams would completely stop what they were doing to watch him," said former teammate Bill Bathe. "He had the most unbelievable God-given talent, whether steroids made him better, I don't know." During a game in Vancouver, when he strolled to the plate, the scoreboard displayed the name "Roy Hobbs" above his statistics. Even opposing ballparks clearly appreciated his talent. So did Canseco.

"I've been given a lot of talent and I'm trying to make the most of it," Canseco told a reporter while playing for Tacoma in 1985. "You can't really let it go to your head or it will affect your play. You have to be consistent. That's what they look for, players who are consistent.

I'm not looking for stats, but I think everybody knows I have the talent to play in the major leagues. I'm just trying to be a consistent ballplayer."

Former Tacoma manager Keith Lieppman attributed Canseco's burgeoning success to Kuehl and mental coach Harvey Dorfman. Both had pushed him to realize his talent. In spurts of tough love, Lieppman said that they harnessed his talent and kept a rein on his attitude. "Both of them really helped him understand the kind of player he could become," remembered Lieppman. "There were a lot of things that got in his way along the way. They kept him together for those years. He gained confidence and that's when he really exploded."

In his sixty-game stint in Tacoma, he clubbed eleven home runs, drove in forty-seven runs, and cemented a batting average of .348. Those were more than enough reasons for the A's to promote him to the major leagues. In September, Canseco, along with minor leaguers Curt Young, Bill Krueger, Tim Conroy, Charlie O'Brien, and Steve Kiefer, received the call-up from Tacoma.

Canseco made the cross-country flight to Maryland, where the A's played a series in Baltimore. When he arrived in the clubhouse at Memorial Stadium on September 2, manager Jackie Moore offered him a standard rookie pep talk. During the game, Moore told him to grab a bat and pinch hit for catcher Mickey Tettleton. Facing right-handed reliever Ken Dixon, however, he whiffed on three pitches in his first major league at-bat. A week later, Canseco made his debut before the Oakland crowd at the Coliseum. And he didn't disappoint. *Crack!* He drilled a hanging slider off Texas Rangers' starter Jeff Russell for his first home run. The eye-opening blast landed at the top of the green tarp, 450 feet away, and rocked the coliseum. The Rangers players were awestruck, but the A's weren't. "It wasn't surprising to us," said Moore. "We saw him in spring training and heard the reports."

He blasted awe-inspiring shots throughout September. At Chicago's Comiskey Park, he launched one that landed on the seventy-five-foot-high roof and hit the base of the light tower. His never-seen power left teammates shaking their heads. "That thing was a blast," former A's infielder Mike Gallego told the *Oakland Tribune* after the game. "It was a line shot, not a high fly. That guy has so much power he doesn't know what to do with it." That homer gained another admirer, Tony La Russa, the manager of the White Sox, who watched him circle the bases from the dugout. Canseco played in twenty-nine games, batted .302, and belted five home runs during his brief call-up. So incredible was his performance that he was crowned the American League Player of the Week by virtue of a .491 batting average and four home runs. In three levels of play, he slammed 41 homers and collected 140 RBIs in 147 games, while maintaining a batting average of .322. Nineteen eighty-five propelled him to greatness.

"He didn't make much contact in the minor leagues before that year," said former teammate Steve Ontiveros. "He never had eye-opening numbers before 1985."

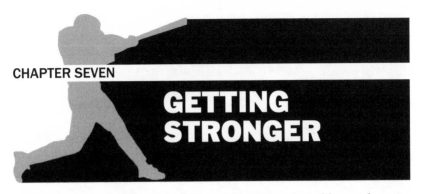

CHAPTER SEVEN

GETTING STRONGER

"He was obsessed with weight lifting. After games, I would come down to the clubhouse and everyone was gone, but he was bench-pressing all by himself. In those days, we had a couple pieces of weight lifting equipment. The guy was devoted to it. I've never seen anything like that."

—Former Huntsville Stars radio play-by-play broadcaster Rick Davis
July 2007

McGwire couldn't savor the moment. After grinding through an energy-sapping, endless travel schedule with University of Southern California and Team USA, he limped into Modesto, California. The year-round schedule had drained his mind and body. Exhausted and also nursing a pulled hamstring, he hoped for a more storybook baptism into professional baseball. Adapting to the slower pace and sweltering climate of the Central Valley, which was hundreds of miles from the adrenaline rush he felt during the Olympic Games at Dodger Stadium, McGwire recognized the challenge. "He was wiped out," recalled former Modesto coach Grady Fuson. "That traveling schedule and the amount of games they [Team USA] played during a short period of time just zapped those guys. His body was really fatigued."

The buzz surrounding the first-round, deep-pocketed, and highly regarded prospect gripped the clubhouse. Several players, including center fielder Rocky Coyle, anticipated his arrival and greeted him with some light-hearted fun but also a dose of reality. Coyle and some players grabbed an old Copenhagen tin can, tape, and yarn. Out of those materials, they manufactured a mock silver medal and hung it on his assigned locker before he arrived. Since heavily favored Team USA settled for a silver medal by losing the gold medal game to Japan, they felt the prank would generate laughs in the clubhouse. When McGwire strolled in, several players sarcastically welcomed him by showering him with the Olympic chorus. Once at his locker, he spotted the artificial silver medal. It read, "Don't Be Afraid To Bring Home The Gold, Bitch."

"We were like, 'hey, buddy, welcome to real baseball,'" said Coyle, who had spearheaded the hazing. "He came in and politely greeted everyone."

His arrival planted a smile on the face of Dan Kiser, the general manager of the Modesto A's at the time. Kiser understood the jumbled relationship between an affiliate and a franchise. The way players are hastily shipped like goods from one city to another one can cause headaches for affiliates. That such as prized prospect of McGwire's caliber would energize the lineup and swell ticket sales excited Kiser. He crossed his fingers, though. "Until they actually arrive, you never know that you're really going to have them," said Kiser. "We were anxiously waiting to see him. Whenever a number one draft pick comes in, that's obviously something the fans get excited about. There was a lot of talk about him."

Steve Gokey served as the team's inspirational coach and also had been in the locker room when McGwire first arrived. Although Gokey had heard the reports of McGwire's hitting feats at USC, he feared that the fame attached to such accolades would interrupt the team's camaraderie. He wondered how McGwire would blend with the other players. "You never know what you're going to get," admitted Gokey. "Are you going to get a jackass? You get a guy who's coming off the Olympics and a first round pick, and you never know. But he was very good with teammates and fit right in."

And Gokey made sure of that. His role on the club was to boost morale and keep players loose. When he spotted a player mired in a slump, he encouraged him. He was also notorious in the California League for ragging on umpires from behind home plate, which got him tossed out of his share of games. The always animated Gokey loved life and baseball, but he had every reason to bark at both. Gokey was blind. His condition, however, didn't rob him of his passion for the sport. From the dugout, his uncanny instinct and senses — without the privilege of gazing at a majestic home run — was unrivaled. From the sound of the ball exploding off a bat, he could sense a home run. By the sound of the ball meeting the catcher's glove, he could locate the pitch.

Gokey soon became an integral part of the team and immediately connected with McGwire and his girlfriend at the time, Kathy. "We hit it off right away," remembered Gokey, who still resides in Modesto. "When he found out I was blind, he zeroed in on me. He was always nice to me and we had a great relationship. He was a lot of fun to be around." Kathy also connected with Gokey. On road trips, she grabbed his hand and helped him find his way around hotels. "She was a very sweet lady," said Gokey. "One time, McGwire ragged on me and said, 'Gosh, we're in this hotel in Bakersfield and my girlfriend spends more time with you than me.'"

On the field, though, McGwire wanted to prove he could hold his own in professional baseball. With the pressure associated with being the A's prized prospect, he pressed and struggled immediately. The coiled batting stance and compact swing that helped him become the nation's most sought after slugger abandoned him. Transitioning from the lively aluminum bat he used in college to a wooden one, which welcomed him in Modesto, was also a challenge for McGwire. His tired swing couldn't match the blazing fastballs in the California League. Karl Kuehl, the A's farm director at the time, spotted his flaws at the plate.

> He had a real slow bat. He stood too far from the plate and had a big hole inside. Any kind of heat, he couldn't handle. He had hitting mechanics that worked for him at the college level, but when you come to professional baseball you're seeing better pitches more often. Pitchers began pounding him in with fastballs.

Modesto manager and former catcher George Mitterwald quickly recognized that if the twenty-year-old were to survive in professional baseball, he would have to adjust. According to Mitterwald, McGwire stood too far away from the plate and too deep in the batter's box. Mitterwald tried to convince him to move closer to the plate. While McGwire tinkered with it during batting practice, he wouldn't apply it during the game, though. "He had a lot of flaws, but we knew he had potential," remembered Mitterwald. "During the season, I tried to get him to move closer to the plate, but when I was playing, I had a career average of .236, so he never really listened to me. In the college game, if you hit the ball off the end of the [aluminum] bat or get jammed, you might still get base hits, but with the wooden bat, you may not."

Mitterwald also attributed McGwire's struggles to his pulled hamstring, a muscle that hitters depend on for leverage and power. Because of the injury, Mitterwald inserted him as the designated hitter in games. Still, pitchers successfully stifled McGwire with inside fastballs. Kiser pointed to the higher caliber of pitching in the California League to explain his adversity at the plate. "At the college level, you get one guy with major league velocity every three or four games, but when you come here, you see it every night," said Kiser. "If you press a little bit, it's not hard to go 0 for a week. I'm sure that was a tough adjustment for him."

Modesto shortstop Brian Guinn played for the University of California, Berkeley, and competed against McGwire in the Pacific-10 Conference before both were drafted by Oakland. Though Guinn watched him clobber some thunderous home runs for USC, he, too, spotted opposing pitchers blowing him away with heat. "He couldn't hit an inside fastball to save his life," remembered Guinn. "His bat was a little slow and he had to make some major adjustments."

Back in Oakland, A's scouting director Dick Wiencek, who had convinced the organization to sign McGwire and bestow upon him a $145,000 signing bonus, began hearing the grumblings from his colleagues. Despite McGwire's struggles, though, Wiencek believed he would turn things around. Having watched other collegiate players scuffle trying to adjust to the wooden bat when they first arrived, he felt it was only a matter of time before McGwire felt comfortable and produced. Wiencek, a legendary scout who signed a record seventy-two big leaguers throughout his fifty-eight-year career, faced his doubters. "Everyone was jumping on me about why the hell I picked him first," said Wiencek. "But I told them that if he doesn't do well next year, I'll admit I made a mistake. For a while, I was getting second-guessed."

When McGwire would actually muster his first professional home run was anyone's guess. That curiosity prompted several players to participate in a pool and place bets on when he would club his first homer. Watching him scuffle so much, one teammate suggested he would hit it during a softball league in 2010. One player who befriended McGwire and played golf with him during the off-season, Ron Cummings, suggested August 25 of that current year; McGwire ended up hitting a home run one day later. "He was pretty worn out," said Cummings. Trying to prove that he belonged wasn't McGwire's only hurdle. He was also frustrated by learning how to successfully man third base. With the A's leaning toward prospect Rob Nelson as their future first baseman, they planted McGwire there for the time being; he, however, was uncomfortable from the start. With his six-foot-five, lanky frame patrolling the hot corner, a position demanding quick reflexes, he looked clumsy. "Once he got there, we figured he was going to take over first base, but to our surprise, they put him at third base," said Guinn.

Guinn, who manned shortstop a few feet to McGwire's left, remembered having private discussions with him between innings and during pitching changes about McGwire's anxiety over playing third base. "He hated it," said Guinn. "He was new at the position, so he made a bunch of errors. He didn't want to fail and there was a lot of pressure on him. I remember him asking me to help him out with ground-balls to his left, and I told him, 'If you give me some of that bonus, I'll catch everything.' He laughed. I was trying to keep him upbeat."

Pitcher Greg Cadaret said McGwire mostly possessed the athletic ability to play third. His frame, however, robbed him of the quick reactions required to smother sizzling grounders. "That was a nightmare for us pitchers," joked Cadaret. "As tall as he was, it took him three seconds to dive for a ball. His talent wasn't as obvious as José's when he first got there."

Kiser also figured McGwire's defensives lapses followed him to the plate. When he did cleanly glove balls, he threw erratically to first base. The errors piled. "Being that tall, he just didn't have the quickness. On a groundball, it took him too long to get to the ground and dive for balls," said Kiser. Even though McGwire didn't see a future at third, he worked hard. He asked coaches to drill smoking grounders around the bag. In time, his determination paid off. Mitterwald applauded his efforts and said McGwire played adequate defense. "The hardest play for a third baseman is that slow roller down the line where they come up and throw side arm to first base," said Mitterwald. "He worked hard on that play every day."

Embracing teammates from different parts of the world also expanded McGwire's horizon. After growing up in the affluent, suburban city of Claremont, he teamed with a melting pot of ethnicities in Modesto. Several teammates ragged him about his hefty signing bonus and pampered upbringing. But McGwire only wanted to be considered one of the guys. "Once he got around a whole different culture of players and backgrounds, he had to grow up," said Guinn. "Some of the Dominican players took well to him. He tried to hide the fact that he received a lot of money because he didn't want to flaunt it, but we teased him so much, he couldn't help it. He was just trying to fit in."

McGwire labored through sixteen games in Modesto. During his short stint, he hit .200 with only one home run and a single run batted in. He wore his frustration on his sleeve, and it exuded from his body language. He leaned on teammates for support. "When everything was going well for him, everything was fine, but when it wasn't, he showed his emotion more than anyone else," confirmed Guinn. Teammate José Tolentino said McGwire's first taste of the minor leagues seasoned him. "He was a very polite sweetheart and soft person, but he battled with the toughness of minor league baseball," said Tolentino.

McGwire's frustration didn't stop his club from winning. In a magical season, the Modesto A's surprisingly captured the California

League championship. In the championship series against Bakersfield, McGwire hammered a home run in game four. "I still remember that home run," said Grady Fuson. "He struggled. A lot of people claimed it was because of the wooden bat, but to me, it really wasn't. He hung in there and became a big reason why we ended up winning the championship that year."

McGwire couldn't recuperate from his taxing season for very long. Shortly thereafter, the A's instructed him to report to their Instructional League in Scottsdale, Arizona, during the winter. It was at Scottsdale Community College where the A's hoped to shorten his swing, which "he wasn't ready to buy into," according to Kuehl. They also still hoped he could improve his defense at third. With several coaches flown in to tutor him, he worked on range and reflexes. Coaches pushed him and challenged his work ethic. While he toiled through the drills, he never quite embraced the position. "We worked him so hard on defense, there were a lot of days when he said, 'I'm not coming back tomorrow—I'm quitting. I don't need this. I've never had to work like this before to ever do anything in athletics,'" recollected Kuehl.

After Instructional League, he returned to California and married Kathy on December 29, 1984. When McGwire reported to spring training in February, he bumped into Tolentino, a slick fielding first baseman whose charm and handsome features made him popular with the ladies. The previous season, in 1984, he had dominated the California League. Tolentino's hitting terror earned him a promotion to Double-A Albany. He claimed he was bumped up to create room for McGwire, who ended up earning a championship ring for his short stint. After Modesto snatched the California League championship, though, many teammates felt the ring should have been awarded to Tolentino, who headlined the lineup most of the season—not McGwire. "Everybody was making fun of him because they felt the ring belonged to me," said Tolentino, who had the misfortune of trying to claw his way through the organization behind other infield prospects such as Nelson and McGwire. "But he quietly came up to me and asked me, 'Do you want the ring? You deserve it more than I do.' He was that kind of guy."

Guinn said McGwire looked more relaxed during his first spring training and spending the entire time with other players helped him. "He had a little different focus," said Guinn. "He learned a lot during that spring." Grady Fuson worked with McGwire throughout the spring and began seeing improvements in his game. Those promising signs relieved Fuson, who caught glimpses of the player they had drafted. "I spent a lot of time with him in infield drills," said Fuson. "I saw his progress and how his path was turning. Once Mark got a foundation in hitting, his rhythm, timing, and recognition became impeccable."

At the conclusion of spring training, the A's shipped McGwire back to Modesto. The organization hoped spending a full season in Single-A would bolster his confidence and erase his doubts. He couldn't have chosen a cozier ballpark. The hitter-friendly dimensions at Modesto's John Thurman Field enticed power hitters. With the center-field fence only 370 feet from home plate and the power alleys 345, lazy fly balls frequently found their way over the fence. The ballpark and McGwire seemed like a perfect match. Additionally, working out during the winter strengthened his bat. Mike Cobleigh, an assistant to the general manager, noticed his increased size. "He came back a little bigger that year," said Cobleigh. "Back then, players had a lot supplement drinks. Most of them are still legal, but some of them had been since banned."

Away from the gym, McGwire and Kathy forged relationships with several residents and local businesses around town. McGwire was also active in the community and made appearances in booster club gatherings and high schools. Cobleigh said McGwire was accessible to the community. "He made some friendships here," said Cobleigh. "He would sign autographs for people and if we needed a player to go to a school, he was very good about that. He would go out to dinner with fans and had a real good sense of involvement. He wasn't stuck on himself and didn't have an ego." Long-time season ticket holder Darlene Westley saluted Kathy as one of the active players' wives. "She played an important role in setting up a baby shower for my daughter," said Westley, who hosted spaghetti dinners and barbeques for players throughout the season.

On the field, McGwire began channeling his power into games. A visit from the A's roving minor league hitting instructor Bob Watson also shortened his long swing. Watson, who flew back and forth between Alabama and California during the season tutoring hitters, spent hours with McGwire. "We did hitting drills day in and day out," said Watson. "I probably spent 1,000 hours with him on his swing and approach. He really learned how to speed up his bat." McGwire absorbed Watson's advice, and it showed in games. "He went on a big-time hitting streak and he was locked in," said Guinn. "He found something that worked for him. He was figuring things out. He was always able to hit the breaking ball.

McGwire wasn't the only redhead in the Modesto clubhouse. His younger brother, J.J., frequently visited the Central Valley. The fifteen-year-old ferocious linebacker starred for Claremont High. After a bizarre BB gun accident that blinded his right eye, he dove into bodybuilding. On his fitness training website, McGwiresfitness.com, J.J. detailed his romance with weight lifting. "At the age of thirteen, I found that my true passion and calling was in weight lifting and body-building. At age twenty-three, I was so involved in bodybuilding that I began to compete. This passion for weight lifting took me into a career that has become my lifelong endeavor," J.J. wrote.[1]

McGwire's childhood friend Scott Larson hailed J.J. as a football standout who fell below the radar after the eye injury. "Prior to the injury, he was well on his way to making a name for himself on the football field," Larson said in an email in December 2007. "After the injury, I saw little to none of him. The injury shattered his dreams and really dislodged him from his social circles. Bodybuilding allowed him to stay in the presence of his brothers in a useful light."

With his older brothers Mark and Dan, a Seattle Seahawks' quarterback, bursting into professional sports, J.J. had much to live up to. He soon bench-pressed his way into a hulking physique, and when he strutted in the clubhouse in 1985, it sparked curiosity in players. He perused the clubhouse and casually discussed steroids with players. One of McGwire's teammates in Modesto, who preferred anonymity, quickly figured things out. "He was about six foot two, 230 [pounds] and nothing but muscle. A select group of players would inquire. He was around there for a reason. As players, we knew what was going on, but it was an unwritten rule that you never said anything. So Mark may have not gotten as deeply or heavily into it [steroids] by '88, but he was introduced to it at an early age."

At the plate, McGwire generated a promising season. In 138 games, he batted .274 with 24 home runs and collected 106 runs batted in, leading the league in home runs and RBIs. For those efforts, he was also crowned the California League's rookie of the year in 1985. His improvement pleased the A's, who were also glistening when the twenty-one-year-old Canseco overshadowed the farm system by demolishing three levels of baseball that year, capturing *Baseball America*'s Minor League Player of the Year. The next season, in 1986, the A's dropped McGwire onto the same route Canseco paved the year before, starting in Double-A Huntsville.

Nineteen eighty-six. Huntsville Stars batboy David Sharp scurried through Huntsville International Airport. It was a new baseball season for the city and the fifteen-year-old Sharp, escorted by his mother, came to get his first glimpse of the team. The players were leaving spring training in Arizona and were tapped to play Double-A in Huntsville. The previous season, Canseco roared through Huntsville and captivated Sharp, and Sharp now anticipated another touted prospect—Mark McGwire. McGwire was not a foreign name for Sharp.

During his spare time he collected baseball cards and prized his 1984 McGwire Olympic rookie card, produced by Topps Trading Cards. Because of that fascination, he couldn't wait to meet him. As the players rested in the lobby and waited for their bus, Sharp ran into Stars' outfielder Rocky Coyle, a returning player from the previous season. "Which one is McGwire?" Sharp asked him. Coyle pointed to a mild-mannered, modest-looking redhead. "That's him over there—sitting by himself." Sharp, now a thirty-six-year-old baseball coach in Huntsville, to this day claimed his first encounter with McGwire best exuded his character. "The way I saw him at the airport was just how he was," explained Sharp. "He was quiet, subdued, and a very laid back guy. He didn't have that superstar flash to him."

McGwire's presence in the city generated a buzz. When he first trotted into Joe W. Davis Stadium, he was forced to inherit the residue of Canseco's success. "Will you be the next Canseco to rock the city?" asked local reporters. Regularly, he fielded questions littered with Canseco. He downplayed the comparison. "I'm not going to be the next José Canseco and I'm not a home run hitter," he told *Huntsville Times* beat writer Bob Mayes in 1986. "I hit the ball into the gaps and am more of a doubles hitter. If people expect me to be José Canseco, they're going to be sorely disappointed."

Coyle remembered hearing the comparisons, but sensed that those distractions didn't alter McGwire's approach on the field. "I didn't see him put pressure on himself to be better than Canseco," said Coyle. "That wasn't a big issue for him. He was trying to get to the big leagues, so it was business as usual for him."

McGwire's modesty, however, didn't soften his bat. He roared to open the season. During his first twenty-seven games, he hit .303 and, at one point, homered in five consecutive games. He also boasted a ten-game hitting streak. His torrid hitting pace was capped by a game against the Orlando Twins in late April; that game, he crushed a three-run homer and drilled a run-scoring single to provide all of Huntsville's runs and help fuel them to victory by a score of 4-3. Those statistics helped twenty-one-year-old McGwire garner Southern League Player of the Week honors. On May 8 McGwire ripped four hits and drove in five runs to lead the Stars past the Chattanooga Lookouts, 14-8. Because of McGwire's immediate success, word quickly spread that his stay in Huntsville would be brief. "Everyone knew he was going to hit—there was no doubt about that," said Don Mincher, the former general manager of the Huntsville Stars. "He hit balls a long way."

Coyle, who consoled a frustrated and confused McGwire with Modesto in 1984, marveled at his development two years later. "He was a whole different player," said Coyle. "When he had that full season in Modesto, I saw a huge improvement. They just left him alone and he hit. That's when he really started to mature."

Although McGwire claimed he wasn't a power hitter, his long, booming home runs proved otherwise, as did his fascination with weight lifting. Most players in the organization understood weight training had elevated Canseco's game, transforming him into a minor league legend. And while McGwire tinkered with weights in college, he dedicated endless hours to building his physique in Huntsville. "He was obsessed with weight lifting," said former Stars' radio play-by-play broadcaster Rick Davis. "After games, I would come down to the clubhouse and everyone was gone, but he was bench pressing all by himself. In those days, we had a couple pieces of weight lifting equipment. The guy was devoted to it. I've never seen anything like that."

Sharp, too, recalls McGwire's passion for the weight room. He religiously stalked the small bench press stationed in the middle of the locker room and impressed teammates with the amount of weight he could lift. "I remember [Rocky] Coyle jokingly telling him, 'you know, we had a guy last year who could lift about that much' . . . referring to Canseco," Sharp said. "He actually lifted more than José did."

Coyle also lifted weights with McGwire in his hotel room on the road. He points to Huntsville as the stop where McGwire intensified his workouts, the dawning period of him sculpting his physique. "When he got there, he really started to get into weight lifting," said Coyle. "You could see him getting stronger. He had a duffle bag filled with weights and he would take it on the road."

Cadaret said McGwire had bought into the A's conditioning and weight lifting program, and his body started to change. "He was getting stronger," said Cadaret. "He was just a naturally big-boned guy without a lot of weight room strength. He had big forearms, big hands, but not a lot of upper body. He started to lose his baby fat, thin out, watch his diet, and really start to take care of himself. His body started to change."

His muscles couldn't help him feel any better at third base, though. Complicating matters was the stadium's rocky infield dirt, which made it difficult for infielders to field clean hops. That combination made for grueling games for McGwire. "It was a tough surface to play on," recalled Guinn. "It had hard and soft spots, so you couldn't get a true hop." Davis saluted McGwire's hard work to improve his defense at third base, but he noticed his heart wasn't there. "He wasn't a third baseman—but a backstop," recalled Davis. "When a ball was hit at him, he let it bounce up and hit his chest and then threw to first base. He wasn't really happy about playing there, but he tried really hard."

Fans bashed McGwire for his defensive miscues. Even though he wasn't eagerly embracing his position, fans couldn't comprehend the A's long-term plan for him, which didn't guarantee immediate success in Huntsville. "The fans didn't appreciate his defensive ability," said Don Mincher. "His range wasn't there and he had some problems. Some recognized very quickly that if he was to sustain defensively, he was going to have to move to first base."

McGwire's bat did cause enough havoc in the Southern League to warrant an abrupt promotion. In fifty-five games, McGwire launched ten home runs and amassed fifty-three runs batted in. His .303 batting average and fifteen doubles also bolstered his resume. McGwire's consistency at the plate gave the A's more than enough reason to elevate him to a higher caliber of baseball. In June, the A's sent him to Tacoma, Washington, where he would play in the Pacific Coast League for the A's Triple-A affiliate, the doorstep of the major leagues. "The plan was definitely not move those guys [Canseco and McGwire] in the middle of the season, but they had nothing else to prove in Double-A," remembered Kuehl.

When McGwire planted his feet in Tacoma, he arched more eyebrows. Catcher Bill Bathe, who looked forward to teaming with the prospect, greeted him in the clubhouse and recognized his strength. "Back then, he wasn't as big as he became later in his career, but whenever you'd shake his hand in the clubhouse, you'd say, 'Oh my God . . . this guy has serious power' —just by his natural handshake," remembered Bathe. "And then you'd watch him in batting practice and the way he would launch balls and you'd be like, 'this guy has some pop.'" Bathe had watched McGwire hit in Arizona for spring training and was impressed by the maturity McGwire carried to the plate and his studious approach during batting practice. "He had a great mindset and tremendous power," said Bathe. "He was hitting home runs where most players didn't hit them. You knew he had a lot of potential."

In his first game in the Pacific Coast League, McGwire blasted a home run, maintaining his torrid pace. By July, he was leading Tacoma with a .337 batting average and accumulated seventeen runs batted in over only twenty-five games. On July 14, he clobbered two solo home runs to lift Tacoma past the Phoenix Firebirds, 7-4. One observer, Tacoma assistant general manager Ron Zolo, raved about McGwire's hitting exploits, including his power to the opposite field. "I remember him just going with a pitch and hitting a home run to right field," said Zolo. "You could tell he was going to play in the big leagues." Tacoma general manager Stan Nacarrato, who had scratched his head over the ridiculous number of balls Canseco lost over the fence the year before, confronted the same financial worries with McGwire. "I'd come out of my office and watch him take batting practice and wondered how poor we would be today," Nacarrato said with tongue in cheek. "He left lots of smiles and was an asset here."

Keith Lieppman was McGwire's manager in Tacoma. As a seasoned member of the organization's managerial staff, the thirty-five-year-old Lieppman monitored his early struggles breaking into the minor leagues, but began seeing glimpses of the caliber of player he would become. "He hit one off this big monster in centerfield, some 450 away," said Lieppman, who's now the A's director of player development. "It was a tremendous shot. At that time, he started doing things power-wise that I'd never seen before."

Lieppman, who also managed Canseco in Tacoma the year before and tossed batting practice to both before games, admired their spectacular display of power and how it impacted games. "They were of a different ilk—different animals," Lieppman said. "You could feel their presence. You had to be very careful not to leave yourself exposed over the screen. Some guys can hit them in batting practice, but can't in the game—those guys learned how to do it in a game." In seventy-eight games, McGwire boasted a .318 batting average, slammed thirteen home runs, and drove in fifty-nine runs. "He became much more efficient," said Kuehl. "He didn't really change his swing, but it was getting to the point where he just didn't miss mistakes. He made improvements as his career went along, no doubt about that."

Back in Oakland, meanwhile, hot-hitting second baseman Tony Phillips strained his knee on the base paths, forcing him on the disabled list a week later. With the A's in dire need of an additional infielder, they called up McGwire. The abrupt promotion was disappointing news for Tacoma, which was battling for a wild-card berth in the Pacific Coast League and hadn't made the playoffs since 1982. The following week the club was scheduled to finish off the season in Hawaii. McGwire's call-up meant he wouldn't make the trip.

"We're disappointed as hell to be losing McGwire now; I can't lie about that," Naccarato told the *San Jose Mercury News* in 1986. "But I understand where they [the A's] are. They're fighting for third place, which would salvage a tough season for them. . . . Whatever I think isn't that important, anyway. We just have to go on. Our fans are going to be a little ticked."[2]

Not McGwire, though. On August 20, McGwire boarded a plane and traveled to Baltimore, where the A's were playing a three-game series against the Orioles. Scheduled to play third base against crafty left-handed starter Mike Flanagan, McGwire's debut would give way to Mother Nature as the game was rained out. The gloomy weather couldn't keep the happy-go-lucky twenty-two-year-old from holding court with reporters in the clubhouse. During the rain delay, reporters probed him about the twenty-five errors he committed at third base in the minor leagues. "The toughest thing is knowing when to use my arm," McGwire told reporters. "Sometimes I don't throw the ball as hard as I should. I'll just throw the ball too softly."

Two games later, on August 22, McGwire fittingly made his entrance at New York's Yankee Stadium, baseball's most legendary platform. Dubbed the House that Ruth Built after iconic slugger Babe Ruth rocked the Bronx and compelled the team to build Yankee Stadium, it opened in 1923 and its storied history flashed a series of baseball greats. Plaques honoring such late Yankee greats as Babe Ruth, Mickey Mantle, Joe DiMaggio, Lou Gehrig, and Roger Maris all headlined Monument Park located beyond the left-center-field fence. Before the game, McGwire strolled by the monuments.

McGwire, however, had to steer his focus on the field. A's manager Tony La Russa started him at third base and inked him seventh in the batting lineup, two spots behind Canseco, who was mired in a 0-for-33 slump. Besides a deep drive to left-center field, McGwire was hitless in three at-bats in the game. His critical mistake at third base, though, generated the most interest in the clubhouse. With the A's leading by a score of 2-1 and a runner on second in the bottom of the fourth, Dave Winfield ripped a two-out single to left off A's starter Joaquin Andujar. Canseco, who charged in from left field and fielded the ball, fired a bullet toward home plate, appearing to be way ahead of the runner. But the rookie McGwire overzealously snagged the throw near third base, allowing the runner to score. His decision to cut off the throw baffled teammates. Agonizing over his decision, too, he wanted to smother his face with his glove in embarrassment. "Nobody said anything, it was just a reaction thing," McGwire admitted to reporters after the game. "Right when I did it, I knew I shouldn't have."

During the final game of the series, McGwire righted his blunder. Although he began his career going 0-for-6, he took good swings and launched deep drives. His swings didn't translate into hits until he ironically faced his father's dental patient back in Orange County, Yankee veteran starter Tommy John. In the early 1980s, John stumbled into McGwire's dad at a celebrity golf tournament in Southern California. And when John was traded from the Yankees to the California Angels in 1982, he became one of John McGwire's patients. With John entering into the twilight of his career and McGwire bursting onto the scene, against the odds, fate orchestrated the match up.

"Tommy use to sit in the chair," Dr. McGwire told the *Globe and Mail* in 1987. "And I'd ask him how he planned to pitch to my son when he broke into the big leagues. And Tommy would say something like, 'real slow.'"

On August 24, a Sunday afternoon, in front of a crowd of 31,796, McGwire battled John. Leading off the top of the second inning, McGwire banged a single to center field for his first major league hit. In the sixth inning, he scorched a run-scoring double to left off John for his first RBI, capping a three-hit game. "What the heck, they found the holes pretty good today," McGwire told reporters after the game.

Years later, when John was asked about coughing up McGwire's first two hits of his career, he responded, "When your dentist's kids start hitting you, maybe it's time to start thinking about retirement." McGwire had only begun. The next day, McGwire marched into Detroit's Tiger Stadium, a familiar spot. When McGwire toured the country with Team USA in 1984, he homered in the historic venue. During batting practice, McGwire peppered the upper deck with booming blasts. But facing the wiles of a poised veteran right-handed pitcher such as twenty-eight-year-old Walt Terrell, who was scheduled to start for the Tigers, is another story.

Before his call-up, the A's planned on using McGwire mainly against left-handed pitching. After brooding over the line-up card in his office before the game, however, La Russa wanted to see how he would respond and tapped him to start. After twice striking out against Terrell during the game, McGwire rewarded his manager in the top of the fifth inning. He blasted a colossal two-run home run that cleared the 440-foot sign in dead center field, 450 feet from the plate. The buzz about McGwire's first major league home run and its distance rippled through the dugout. At the time, McGwire was one of only four players since 1973 to clear baseball's most spacious grounds. "I don't know if I've hit one farther, I really can't say," McGwire told reporters after the game. "I don't judge them. They had been working me away with sliders, but this pitch was up. . . . I know that's a death valley out there like New York, so I just started running. Then I saw it go out. It's good to get all the firsts out of the way."

A's hitting coach Bob Watson, who had tweaked his batting stance a year before in Modesto, proudly applauded McGwire's efforts. "I knew he had power," Watson told the *San Jose Mercury News* after the game. "But I can't honestly tell you I thought he'd hit a ball 440 for his first major league homer. That's about a $6 cab ride out there."[3]

McGwire clubbed three home runs the remainder of the season, also victimizing Baltimore's Scott McGregor and Chicago's Ray Searage. With fifty-three at-bats under his belt, he also batted .189 and drove in nine runs. In three levels of professional baseball in 1986, McGwire batted .270 with 26 homers and 121 RBIs.

"He had great power," remembered former A's radio play-by-play broadcaster Lon Simmons. "At that time, he was big, but wasn't as impressive size-wise as he became to be when he matured." One A's coach, however, felt McGwire needed more polishing in the minors. "I didn't think he was ready for the big leagues," said former A's strength and conditioning coach Dave McKay. "But I was thinking a lot about his play at third base. He had some throwing problems in the minors and it looked like that was going to be a position he was going to have some trouble playing at the level we preferred. I definitely didn't stand up and say, 'Hey this guy is going to rake up here.' That goes to show you that coaches make mistakes, too."

McGwire was still a work in progress for the A's, however. During the off-season, they sent him to play winter ball in the Dominican Republic. Playing for league powerhouse Licey Tigers, McGwire was expected to hone his skills at third and get more at-bats to prepare him for the following season. That Triple-A manager Lieppman was scheduled to manage the club during the three-month season and monitor his development confirmed the A's plans. Those plans, though, were short-lived.

Although McGwire had previously traveled domestically and internationally, he couldn't adjust to the lifestyle and mediocre playing facilities of Latin America.

Because of local energy constraints, only two banks of lights were used during evening practices, making it hard to see the ball. Unpredictable bounces caused by lumpy infields hurt his game at third base. Also, the luxuries and amenities he enjoyed in America eluded him. Life in the Dominican took its toll on McGwire and his play, as it was a far cry from the cozy suburb of Claremont where he grew up. "I didn't like it," McGwire told reporters the following spring in 1987. "I wasn't playing very well. I wasn't improving my game. I wasn't happy."

McGwire bolted early and returned to California. "He hated the experience and walked after about a month," said Lieppman. "He just didn't want to be there." Catcher Terry Steinbach, who also made the trek, said that McGwire wasn't the only player hassling to adjust. He claimed the 160-plus game schedules both played earlier had drained them. "We were fried and neither of us did well there," said Steinbach, who lasted a month longer than McGwire. "After the season, we went home for literally six days and then went to the Dominican. Both of us were probably hitting below .200."

McGwire's abrupt departure, however, didn't bode well with Oakland. In fact, by leaving early, he unintentionally focused even more attention on Rob Nelson, who gutted it out for the entire winter ball. "Once he left, he left a bad taste in the organization's mouth, because they provided him an opportunity to play all winter and with at-bats to get him ready for the big leagues," said Lieppman. "So when he left around the first of November, it set the tone that Rob Nelson was going to be the number one choice to win the job in the spring. It didn't look like he was going to make the club." The risk of smudging his hard-working reputation was worth it for McGwire, who figured if he impressed manager Tony La Russa during spring training, he could still make the club. No matter how disappointed the A's were about his decision, he realized they couldn't ignore a monstrous spring.

NOTES

[1] Jay McGwire, "About Jay," *McGwire's Fitness*, http://www.mcgwires fitness.com/aboutjay.htm. Author note: Emails and phone messages to J.J. were not returned.

[2] Bud Geracie, "Tacoma-Oakland Shuttle Brings McGwire," *San Jose Mercury News*, August 21, 1986.

[3] Bud Geracie, "McGwire's First HR in Majors Is a Monster," *San Jose Mercury News*, August 26, 1986.

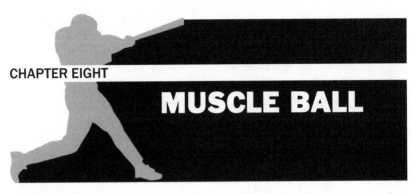

CHAPTER EIGHT

MUSCLE BALL

"Karl and Dave ran a military-like camp in the minor leagues, to get the players physically stronger than any other team. I think that was one of their objectives—to be the strongest organization in baseball. It was a grind."

—Former A's outfielder and first baseman Doug Jennings
August 2007

Oakland Athletics' farm director Karl Kuehl's baptism into professional baseball began as an inquisitive, eighteen-year-old outfielder in the Cincinnati Reds organization in 1955. Though his journey never landed him in the big leagues, he acquired enough instincts to serve in behind-the-scenes capacities, such as molding talent, for three decades as a major league scout. Kuehl relished dissecting a hitter's bat-path and identifying his holes at the plate—the old-fashioned batting vernacular. After watching one swing, he could spot flaws and offer remedies.

When Kuehl was playing, he stumbled upon a wrist-building piece of training equipment at a local store in his hometown of St. Petersburg, Florida. Out of curiosity, he purchased the device and casually squeezed away during his spare time. He soon noticed a change in his forearms; they ballooned. After carrying his swelled forearms and taking hacks in the batting cage, Kuehl noticed another development: the ball suddenly jumped off his bat. He immediately attributed his rejuvenated swing and increased power to his hardened forearms. That revelation has positioned him as one of baseball's most vocal ambassadors for hand, grip, and wrist strength and he injects those principles to his minor leaguers. Now a Cleveland Indians' special assistant, Kuehl still carries a presence. When he swaggers into a clubhouse, players abruptly clench their fist and flex their forearms, searching for his approval. "Hand strength is critical and the forearm is what makes

91

those muscles work. It's all about grip strength for hitters," explained Kuehl.

Kuehl was onto something. His discovery drove him to study other muscles that were an integral ingredient to a hitter's swing, such as triceps and back; according to Kuehl, these muscles, along with forearms, are the hauling muscles of a swing. He encouraged his players to concentrate on those muscles during weight lifting, which could maximize power at the plate. They, too, began noticing the benefits. Kuehl was ahead of his time. Though strength training was frowned upon in the 1970s, he was one of the few who endorsed it. That philosophy led him to another discovery: when he walked into several clubhouses over the years, he noticed the staggering disparity between major league players' physiques and minor leaguers'. "Those minor leaguers couldn't measure up," observed Kuehl. "Strength was a factor."

Kuehl's observations began taking shape. In the late 1970s, Kuehl spotted players, such as Roy Smalley, Lance Parrish, and Brian Downing, thriving in the majors, who all pointed to weight lifting as their secret for maintaining peak performance amid a rigorous 162-game schedule. Their endorsements were enough for him to enforce a groundbreaking strength-training program for the A's minor leaguers shortly after he inherited the role of farm director in September 1983. Kuehl claimed that the mandatory program promoted strength training—not bodybuilding. Not many of his colleagues applauded Kuehl's unorthodox thinking and scoffed at him instead. They believed that too much muscle could rob a player of the athleticism and flexibility required for baseball. Kuehl hoped to prove his doubters wrong. "They laughed at me," said Kuehl. "Clubs certainly weren't encouraging it, but I knew that we didn't have any player in our system that wouldn't benefit from it."

One person who certainly backed Kuehl was A's athletic trainer Ted Polakowski, who was hired by the A's in 1984. He assisted Kuehl in structuring and transmitting the vision into the organization. By aiding Kuehl, he fended off the criticisms heaved by baseball circles, but still provided unwavering support. "We were very criticized," said Polakowski. "In those years, that was our forte; no other teams were doing it. While a lot of those practices are accepted now, weight training wasn't accepted back then. It was almost a taboo."

That didn't stop Kuehl, who channeled his vision into his first Instructional League with the A's at Scottsdale Community College in Arizona. He rented bench presses, barbells, exercise tubing, and dumbbells, and stored the equipment in the visitors clubhouse at Phoenix Municipal Stadium, the A's spring training complex. He soon persuaded Scottsdale Community College to allow his players full access to its weight room during spring training. Over time Kuehl's embryonic program evolved into the most meticulous in minor league baseball. Driven by fierce accountability, he obsessively monitored player's body fat and measured chest, biceps, and forearms. Snapshot photos of players were taken before and after the season to gauge progress. Kuehl explained:

> I wanted to know where guys were, so I wanted some measurements. We actually started out measuring our pitchers. The thing we discovered out almost immediately was that if a guy had a 14 1/2 inch bicep, for example, and it suddenly decreased below his norm, those were the guys who had atrophy and were breaking down. Back then, we were finding our way and the only way to do that was with measures.

Those measurements advanced his program. By 1985, the A's philosophy echoed throughout their farm system. That year, *Baseball America* ranked the A's minor league system as the third best in baseball, only behind the Yankees and Mariners. It was a vast improvement from ranking sixteenth the year before. While some players reluctantly participated in the program, others bought into the system, dedicating their entire off-season to prepare for spring training. The catchphrase "Make the sacrifice during the off-season to become a winner during the season" was embedded into players. "The industry began to change," said Polakowski, who graduated from Arizona State in 1984 with a degree in sports medicine. "Years ago, players came to spring training to get in shape. Now players were coming to spring training already in shape."

Kuehl prodded players into impeccable shape and pushed them to greater conditioning during the off-season. Some players embraced the system, but others felt victimized by it. One former player, who preferred anonymity, described the pressure.

> Karl use to come around the clubhouse the first couple days of spring training and would watch you take your shirt off to see if you came in shape or not. If you didn't and were fat and out of shape you were released or traded. The message was sent very early that it was unacceptable to report to spring training out of shape. There was an unwritten rule that you do your work in the off-season and if you don't cooperate, you wouldn't be in the organization very long.

In 1984, Kuehl also lured Phoenix-based power lifter John Kanter, whose son John, Jr., was a second baseman in the A's system. Kanter, who had shattered power-lifting records throughout the country, was responsible for teaching strength training and nutrition to herds of minor leaguers in Phoenix. "Out of all the guys that would come, I never saw Canseco, but the next year he walked in twenty pounds heavier," recalled Kanter, now a sixty-seven-year-old trainer. "Everybody wondered what the hell happened. He looked like a balloon."

According to an A's former minor leaguer, several players used performance-enhancing drugs during the 1980s. "They taught that you needed to do something extra, because people are going by you," said the former A's farmhand. That's what frustrated Kanter. Although he encouraged players to buy into his drug-free lifting principles, he battled a rising trend. "Guys like Canseco were getting big without training; just fooling around in the gym. That's what was so negative about it. I was battling the drug scene and all the cheating. You had to be very naïve not to know what was going on." Once other players spotted Canseco getting bigger and more successful, others followed according to Kanter. "I've never touched a steroid in my life. The steroid guys I lifted against for years in national world competition, eleven of them are dead. Their livers and kidneys are gone. I'm sixty-seven and I'm still working out."

Former A's catcher Terry Steinbach shattered home-run records for Minnesota's New Ulm High School and later starred for the University of Minnesota, where he was named Big Ten Player of the Year in 1983. His performance prompted the A's to select him in the ninth round of the 1983 amateur draft. Growing up in Minnesota, Steinbach remembered the stigma attached to weight lifting in baseball. In the late 1980s and early '90s, Steinbach believed more emphasis was placed on weight training and noticed players becoming stronger. And the A's, he reflected, were the pioneers of the weight-training movement in baseball.

> When I was in high school and college, the consensus was that "no baseball player should lift or you're going to get too tight and won't be able to swing." But when players started to get paid more and didn't have to work full-time during the winter, they went home and hired strength and agility coaches. And if you look at today's players, it's almost a norm to have your own personal trainers and go to specially designed facilities to get them in peak performance shape for baseball. Oakland was the first club to have a strength coach. It was a changing era.

David Wilder spent five seasons in the A's organization, beginning in 1982. A former outfielder, he climbed his way through the minor leagues before being packaged in a trade to the Chicago Cubs for starting pitcher Dennis Eckersley in 1987. With stops at minor affiliates

Idaho Falls, Modesto, Huntsville, and Tacoma, Wilder experienced first hand how the A's groomed their players and blazed a new culture in baseball. He valued Kuehl's efforts.

> Single-handedly, they were the first organization to make it a point that weight lifting was something that's good for you under supervision. They pushed that a baseball player can benefit from becoming a stronger athlete. It was a whole different culture; we participated in aerobic classes and stretching and not having a gut. It wasn't about being bulky; it was about athleticism and strength.

Lifting weights and gaining strength is where conditioning coach Dave McKay stepped in. Before retiring with the A's in 1982, the scrappy, switch-hitting, infielder batted .229 and mustered only twenty-one home runs during his eight-year career with the Twins, Blue Jays, and A's. Aside from those mediocre numbers, however, McKay was an oddity among teammates. He compulsively incorporated weight lifting into his baseball life; he believed weight lifting made him durable enough to overcome injuries and endure the long season. Though players ridiculed him and downplayed its advantages, McKay stubbornly chased his addiction and claimed it gave him a psychological edge. "I just always felt like I had to be in better shape than the other guy," admitted McKay, who currently serves as the first base coach for the St. Louis Cardinals. "Once I got out of the game, I started getting into bodybuilding a little bit."

Shortly after retirement, the thirty-four-year-old Phoenix resident was hired by A's general manager Sandy Alderson as the strength and conditioning coach. Alderson assigned him to travel with the club and develop workout regimens for players throughout the season. Though Alderson had only entered the industry in 1981, the Harvard Law School graduate was savvy enough to recognize how weight lifting had bolstered Chicago White Sox catcher Carlton Fisk's power surge in the mid-1980s. In 1983, the thirty-six-year-old Fisk met Chicago-based chiropractor Dr. Phillip E. Claussen, who helped him overcome a chronic stomach muscle strain through weight training. Both became workout partners during the winter, and Fisk soon became a strong advocate for weight lifting. From that point, Fisk's home-run totals soared from twenty-one in 1984 to thirty-seven in 1985. Those increases intrigued Alderson. "He was an older guy and started lifting weights during one off-season," Alderson said of Fisk. "His sudden resurgence of power was attributed to the fact that he lifted weights. That caused me to ask, 'Why aren't we doing weight training?' Being new to the industry, my attitude was, 'Why not give it a shot?'"

And the franchise did. Alderson anointed Kuehl and McKay to school players in the world of strength and endurance. McKay admitted that the strength training exercises he initiated in the early 1980s have faded over the years and have taken a back seat to more advanced baseball-targeted ones used today. Today, in fact, he cringes at some of the workouts he once endorsed. "We were the black sheep. It was real close to the first time players started lifting," recalled Dave McKay, who later teamed with Canseco to author *Strength Training for Baseball*.

> Everyone felt we were doing more damage than good for our players. So there were things that we learned over time. Through trial and error, we discovered what machines worked and didn't work and which ones were best for a player. In the beginning, we probably did exercises that we wouldn't do today; it was a learning stage at that point. I remember Sparky Anderson saying, "There's no place for weight lifting in baseball," and four years later, they had had a strength coach and a weight room.

McKay claimed he never intended for his affair with muscles to endorse bulk or assist players in acquiring a massive Herculean physique. He said he hoped his advice would proactively prevent injuries and produce a lean, well-balanced physique built for baseball. "It really stemmed from perfect form and technique—not trying to put on size," explained McKay. "We focused on each body part and we almost treated it as rehabilitation. We focused on balance: biceps, triceps, chest, and back, instead of focusing on one muscle group over the other. We stressed balance as much as we could."

McKay insisted he also adamantly discouraged steroid use, a muscle-building drug rippling through the bodybuilding community. McKay confessed, however, that at one point several A's players were exposed to the drugs during spring training in 1985. Through a coach's recommendation, Kuehl had just hired a muscle-bound power lifter to offer training tips to his players. Rumors circulated around camp that he was introducing steroids to players. "He was this Hulk-looking guy and felt like he was in an area where most people didn't understand, so he thought it was easy to slip in and out without people knowing it," McKay said of the trainer. "There were rumors of him using and talking to other players, but that wasn't what we were after."

Mike Ashman, who played catcher for both A's Double-A affiliate in Huntsville and Triple-A affiliate in Tacoma in 1985, recalled seeing the trainer stroll through camp. "It's funny reading some of the quotes from the past where [A's] management was unaware about what was going on," said Ashman. "He would go to the restroom and after he came out, it smelled like a chemical factory."

The trainer's raucous and aggressive style of training also concerned McKay. Because of the way the trainer pushed exhausted players to finish repetitions during circuit training, McKay feared one of his players would overextend and injure himself. "There was a lot of hollering and pushing, and I was thinking, 'hey, these guys aren't body-builders; they're baseball players.' I couldn't have one guy blow out his shoulder trying to do one more chin up."

To block his influence from spreading through camp, McKay claimed he informed Kuehl. Kuehl said he immediately severed ties with the trainer. "As soon as I was informed that this guy was hanging around, I told his friend, 'you have to get him out of here—I don't want him around,'" confirmed Kuehl. "He lasted two weeks, at the most. We wouldn't let him back."

His program continued, but Kuehl realized he couldn't control what activities players engaged in away from the ballpark. Two of his touted prospects, Canseco and McGwire, savored their time in the weight room at Scottsdale Community College. "We had other kids that participated, too, but nobody got after it the way they did," remembered Kuehl. "I used to have them doing wrist curls and they lifted more than anyone else." Ted Polakowski, the director of Arizona Baseball Operations for the A's, also recalled how both spent countless hours in the gym. "If it was early work or late afternoon work, José and Mark were always there," recalled Polakowski.

Some former minor leaguers in the organization recalled no such emphasis on weight training, however. They claimed that it was only after Canseco beefed up his frame and displayed astronomical power in Huntsville, Tacoma, and Oakland in 1985 the A's preached its value. Former Huntsville Stars outfielder Rocky Coyle, who fans still dub the "Mayor of Huntsville" for his gutsy play in 1985, recalled:

> It was not there. We didn't experience that until after Canseco's phe-nomenon. We did push up and sit ups, but if you lifted weights it was only on your own. That's why José went to Miami and got that [ste-roids]. If there was more guidance and they were so responsible then none of that steroid stuff would have been there. They were a good organization, but they weren't prepared for steroids. I never got one program from one of them. Everyone got on Canseco's bandwagon and wanted to take credit for him.

Former first baseman José Tolentino, who played five seasons in the organization before he was traded to the Texas Rangers in 1987, admitted that players began toying with weight lifting in the organization. Canseco's legend, however, propelled its popularity within the organization. "The A's adopted the philosophy of weight lifting from Canseco," said Tolentino. "A lot of people want to take credit, but Canseco was the one who started it in Modesto. They adopted it because they saw him. That was already a culture coming around, but he was the first one. I wish I could have caught that train, too. A lot of us wish we would have."

Outfielder Ron Cumming played for Single-A Modesto in 1984. While he admitted to being exposed to weights during spring training, it was never mandatory during the season. "At that time, none of us were doing any of that during the season," said Cummings. "Oddly enough, there was still an underlying taboo against weight lifting in baseball. While there was some power running and weight lifting during spring training, those six weeks wouldn't do a lot of good for an entire season."

If Canseco pioneered a weight lifting revolution in the franchise, though, he did it on his own, McKay asserts. He claimed Canseco stubbornly drifted from team weight-training workouts he implemented and chose to branch out into bodybuilding. McKay had difficulty then guiding him through a structured program. An even greater concern for McKay was Canseco's prolonged absences from the gym. When he did finally stroll into the weight room, he stubbornly worked out with heavy weights. That concerned McKay and prompted him to inform Sandy Alderson that Canseco had his own agenda. "I worried about him because he would do his own thing," said McKay. "He wouldn't lift with the guys; he would pick his own time. No matter what you'd tell him, he was going to do his own thing."

That forced McKay to use other tactics to keep him on track. "I would have to walk up to him and say, 'José, it looks like you're losing some size,'" said McKay. "That would get his attention and he might show up the next day." On the road, McKay woke up early, grabbed the hotel's breakfast menu, checked off a breakfast dish, and hung it on Canseco's door for a 9:00 AM wakeup call. "They [room service] would knock on his door and he would say, 'I didn't order breakfast,'" said McKay. "He knew what I was doing because I wanted to get him up, otherwise he'd sleep in."

Lifting weights was only one element to shape A's players. Fitness guru Mack Newton complemented the program. A tae kwon-do instructor since 1966, Mack had operated several martial arts studios in Chicago before migrating to Phoenix in 1985. After arriving, Newton hoped to establish himself around the community and wrote a weekly fitness column for the *Phoenix Gazette*. He never thought that one of his columns would pique the interest of Sandy Alderson, who was in town for spring training. After reading the column, Alderson was so intrigued that he sent A's assistant trainer Larry Davis to interview Newton and convince him to offer his fitness principles to players. Since Newton had already trained a few minor league players, he agreed and came to Scottsdale to work with the minor leaguers. Newton soon became a part of the A's coaching staff. "It quickly blossomed," said Newton, who became baseball's first conditioning coach. "They just believed they could make themselves better by bringing on someone like myself to improve their core strength and flexibility."

A charismatic but unbending disciplinarian, Newton took his craft seriously. Anointed by Alderson, a former member of the United States Marine Corps who served in Vietnam, to train his players, Newton taxed players with strenuous stretching exercises and flexibility training in the early morning hours before field workouts. During formation, if a player mumbled or interrupted his instructions, he urged them to leave the group. "I was hard-nosed, but tolerant," said Newton. "The bottom line was that they were always going to do things my way. They liked having someone like myself with a quasi-military background, who could control the guys and bring a disciplined approach to the players."

At one point, prima donnas such as Reggie Jackson and Rickey Henderson all faced the wrath of Newton. In 1987, after Newton had already established his stretching routine, Jackson arrived for spring training and began chatting with teammates during stretching exercises. Newton ordered Jackson: "Hold it down, number 44!" Jackson glared at Newton. "He gave me this 'do you know who you're talking to?' look," said Newton. "I told him, 'Listen, hold it down, I'm at work right now; either follow or get out of my formation.'"

Some players rejected Newton's authority and believed his exercises had no place in baseball. In 1986 former A's starter, flamboyant Joaquin Andujar, tried to persuade other players to boycott Newton's instructions. A's manager Jackie Moore warned his players that if they weren't going to participate, they should go home. Andujar eventually participated. "He tried to get me out of there, because it was something he didn't want to do; he thought it was bad for him. In the beginning, everyone was pretty much confused because it was so out of step with the conventional thinking in the big leagues," said Newton, who also focused on a player's mental aspect for winning and staying positive. "With Jackie's influence and by putting his foot down, that was that. Once I knew Jackie was behind me, I took over."

A's players embraced his teaching. When Newton spotted other teams sending trainers to videotape his sessions from the stands at

Phoenix Municipal Stadium, he realized his program's significance. Players such as Dave Kingman and Mike Davis followed his training. For example, Kingman flew his wife to Phoenix so Newton could produce a video for her. "People knew it was the wave of the future," said Newton. "We prided ourselves with our fitness. We had guys taking off their shirts and flexing. Our players wanted to wear tight uniforms so they could look cut."

Enforcing his stretching exercises, Newton forged a tenuous relationship with Canseco, who, he contended, spurned the instruction.

> He didn't take to it well at all. Off the field, though, he related to me very well. He didn't particularly like stretching and structure. And he didn't want anyone seeing him cooperate, and I had no idea why, because off the field we got along. He would frequently apologize for not cooperating with me on the field. Even though he was giving me trouble, he tried to cooperate.

Because of Canseco's reluctance to accept the program, Newton said McGwire would sit near Canseco and encourage him to participate. "He tried to be a better example to him, especially on the stretching part," said Newton.

Cooperating with Newton was not so grueling for McGwire. He valued the conditioning and even lured several family members to participate. "Mark liked the stretching part and did all of the stomach conditioning, leg work, and shoulder conditioning," said Newton.

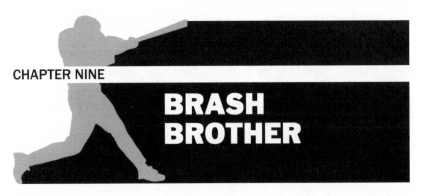

CHAPTER NINE

BRASH BROTHER

"Standing in the cage, his biceps bulging from his short-sleeve shirt, he looks like a middle linebacker who got lost. But with each swing, he sends another murmur through the stands. Each towering shot silences even the crusty old baseball scouts. There is the respect given Canseco that once was given to myths like Mays and Mantle."

—Steve Kelley, *Seattle Times*
March 1986

Nineteen-eighty six. When Cubs pitcher Dennis Eckersley grooved a fastball to twenty-two-year-old Canseco during an exhibition game in Arizona, he couldn't bear to watch. All spring Canseco had dominated him, whacking every fastball and slider he tossed. Canseco's brawny build and Eckersley's fearless demeanor made for an intriguing match up: a clash of brash youth and unflinching experience. Eckersley figured he would go straight after Canseco; Canseco swung as hard as he could. The ball sailed the other way, over the right-field fence. As Canseco circled the bases, a bewildered Eckersley was convinced he was bound for greatness. Eckersley, who started reviving his career in 1987 from Oakland to Cooperstown, remembered pitching to the prodigy.

> It was intimidating. He was just so far ahead of everybody that particular spring training. He was wearing me out and even took me deep a few times. He had this great big strike zone, so I just went right after him. . . . Right away, I knew this guy was going to be the real thing.

Everyone else who laid eyes on Canseco were amazed by his ability, including the A's, who hailed him as "The Natural" on their media guide's front cover in 1986. That Canseco clobbered tape-measure home runs, sped on the base paths, and unleashed a cannon for a right arm convinced many scouts he had the tools to become the next Willie Mays. It was as if the character Ivan Drago, played by Dolph Lundgren in *Rocky IV*, grabbed a bat and had been transformed into a hitter. As the rookie whipped his bat in the batting cage, admirers such as veteran broadcasters Lon Simmons and Amaury Pi-Gonzales reminisced of the 1960s, comparing his power and speed to that of Mays. "It came so easy for him," recalled Lon Simmons, who broadcasted for the San Francisco Giants in the 1960s and covered Mays. "When I first saw him, I thought he was going to establish every offensive record in baseball."

Those glowing reports filtered through the major leagues and reached Merv Rettenmund, a coach for the Texas Rangers in 1985. Even though he had yet to watch Canseco at the time, he was eager to see him play. Rettenmund remembered bumping into a public relations director who raved about Canseco. "He told me, 'Wait till you see this rookie on the Oakland A's—José Canseco—he's the best baseball player ever,'" recalled Rettenmund, who later coached him from 1989 to 1990. "Physically and mentally, he was the best player I've ever seen."

His talent also enthralled former teammate Mike Davis, an outfielder who teamed with Canseco from 1985 to 1987. Though Davis played with stars Dave Kingman, Rickey Henderson, and Reggie Jackson throughout his career, none matched Canseco. "When you first spotted Canseco you knew he was a Hall of Famer if he played long enough," said Davis, who broke in Canseco by taking him bass fishing during his rookie season. "He was on track of becoming the greatest player you would ever see. We'd be on the field and say, 'This cat is absolutely amazing.'"

After admiring his tools, baseball brass from around the league began to buzz about the muscle-popping rookie. "He'll be the first one to hit 70 home runs," Chicago White Sox executive Hawk Harrelson forecasted in 1986. His dependable defense in right field, adequate range, and strong arm convinced many he was more than a one-dimensional power hitter. "When he first came up, he was a very good defensive outfielder," said Mickey Morabito, the A's traveling secretary. "Everyone in the organization was saying he was a five-tool guy."

Canseco confronted such acclaim when he arrived in Phoenix for spring training in 1986. Having given the organization and fans a glimpse of his freakish power during his brief call-up in September the previous year, Canseco was poised for his rookie season, despite choosing to spend more time weight training than hitting baseballs during his off-season. Despite the A's suggestion that he play winter ball for the Licey Tigers in the Dominican Republic, Canseco preferred to sculpt his physique at the Miami Court Club. Packing on nineteen pounds of muscle during the winter, he carried 17 1/2-inch biceps and a 49-inch chest to camp, helping him swing his thirty-six-ounce bat. "I left Oakland at 210, and now I weigh 229," Canseco told the *Sacramento Bee*'s Susan Fornoff during spring training in 1986. "I've gotten stronger in every aspect. My arms are stronger, and I'm a faster runner also."[1]

Some of the A's management, though, felt he arrived to camp too bulky for baseball. "I guess he knows what he's doing, but I didn't think he needed to get bigger," said manager Jackie Moore in 1986. "Enough is enough."[2]

Canonized as the most legendary prospect to arrive to spring training in decades, he faced enormous expectations. Fans expected colossal home runs in bunches from Canseco, because he was being trumpeted and marketed as a machine built for baseball by the media and everyone who followed his exploits. Anything less would cast him as a bust, another player with legendary power in the minor leagues who couldn't carry those feats into the major leagues. "He was built up as 'The Natural,'" said Glenn Dickey, a columnist for the *San Francisco Chronicle* from 1971 to 2004. "He didn't have any experience in the major leagues and he wasn't prepared for the kind of attention he was getting."

Canseco welcomed those expectations, according to Tim Birtsas, an A's left-handed pitcher who was his close friend, roommate, and teammate during his rookie season. Birtsas became acquainted with the Canseco family when he met Canseco's twin brother, Ozzie, while both were pitchers in the Yankee organization. The two pitchers became friends, and eventually Ozzie asked Tim to be in his wedding party. At one time, Birtsas was one of the Yankee's prized pitching arms, but landed in Oakland when he was one of five players traded to the A's in exchange for superstar Rickey Henderson in 1984. "José was very confident in his ability and dedicated to the sport at the time. The A's organization didn't put anything on him that he didn't already expect from himself," recalled Birtsas.

If Canseco feared failure and buckled under the pressures to be a larger than life slugger, one couldn't detect it. His flair and swagger for a rookie, in fact, rubbed teammates the wrong way. Some interpreted his standoffish nature and confidence as arrogance and cockiness. The buzz around camp was that the comparisons of Mickey Mantle and Willie Mays inflated his ego, an aura teammates hoped to contain. One day, in the clubhouse in Phoenix, Canseco sported a tight t-shirt, exposing his bulging biceps. Several teammates suggested he intentionally washed it to make it shrink. Bruce Jenkins, the A's beat writer for the *San Francisco Chronicle* in 1986, spotted his swagger.

Although he tried to fit in, he couldn't help but expose his confidence—
his cocky side. There were times hanging around him when he seemed
essentially very shy. He wasn't terribly forthcoming with us. You knew
this kid was different; he was bigger than everyone else; he was better
looking than the rest of them and was going to get all the women he
wanted. He hit the [ball] further and he could throw it harder. Within
two weeks of hanging around the team and watching him hit in the
batting cage, I knew this guy was completely special.

Former A's third baseman Carney Lansford, who played with
Canseco in 1986, confirmed his arrogance. "He was very brash," said
Lansford. "He certainly didn't lack for confidence, that's for sure."
Former teammate Bill Bathe believed that Canseco walked with an
aura once he transformed his physique and improved his play. "Once
he really discovered who he was and built himself up and started
hitting the ball, he had a cockiness about him," said Bathe, whose
brother, Bob, roomed with Canseco in the minor leagues.

Still, adjusting to the major league lifestyle and fielding an array
of questions on a daily basis can take its toll. As a featured player on a
struggling club, the spotlight beamed on Canseco. From every angle,
reporters wanted a piece of him. He soon began feeling the effects that
accompany stardom, with fans and reporters hounding him and interrupting his private life, sapping all his energy. As a rookie, he didn't
indulge reporters with long-winded answers. Being asked the same
questions bugged him. That was evident when he lashed out at a reporter in the clubhouse after one exhibition game. "You've got five
minutes," Canseco barked at the reporter. "I'm just here to play ball,
not to be bothered by things that don't have anything to do with the
game. I don't mind being the center of attention, but it's getting ridiculous. Everything. It's carrying over into my private life."

Before the season, most experts projected him as the favorite to
capture the American League Rookie of the Year award, a hefty honor
considering the other crop of talented rookies such as Angels' first
baseman Wally Joyner, Rangers' outfielders Oddibe McDowell and
Pete Incaviglia, Mariners' second baseman Danny Tartabull, and Indians' outfielder Cory Snyder.

Canseco immediately reminded everyone why he was so touted.
His entertaining batting practice sessions became the highlight of camp.
Teammates and opposing players watched in awe as he drilled monstrous blasts over Phoenix Municipal Stadium. Suddenly batting
practice became a fireworks spectacle rather than a pre-game ritual.
Some teammates sarcastically blamed Canseco for losing so many baseballs that the team wouldn't have any balls left to practice. Jackie Moore,

Canseco's first manager in Oakland, said he feared for the safety of infielders and pitchers when he strode to the plate.

> We were in awe. There was a street that ran past the left-field fence at Phoenix Municipal Stadium, and when he took batting practice you heard tires screeching and balls denting cars. It was almost a dangerous situation. Hell! That type of power had never been with us before. He had that unusual open batting stance and because he closed up toward the pitcher and hit straight away, I thought he was going to hurt someone. There was always a fear in my mind of: 'what's going to happen if he happens to hit a ball right back at the pitcher?' As hard as he hit the ball, there's no way to react to it.

When conditioning specialist Mack Newton beheld one of Canseco's mythical blasts at Phoenix Municipal Stadium, he felt that the home run transcended human strength. With two pine trees planted on a hill looming behind the center-field fence, Canseco awed observers. "He hit a ball that cleared the fence, cleared the hill, and cleared the trees. We had no idea where it went," marveled Newton. "His power, sometimes, was beyond belief. It was unreal, humanly impossible. It was like standing under [Kareem] Abdul-Jabbar when he threw down a sky-hook."

Canseco wasn't the only rookie to generate headlines in the Bay Area. Across the Bay, in San Francisco, a charismatic, sweet swinging, left-handed first baseman, Will Clark, thrilled fans and sparked comparisons of Ted Williams. A graceful gap hitter with impressive power to all parts of the field, the slick-fielding standout shined at Mississippi State before the Giants snatched him as the second pick in the country during the 1985 amateur draft. With thirty-five years having passed since Willie Mays and Mickey Mantle arrived and split allegiances in New York, Canseco and Clark drew their own fan bases on each side of the Bay Bridge. "In this particular market, it may not have been quite as big of a story as it would have been elsewhere, but Will Clark was the best young hitter anyone had ever seen at the time. The Giants had the best young hitter and the A's had the best young power hitter. It was amazing times on both sides of the Bay," Bruce Jenkins explained.

Canseco generated a stir by blasting five home runs during spring exhibition games. His impressive performance convinced manager Jackie Moore to start him in left field and plant him fifth in the lineup on opening night at the Oakland-Alameda Coliseum on April 8. Batting fifth meant protecting veteran clean-up hitter Dave Kingman, who blasted sixty-five home runs for the A's over the previous two seasons.

Often perceived as moody, antagonistic, and distant in the clubhouse, the thirty-six-year-old Kingman garnered a plethora of press coverage during the 1970 amateur draft when the San Francisco Giants selected him first in the country. Touted as the nation's top collegiate power hitter at the University of Southern California, the former pitcher was facing the twilight of his sixteen-year career in 1986. Some wondered if the veteran would take Canseco under his wing and guide him through the perils of rookie stardom.

"Kingman had been through it," said Jackie Moore, currently the manager of the Round Rock Express, the Triple-A affiliate of the Houston Astros. "He was a guy that received a lot of publicity when he was coming up, and by being through it, he explained it to him and tried to be as much of an influence he could."

Some argue, though, that Kingman's fingerprints on Canseco were vague and he didn't spend much time mentoring the rookie. Also the strong-willed rookie developed a reputation as being a loner and for steering his own ship. "Kingman did have some influence on him," former A's beat writer John Hickey said. "But I wouldn't think it was all that significant. Canseco was always his own guy." Teammate Bill Bathe, who lived in Canseco's apartment complex in San Leandro, California, admitted he never observed such a relationship between the two sluggers. "I never saw it, and I think that's because Canseco was in a class all by himself," said Bathe.

What Bathe did remember was their explosive rounds of batting practice before each game. Canseco and Kingman entertained early arriving fans by belting booming tape-measure home runs. The Canseco-Kingman show raised eyebrows throughout American League venues. "They were in the same hitting group and if you were shagging in left field, you were lucky to get one or two balls because they were launching them right and left," said Bathe. "It was worth the price of admission just to watch."

Though Canseco amazed with enormous blasts before each game, his first home run of the season barely cleared the fence. On April 10, the third game of the season, he muscled a change-up off Minnesota Twins starter John Butcher in the bottom of the seventh at the Oakland-Alameda Coliseum. The blast, which a leaping center fielder Kirby Puckett nearly snatched at the wall, propelled the A's past the Twins, 3-0, salvaging the final game of the series. As Canseco barged into stadium after stadium, his batting practice displays generated a buzz around the cage. Players stopped stretching. Fans grabbed a seat. Everyone stopped and watched. "It was absolutely amazing," Mike Davis recalled. "It was the first time I ever saw a kid take batting practice, and the fans giving him a standing ovation when it was over." Strength coach Dave McKay admired the blasts. "You couldn't imagine balls traveling further," marveled McKay. "He lived for exciting the fans."

Despite his success, Canseco soon discovered the climate and elements at his home field, the Oakland-Alameda Coliseum, knocked down many of his deep drives. He believed that playing half of his games in Oakland smothered his home-run totals throughout the season. On the road, he relished the hitter friendly confines of Boston's Fenway Park; how the ball carried there; and the inviting left field monster, a thirty-seven-foot-high wall, 310 feet from home plate, whose dimensions right-handed sluggers lusted after. As a rookie, he hinted of one day playing for the Red Sox. Instead, he watched many of his potential home runs victimized by the conditions and dimensions at the coliseum. In July, *Miami Herald* journalist Joel Achenbach flew to the Bay Area to write a story on Canseco. "It's a dead ballpark . . . heavy air," Canseco told Achenbach. "I do not enjoy playing in this ball park. . . . Ball don't carry. . . . I'm cold. It's overcast everyday."[3]

The hecklers in the right field bleachers didn't make playing in Oakland any easier, either. He claimed fans taunted him with a long list of slurs about his Cuban heritage: from his work ethic, his emigration from Cuba, and, ignorant of his Americanization, the Spanish dialect. Canseco endured the barrage and shrugged it off. "They always do that shit. I don't pay no attention to those fools," Canseco revealed to Achenbach. "These fans out here aren't true fans." Canseco later retracted his comments. "The majority of them are fine. But a lot of these kids just come out here to drink, get high. They're jealous of the ballplayers."

A's fans didn't have much reason to cheer, though. By late June, the A's were in last place and desperate for answers. Their 29–45 record convinced general manager Sandy Alderson to fire manager Jackie Moore and tap bench coach Jeff Newman as his replacement until he discovered a suitable successor. Ten games later, he found one: Tony La Russa, an articulate forty-two-year-old lawyer who had recently been fired by the Chicago White Sox. La Russa was named the new A's manager on July 2. Having led the White Sox to a division title in 1983, La Russa brought impeccable game preparation and a winning attitude to the A's. He also lured his pitching coach in Chicago, Dave Duncan, to coach with him in Oakland.

That wasn't the A's only move in July. The A's also signed Canseco's brother, Ozzie, who struggled as a pitcher in the New York Yankees' organization, to a minor league contract. Ozzie wanted to follow in the footsteps of his brother and become an everyday player, but the Yankees wanted him to stick to pitching. The disagreement prompted Ozzie to ask for his release, so they obliged. Ozzie grabbed his bat and reported to the A's Single-A affiliate in Madison, Wisconsin. "I talked to people that told me he had a shot as a pitcher for the Yankees," teammate Greg Cadaret said of Ozzie. "But he saw all the success his brother was having and wanted to be like him."

The joy of Ozzie joining the organization capped a promising first half for Canseco. Smashing a league leading twenty-three home runs and amassing seventy-eight RBIs by the All-Star break convinced Kansas City Royals manager Dick Howser to select Canseco to be a reserve player on the American League All-Star team. Heading to Houston for the fifty-seventh All-Star Game, Canseco looked forward to rubbing shoulders with other stars. "It's going to be fun to be there and maybe talk to some of the guys," an excited Canseco told the *Oakland Tribune*.

When Canseco stepped inside the Astrodome, reporters from around the country swarmed him. Having heard of his legendary power and feats, they bombarded him with interview requests and questions. Canseco indulged them with an electrifying batting practice during workouts, crashing one ball into the fourth deck.

Canseco wasn't the only rookie tapped as an All Star, however. Wally Joyner, a twenty-four-year-old, baby-faced first baseman for the California Angels captured the hearts of Southern California, becoming the first rookie ever to be voted by fans to start the All-Star Game. The smooth swinging left-handed slugger hit .313 and pounded twenty home runs by the All-Star break, making him the leading candidate to earn the American League Rookie of the Year honors.

Fans so embraced his performance and popularity that they christened the right-field stands at Anaheim Stadium "Wally's World." What made their closet rivalry more intriguing was when Canseco and Joyner represented the American League in the home-run derby, one of the feature attractions of the All-Star festivities. The competition pitted All Stars from both leagues facing off to see which league could hit more home runs. "I can't keep up with the guy, and I don't even try," Joyner said of of Canseco during the All-Star festivities at the Astrodome. "My goal is not to lead the league in homers. Just look at me. Do I look like a home run hitter?" Joyner was referring to his slim 6-foot-2, 185-pound frame.

Joyner did more than keep up with Canseco. During the derby, he blasted four home runs; Canseco hit only one. The National League power hitters edged the American League, 8-7. Canseco hoped to showcase his power during the game. With friends and family gathered at Canseco's father, José, Sr.'s home in Miami glued to the television set anticipating his entry into the game, manager Dick Howser told Canseco to grab a bat in the top of the ninth. If Frank White reached base, Howser imparted to Canseco, he would pinch hit for the pitcher. But when White flied out to end the top of the ninth, the chances of Canseco swinging his bat in the game evaporated. Canseco didn't play. "Leading the league in home runs and runs batted in, you'd think I'd at least get a swing," a disappointed Canseco told C.W. Nevius of the *San Francisco Chronicle* after the game. "I know my father was real disappointed."[4]

His frustration carried into the second half. As July gave way to August, Canseco hit a wall. He was homerless for sixteen games and drove in only five runs during that span. Shortly thereafter, he encountered the worst slump of his brief career. On August 8, Canseco began a string of forty hitless at-bats, the longest hitless skid in the majors that season. No matter how far he'd hit the ball during batting practice, he couldn't transfer those hits into the game, hitting only .158 since the break. His strikeout totals soared, too, making him on pace to break the single season strikeout record of 189 established by the San Francisco Giants' Bobby Bonds in 1970.

Although every ballplayer experiences a slump from time to time, this one was agonizing for the rookie. For the first time Canseco seemed unsure of his abilities. At times, he appeared lost at the plate, but somehow his confidence managed to weather the storm. "That slump must have crushed him," former A's beat writer John Hickey said. "But he never lost his sense of humor and his perspective on things. He did a lot of growing up during that time, and through it all, he kept his head up." His slump, which included fifteen strikeouts and only four balls hit out of the infield, finally ended on August 23, when he smashed a game-winning double off of Yankees closer Dave Righetti in the ninth inning at Yankee Stadium. "It's frustrating to anyone," a relieved Canseco told reporters after his hitless streak ended. "I felt I took it in stride. I know I can play here in the major leagues. I know I can hit home runs and drive in runs."

Away from the field, the demands and rigorous schedule of the major leagues began taxing Canseco. He had lost fifteen pounds from the beefed-up frame he carried to spring training. He looked forward to the off-season so he could return to Miami, spend time with his family, and resume his workouts. "I'm tired, I'm worn out, I'm fatigued," Canseco told the *Miami Herald* in 1986. "I've never played so many games in a row. . . . I feel like I'm losing strength every day."[5]

His relationship with older teammates also grew tired. How he prepared for games and his nonchalant work ethic irritated them. They were puzzled by his lack of drive and avoidance of the extra work required to elevate his game. "The part that may have upset the veteran players was that with all the ability he had, he didn't want to work," Davis said. "He was bigger and faster, and he threw better than anyone in the outfield, but all he wanted to do was be a designated hitter. It just didn't match."

Former teammate Steve Ontiveros called Canseco fun and labeled him a "good" guy, but also recognized their frustration. "He would do some things that drove the older players nuts for a rookie," said Ontiveros, a pitcher for the A's from 1985 to '88 and 1994 to '95. "He did a lot things on his own—for his own good." Canseco's instant popularity and good looks, however, may have aroused jealousy among teammates, according to Jackie Moore, who viewed Canseco as misinterpreted. "A lot of people thought he was standoffish and brash for a rookie," said Moore. "But keep in mind that he was a young player coming into an older club and he was getting all of the publicity and I think that rubbed some of the older players in a difficult way."

Team photographer Michael Zagaris connected with Canseco and appreciated his loose demeanor. "He had an easy going, 'I don't give a fuck' manner, but not in a bad way. He was happy-go-lucky; he was laid back and in his own world," said Zagaris. "Personally, I loved him." Girls also adored him and hunted him down. Teammate Mike Davis said everywhere the team traveled, flocks of women followed him and wanted to meet him. "The guy was good-looking, charming, and had a personality; he had a lot going for him," said Davis. Zagaris, who had accompanied the most celebrated of rock stars around the world, said the cluster of beautiful women he lured reminded him of those times. "He was a matinee idol," said Zagaris. "Traveling with Canseco was like going out with Led Zeppelin and the Rolling Stones."

The relentless attention was staggering for Canseco and his onetime girlfriend, Anna McCarter, who rented an apartment with Canseco in San Leandro, minutes from the Oakland-Alameda Coliseum. Things would get so heated that she would feel compelled to intervene. "It was overwhelming for him. We would be driving around after games and there were women and panties on the antennas of the car . . . I can remember driving to games and girls putting notes on the car and me not even reading them; just throwing them on the floor. Girls would come up to me and say, 'that's José's car!' and I would say, 'but I'm his girlfriend and I live with him and he doesn't need your letter.' One time, a girl confronted me and Dusty Baker's wife, who was with me, told her, 'you better back up.' . . . It's almost pathetic. I mean, we weren't married, so he could have done whatever he wanted, but the girls didn't make it any easier."

Canseco didn't make life easier for American League pitchers. Canseco wrapped up his rookie season by hitting .240 and blasting thirty-three home runs, while driving in 117 runs. Those totals helped him squeak past Wally Joyner to capture the American League Rookie of the Year award. Having received sixteen of the twenty-eight first place votes by the Baseball Writers Association of America, Canseco had four more first place votes than Joyner, who batted .290 with twenty-two home runs and 100 RBIs during his rookie campaign. "My statistics overshadowed Joyner's," a confident Canseco told the Associated Press from his Miami home after receiving the news. "Especially in the home run category. But he was popular with the writers, and his team won the division, which gave him an advantage."

Beat writer John Hickey confirmed his selection. "Joyner had good numbers, but Canseco created more buzz. He was this personable, good looking, and strong guy who hit monstrous home runs. Canseco generated more headlines than Joyner."

While his family celebrated his accolades in Miami, Canseco eyed an even more productive sophomore season, so he pumped iron all winter and planned on arriving to spring training at 235 pounds. "I'm maybe halfway there," Canseco said after the season. "I'm just scratching the surface. When I put together everything I'm capable of doing, hitting consistently, and fielding better, I'll be much more of a player."

The A's, meanwhile, were a much better team. With La Russa at the helm, the A's boasted the American League's third best record (42–30) after the All-Star break and found themselves in third place. The talent-laden farm system had also been paying off. In August, another avid weight lifter, rookie Mark McGwire, showed up and displayed promising power.

Canseco blasted softballs in Miami all winter long.

NOTES

1. Susan Fornoff, "Canseco Creates A's Sensation," *Sacramento Bee*, March 2, 1986.
2. Mark Whicker, "Canseco: A's Have a Hero at Work," *Philadelphia Daily News*, April 7, 1986.
3. Joel Achenbach, "From Out of Left Field," *Miami Herald*, September 21, 1986.
4. C. W. Nevius, "Glum Canseco Was Left Holding the Bat," *San Francisco Chronicle*, July 16, 1986.
5. Peter Richmond, "Canseco Shrugs Off Highs and Lows," *Miami Herald*, August 25, 1986.

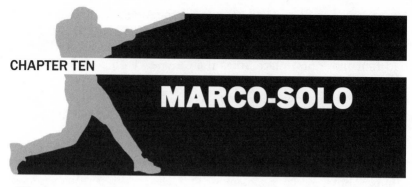

CHAPTER TEN

MARCO-SOLO

"He was so incredibly sweet, innocent, naïve, and accommodating. . . . He couldn't believe the fuss we were making over him. It's like he had no concept about what he was doing. I even referred to him in print as 'Satan's Nightmare,' because there was such goodness about him."

—Former A's beat writer Bud Geracie
August 2007

Nineteen eighty-seven. McGwire knew he had something to prove when he reported early to spring training in Scottsdale. Though he impressed Athletic's general manager Sandy Alderson with his on-base percentage and power during his call-up the previous August, McGwire's abrupt departure from winter ball in the Dominican Republic against the A's wishes cast him in an unfavorable light. That the A's acquired thirty-nine-year-old veteran third baseman Ron Cey during the winter added more pressure. With first base prospect Rob Nelson and hot-hitting Carney Lansford, a staple in the infield, in the mix, there was a chance McGwire would open his season with Triple-A Tacoma. McGwire welcomed the challenge. "I don't think you win a spot on the team during winter ball," McGwire told reporters when he arrived for spring training. "You win it in spring training."

Manager Tony La Russa would provide McGwire an opportunity to produce an eye-opening spring. La Russa prized McGwire—dating back to 1984, while he managed the White Sox. Before a game in Detroit, he watched McGwire, who had been touring with Team USA and played exhibition games at major league venues across the country, club an opposite-field upper-deck shot in Tiger Stadium. Since that blast, McGwire had been on La Russa's radar. "From the first day he showed up in spring training, there was no better looking hitter in camp," La Russa said in 1987. "Even when he started slow he was doing the right things. Early in the spring I wanted him to concentrate on playing his way onto the team, and didn't want him to worry about other things."

An added worry La Russa refused to lay on McGwire was playing first base, a position he had felt comfortable playing at University of Southern California. Though McGwire displayed erratic defense at third base for two years in the minors, he progressed enough that the organization was open to him continuing to patrol the position. La Russa also thought that if McGwire had to adjust to another position during spring training, the extra work might rob him of his concentration at the plate. Coaches had spent countless hours transforming him into a third baseman; switching him to first base wasn't an option at that point. "He'd bring a little baggage to first base and I don't want to mess with him," said La Russa during spring training. "If I want to get him more at-bats this spring I might send him to the outfield."[1]

Rene Lachemann joined the A's coaching staff in 1987. After spending two seasons as Boston Red Sox first base coach and garnering a World Series appearance in 1986, he inherited that role with the A's. As players, Lachemann and McGwire blazed similar paths to the big leagues. Both had went to USC, then signed and later played with the A's, though the team was based in Kansas City when Lachemann signed in 1964. McGwire was no stranger to the Lachemann family. Rene's brother, Marcel, had been instrumental in luring McGwire to sign a letter of intent to pitch for USC in 1981. Six years later, Rene greeted the power pitcher-turned-slugger in spring training. Lachemann recalled uncertainty clouding over McGwire that spring. "When he started off, he didn't really have a position," said Lachemann. "We were working with him at third base and the outfield. He wasn't even looked at as a starter; we were trying to find a place for him to play."

Beat writer John Hickey, too, observed that the A's were in no hurry to force him into the lineup. "When he came up, they didn't think he was going to make the team," said Hickey, who covers the Mariners for the *Seattle Post-Intelligencer*. "He was more less an afterthought. They looked at him as a guy that might come up in 1988." McGwire shattered those plans, though. His sizzling bat impressed the A's. Batting .322, clubbing three home runs, and driving in twenty-three runs in exhibition games during the spring, he earned himself a spot on the opening day roster. La Russa wanted his bat in the lineup but had to shuffle his infielders for that to happen. Carney Lansford, the A's former team captain and third baseman, described the bizarre platoon system La Russa orchestrated to solidify his lineup. In 2004 Lansford said tongue-in-cheek:

Tony had this brilliant idea of moving Mark over to third base and me over to first against left-handed pitching. Both of us hated it. Mark hated third base and I hated first. We were like, "what are they thinking?" Mark used to tell me, "You're a great third baseman and I feel really comfortable at first base—why don't they just move us back?"

Rob Nelson, who also batted over .300 during the spring, made the club as well. Some suspected that Nelson would have to play his way out of being the everyday first baseman, despite alarmingly losing twenty pounds while playing winter ball in the Dominican Republic. "I was so sick down there so often," Nelson told the *San Jose Mercury News* in 1987. "They wash the food with water down there . . . it seems like I was getting sick twice a week. I just kept losing weight and there was nothing I could do."[2]

Heading east to open the season in Minnesota for a three-game series against the Twins, the A's started Nelson at first base while benching McGwire. Not for long, however. Nelson succumbed to a miserable slump at the worst time. For him, going 0-for-4 on opening night set the tone for a grueling two-week span. In seven games he batted .167 and struck out in half of his twenty-four at-bats. By late April, the A's sent Nelson back to Triple-A Tacoma. "Eventually when Nelson didn't work out, Tony moved Mark back to first base. Everything fell into place after that," said Lansford.

Not that McGwire robbed the position from Nelson. He struggled, too. In the first two weeks of the season he only batted .136, but the quality of his at-bats was impressive enough for La Russa to appoint him the everyday first baseman. By April 20, McGwire found himself patrolling first base for good. McGwire appreciated La Russa's nod of confidence. The security helped him to relax instead of pressing during his sporadic at-bats. He had always been an everyday player and felt the consistent at-bats would excel his play. "I've always been an everyday player and I have all the confidence in the world in myself that I can play in the major leagues," he said in 1987.

McGwire rewarded La Russa by blasting nine home runs over the next sixteen games, including five during a three-game series at Tiger Stadium. His sudden power explosion prompted reporters to surround his locker after the series in Detroit. Amid microphones and tape recorders, McGwire found speaking to the press on a daily basis awkward. "I just don't like talking about the things I do," McGwire told a handful of reporters after the series. "So if I stutter a little bit, that's why."[3]

Those pestering questions and his cramped responses on that Sunday afternoon in the clubhouse foreshadowed his season. He never imagined his sudden success would lure so much attention so early on. Team photographer Michael Zagaris observed McGwire's uneasiness as he traveled with the club. "He wasn't a person that was really comfortable in the spotlight," said Zagaris.

McGwire's explosive home-run totals soared each week and would attract more media coverage. If he kept cracking home runs at a record pace, he would inevitably face a mob of reporters after games. The next month in Cleveland his power grabbed national headlines. On July 20, he capped an explosive weekend by belting five home runs in nine at-bats over two games, becoming the first rookie to accomplish such a feat. He also established a new record by scoring nine consecutive runs in as many at-bats. Three and a half months into the season, McGwire had whacked an unprecedented twenty-seven home runs, only six shy of teammate José Canseco's totals as a rookie the year before. Because he hit nineteen of his home runs with the bases empty, teammates called him, "Marco-Solo." "He certainly showed the power he displayed at USC," said former A's general manager Sandy Alderson. "Once he proved he could hit major league pitching, there was no doubt about his power potential."

McGwire's impressive home-run totals became more than a Bay Area story. His home-run rampage headlined media outlets such as ESPN's *SportsCenter*, *Sports Illustrated*, and *Inside Sports*. The redheaded rookie from Orange County became the talk of baseball. "Those were some amazing things he did for a rookie," marveled Rene Lachemann. "He handled the attention as good as any young guy could handle it."

Hoping to relieve him of the mounting pressure, teammates such as Mike Davis tried to distract him from the hoopla, encouraging him to loosen up and enjoy his newfound stardom. For instance, after a rainout at Milwaukee's County Stadium in May, Davis toyed with the rookie. "I tried to throw him in the mud—all 180 pounds of him," recalled Davis. "I grabbed this big guy to show him the love we had for him, but he wasn't having it."

Davis applauded McGwire's head-turning rookie season:

He was a backup to start the season, but got an opportunity to get in the lineup and never came out. He had power to right field that we hadn't seen before and he was hitting for average during that time, too. He also played a solid first base. He put together such a great rookie season and it was a pleasure to be a part of it.

As the season progressed, roommate Terry Steinbach witnessed the onslaught of media coverage zooming in on McGwire. Steinbach said while McGwire did face his share of press coverage when he shattered home-run records at USC, played in the Olympics, and was drafted as the A's first round selection, he wasn't used to this level of exposure. "It was different for him," said Steinbach. "It was really the first time people began saying, 'Hey, check out this guy.' He learned a lot from it. He did some things right, but I bet he would be willing to say he probably did some things wrong during that course of time."

Despite the onslaught, A's traveling secretary Mickey Morabito thought of McGwire as cooperative and polite with reporters. First meeting McGwire in Anaheim shortly after the A's drafted him in 1984, Morabito applauded how McGwire endured the circus. "He knew they had a job to do and handled it really well," said Morabito. "He wouldn't give them a lot and was fairly nice to them. He treated them with respect. That's just the way he was. He didn't really seek the limelight on a lot of things. He handled the onslaught of media very well. He's an intelligent guy."

That was also the claim of longtime and legendary Bay Area columnist Glenn Dickey. His editor at *Inside Sports* assigned him to write a story on McGwire during the off-season, so he traveled to McGwire's apartment in Costa Mesa, California. After the story was published, McGwire bumped into Dickey at a hotel during the following spring training. "When he saw me, he came over and thanked me profusely for the story," said Dickey. "That's the way he was like, and not just with me. He had a reputation of being extremely cooperative."

Former A's beat writer Bud Geracie recalled a game when McGwire smashed two home runs in Detroit. After the game, a cluster of photographers, reporters, and cameramen crammed the locker room and surrounded only his locker. Unaware of the crowd, McGwire faced his locker and dressed for the team bus ride. When he finally turned around and spotted the mob, he was startled.

> There was a genuine look on his face like, "what do you guys want?" You talk about shy; this guy was very uncomfortable, so incredibly innocent, sweet, naïve, and accommodating. Looking back at everything that has happened, it's hard to believe that was genuine, but I believed it then and still do now. He couldn't believe the fuss we were making over him. It's like he had no concept about what he was doing. I even referred to him in print as "Satan's Nightmare," because there was such goodness about him.

Former A's closer Dennis Eckersley noticed his naïve, bright-eyed, and happy-go-lucky temperament. "He was a sweet, green, nice kid who came from a good family," said Eckersley. "He was goofy and corny." To prevent the hoards of media requests from distracting him before games, A's public relations director Jay Alves scheduled a press conference for McGwire before the first game of each road series. This strategy appeased the media and also allowed McGwire to take batting and infield practice with the rest of the team. Despite those efforts, though, the demands taxed McGwire.

Pamela Pitts, an administrative assistant for the A's at the time, noticed the relentless coverage taking its toll on him. Even though he answered even the most redundant questions, he was clearly drained. "He got tired of being asked the same dumb questions over and over," said Pitts, who now serves as the A's director of administration. "It's exceptionally hard to grow up in the public eye and get spoken to by the same people who are always looking for a story. They always want to talk to you. It's extremely difficult when you never get away from being a celebrity. He grew up." By July, he put his foot down. "I'm saying 'no' more now. I'm tired of answering the same questions over and over again," McGwire told *Maclean*, a Canadian weekly news magazine, in 1987.

But being tapped to play on the American League All-Star team accelerated the crush. Private time would have to wait for McGwire, especially since Major League Baseball's fifty-eighth All-Star Game would be held at his home field, the Oakland-Alameda Coliseum. His thirty-three home runs by the All-Star break more than qualified him to be crowned the starting first baseman for the American League. Because Nelson, however, was at first base and Lansford at third to open the season, McGwire's name was left off the All-Star ballot. That didn't stop Boston Red Sox manager, John McNamara, who managed the American League, from selecting him as a reserve player. "Weird's not the word," McGwire told Bud Geracie of the *San Jose Mercury News* in 1987. "It's incredible. No way did I ever picture myself in this situation, being an All-Star. I don't know how to feel, how to accept it. I don't think it's going to hit me until I walk in here with all of those great players."

During the All-Star festivities, reporters and microphones surrounded McGwire. That he was on pace to nearly shatter Roger Maris's single season home-run record laced each question. As did his unexplainable affair with the long ball. In two full seasons in the minors, he smashed forty-eight home runs. Now, in only half of a season in the major leagues, which boasts a higher caliber of pitching, he already had thirty-three.

In 1987, McGwire told the *San Diego Tribune*:

> I honestly don't even want to stop to think about how it's happened or why it's happened. When I do stop to think about it, it's pretty scary to

me. I don't plan things out. I just go out every day and give my best. I think if you do that, chances are that good things are going to happen. But, yes, I'm completely amazed by all of this. You know, I was just trying to make the club. I mean, there was some major doubt.

McGwire's modesty didn't matter to his home fans. When stadium public address announcer Roy Steele announced McGwire's name July 14 during player introductions before the All-Star game, a crowd of 49,671 draped him with the loudest and warmest ovation of the evening as he emerged from the dugout and trotted toward the third-base line. McGwire tipped his hat in appreciation. His adrenaline couldn't translate into hits during the game, however. In two at-bats, he flied out and struck out in a game which the National League edged the American League by a score of 2-0 in thirteen innings.

Behind the fierce coverage attached to his torrid rookie home-run pace, McGwire was one of the hardest working players on the team, according to former A's starter Steve Ontiveros, who teamed with him in 1987–88 and '95. The way he meticulously guarded his diet and prepared for each game impressed teammates.

One thing I admired about him was how hard he worked; he had an incredible work ethic. We wouldn't see him throwing down too many doughnuts. When we're in the kitchen, we're slamming down everything in the morning, coffee and donuts, but he would be making protein shakes. I never saw him eat anything that was bad, or at least, be included in my diet. He was very disciplined in his intake of food.

Perhaps no one noticed McGwire's hard work in the gym more than Steinbach, his roommate. He said McGwire loved his time in the weight room. "I'd call him and ask him what he did today, and he'd say, 'this morning I did legs and in the afternoon, I'm doing calves; then I'm going to do chest and back at night,'" remembered Steinbach. "That was his thing: he liked being there. That was his relief, enjoyment, and relaxation." Hall-of-Fame closer Dennis Eckersley also recalled him spending hours in the weight room. "You'd notice he worked out; he was obsessed with it," said Eckersley. "On the other hand, with Canseco, you got the feeling he didn't have to work as hard."

McGwire's muscles and his intensity pumping iron, however, didn't scare pitchers from brushing him off the plate. Because pitchers sensed the rookie was becoming too comfortable there, they plunked him five times during the season. McGwire's seemingly passive reaction to those daggers, though, concerned some teammates. Each time pitchers nailed him and knocked him off the plate, the mild-mannered rookie politely dropped his bat and trotted to first. That meekness frustrated teammates. As *San Francisco Chronicle* writer Bruce Jenkins explained of McGwire's subdued responses, "Each time he was hit, he was the perfect host: Even with a cocktail thrown in his face, he kept the conversation going." Rumors soon circulated around the league that he was afraid of the ball, and once pitchers brushed him off the plate, his bat was lifeless for the remainder of the game.

Scouting reports around the league wrote of pounding the soft rookie with inside heat above the waist. "Every time he would get hit in the head, Tony [La Russa] would take him out of the game because he figured he wasn't any good for the rest of the game," admitted Karl Kuehl. A game best depicting how pitchers capitalized on the good-natured McGwire occurred on July 5. After Canseco and McGwire hammered back-to-back home runs off Red Sox starter Dennis "Oil Can" Boyd in the bottom of the fourth, Boyd drilled McGwire his next at-bat. McGwire casually tossed his bat and walked to first. When reliever Wes Gardner started the bottom of the eighth inning, he, too, dangerously unleashed a fastball at McGwire's head, denting his helmet. That prompted home plate umpire Tim McClelland to warn both dugouts. A group of A's players, meanwhile, angrily paced the dugout, yelling at Gardner and bracing for a brawl. But McGwire nonchalantly adjusted his helmet and made his way to first, shackling their rage. As Reggie Jackson, who teamed with McGwire in 1987, said, "The man who gets hit has got to start it."

"I remember Tony grabbing his jersey and trying to drag him to the mound," recollects former A's reliever Greg Cadaret. After the game, a group of reporters asked McGwire about his tamed response. "If I'm expecting to get hit and they get me in the head, that's one thing," McGwire explained to them. "I don't think he was trying to hit me. His first pitch was down and away and then he came up and in. If you are going to go after somebody you are going to do it on the first pitch."

Still, teammates insisted McGwire needed to send the league a message. Aside from his safety, if one of those pitches injured him and sidelined him for a long period of time, the team suffered. "When he got hit, he didn't do much," said Lachemann. "He was hit quite a bit, because pitchers tried to pitch him up and in. And he had a problem getting out of the way of the pitch and we kind of worried about him getting seriously hurt. He was a nice, quiet guy in a lot of ways."

As July gave way to August, McGwire's blistering home-run rate tapered off. He hit only five in twenty-six games after the All-Star break. Some players thought the nonstop chatter and pressure of home-run records had finally sapped his energy and concentration. "I think a player would have a lot better chance at hitting 60 or 61 if everybody just left him alone," McGwire clarified to Bay Area reporters shortly after his rookie season. "The constant demand takes a toll. . . . What I went through my rookie season was unbelievable."

Though his power drought dropped him off the pace of the single season mark of sixty-one, he remained poised to break another record. By August 11, McGwire slammed his thirty-eighth home run, tying the single-season rookie record for home runs, which was held by Wally Berger (1930) and Frank Robinson (1956). One more home run would establish a new record and what better place to break the thirty-one-year-old record than in his home, Orange County. When the A's opened a three-game series against the California Angels at Anaheim Stadium on Friday evening, August 14, McGwire's father, John; mother, Ginger; as well as Kathy sat in the stands, yearning to see history.

Angels' veteran starting pitcher Don Sutton grooved a fastball to McGwire in the top of the sixth inning. *Crack!* McGwire's thirty-ninth home run cleared the left-field fence and crowned him the most prolific rookie home-run king ever. McGwire told reporters after the game:

> I thought I hit it pretty good. And when I saw Rene Lachemann do his kick in the first base coaching box, I knew it went out. I'm pretty proud to have done it in Southern California. It was great coming home. I spent the off day with my parents, and this makes it special. They watch us on satellite a lot, but it's better they saw it in person.

Whispers that McGwire could be the first rookie to reach the fifty-home-run pinnacle whirled through the Bay Area. Only ten players had tread upon such a feat, with National League slugger George Foster being the last in 1977. During the final home stand of the season on September 29, McGwire blasted his forty-ninth home run against the Cleveland Indians. Five games remained. For the next two games at the Oakland-Alameda Coliseum, fans anticipated his final at-bats of the season and cheered for him to whack number fifty.

That didn't happen. McGwire then traveled to Chicago's Comiskey Park, where the A's were scheduled to close out the season against the White Sox. Launching that elusive home run wasn't the only distraction for McGwire. Back in California, Kathy was on the brink of delivering the couple's first child. He paced his hotel room and braced for the call. In the first two games of the series, he was homerless. If McGwire were to reach the milestone, he would have to dramatically do it during the final game of the season. Fate, however, had other plans. When McGwire received a call and learned that Kathy was headed to the hospital and going into labor, his goal to break the record took a back seat. In the early morning hours of Sunday, October 4, McGwire phoned A's traveling secretary Mickey Morabito. "He called me and said, 'Mickey, I'm going home—can you get me a flight?' I was able to get him a flight and he went home to be there for the birth of his child. That showed me a lot about him," remembered Morabito.

That afternoon, minutes after McGwire arrived in the hospital, his child, Matthew Ryan was born, weighing nine pounds, two ounces. Born on October 4, three days prior to McGwire's birthday, his newborn launched him into fatherhood. "When I hit forty-nine, I really started to think that it would be neat to hit fifty," McGwire said. "But I've said ever since Matthew was born, that was my fiftieth home run. I consider him my fiftieth home run." Andy Dolich, A's vice president of business operations from 1980 to1994 and San Francisco Forty Niners' president of business operations, recounted, "That endeared him to individuals that weren't just baseball fans. People admired how he walked away from a once in a lifetime opportunity to witness the birth of his son."

Teammate Greg Cadaret respected McGwire's decision, but is still convinced that had he stayed in Chicago and played the final game of the season, he would have reached his fiftieth. "The way the wind was blowing out in Comiskey, he would have hit number fifty," said Cadaret. "All he would have had to do was hit a fly ball." Becoming a father and the most prolific rookie home-run hitter in history satisfied McGwire, though. Those credentials also compelled the twenty-eight members of the Baseball Writers Association of America to unanimously crown him with the American League Rookie of the Year award shortly after the season. Not since Red Sox catcher Carlton Fisk in 1972 had a player become the unanimous choice for the award. "He showed good power from the outset," Carl Steward, *Oakland Tribune* sports columnist, wrote in an email in 2004, "but it wasn't until he hit forty-nine home runs that he was considered someone special."

McGwire finished the season with a .289 batting average, forty-nine home runs, and 118 RBIs. Those jaw-dropping credentials meant lifestyle changes for the baseball star. With McGwire's newfound celebrity, his face was publicly recognizeable and his privacy interrupted. Fame called his name, a price for playing a game he loved. "Nobody predicted that he would do what he did," said former teammate Bathe. "He obviously had immense talent and did well in the minor leagues, but nothing like what he showed up there."

NOTES
[1] David Bush, "Cey Joins A's; Andujar Doesn't," *San Francisco Chronicle*, February 23, 1987.

2   Bud Geracie, "A's Lean to Nelson in Lineup," *San Jose Mercury News*, February 25, 1987.

3   Susan Fornoff, "McGwire's Two Homers Stake A's," *Sacramento Bee*, May 9, 1987.

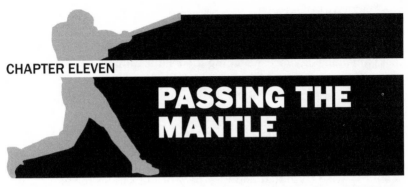

CHAPTER ELEVEN

PASSING THE MANTLE

"When Mark was hitting all those home runs, he used to still say that our season was going to be dictated by what Jose did—not on what Mark did. He talked to Jose a lot. He was a slugger and he liked sluggers. He loved watching him hit."

—Former A's third baseman and team captain Carney Lansford,
June 2004

It was a fitting sendoff for Reginald Martinez Jackson's illustrious career, or so he thought. Since the California Angels hadn't expressed any interest in bringing back the forty-year-old icon after the 1986 season, when the Athletics' offered him the opportunity to finish his career with the same franchise he began in 1967, he jumped at the chance. Jackson loved Oakland, a city where he blazed a trove of memories, and even owned a home fifteen miles from the Oakland-Alameda Coliseum. Powering the Charlie O. Finley–owned "Mustache Gang" era of the Oakland A's to three World Championships, 1971–1974, Jackson hammered 254 home runs during his eight seasons there.

Much had transpired since Finley dismantled the storied franchise, and Jackson, the flamboyant and powerfully built clubber, left Oakland after the 1975 season. With eleven years having passed amid stops at Baltimore, New York, and California, Jackson rose to national prominence and morphed into one of sports' most popular figures, while the A's franchise deteriorated and dwelled in the basement of the American League. Fueling three clubs to eleven division titles in a span of sixteen years (1971–86), Jackson bathed in victory.

Playing for the Yankees, his clutch performances during crucial post-season games molded his legacy. Jackson was at his best when the game was on the line. Earning the nickname "Mr. October" for his momentum-changing home runs during the most hallowed month in baseball, including clubbing three against the Dodgers in Game Six of

123

the 1977 World Series, the candid, fourteen-time All Star thrived in the spotlight.

Ten years later, however, the aging veteran faced what all superstars must one day face: watching their skills diminish and coming to grips with retirement. Although Jackson had never guaranteed retirement, on Christmas Eve 1986, he settled behind a microphone and announced his return to Oakland. "I don't need any presents on Christmas—I got one today," an exuberant Jackson told reporters at the news conference announcing his return.

The A's hoped Jackson's winning presence and veteran leadership would spark a team that hadn't experienced October relevance since 1981. Besides soaring ticket sales that the significance of his sentimental return would bring, general manager Sandy Alderson also savored a statistic Jackson produced. "Reggie was signed as an A's icon, but also because he had a much better on base percentage (.379) in 1986 than our previous designated hitter Dave Kingman (.255)," Alderson wrote in an email in September 2007.

Ticket sales and on-base percentage weren't the only factors, however. By bringing Jackson back, the A's felt he could harness the brash and aloof twenty-three-year-old Canseco, a player whose perceived arrogance and immaturity disturbed teammates. Choosing interviews over outfield drills and showboating in the batting cage were only a few of his antics. The direction Jackson wished to provide for Canseco was the same he provided the previous season, in 1986, for former Angels' teammate, Wally Joyner. That year, Jackson taught Joyner how to handle the spotlight and guided him through the ups and downs of stardom. "Now, I know it's going to be fun for me to be around José Canseco," Jackson said during the press conference. "I hope it's going to be fun for José, too. But I know that watching him hit homers will bring back a lot of pleasant memories for me."

The chemistry seemed perfect. Growing up in Miami, Canseco admired Jackson, donning his number 44 while playing for Double-A Huntsville in 1985. And Jackson, while playing for the California Angels in 1986, was enamored with Canseco's hair-raising power from afar, bringing him back to his valiant youth when he barged into the majors in the 1960s. Both shared Latin descent and spoke adequate Spanish. Jackson was so fascinated by Canseco that when asked his thoughts on the rookie in 1986, he marveled, "He hits 'em where I hit 'em except he's right handed. That's scary."[1]

When Canseco's former minor league teammate, José Tolentino, visited Anaheim Stadium in 1986, he noticed how much Jackson loved watching Canseco take his cuts in the batting cage. There, while the local media was buzzing about rookie sensation Wally Joyner and his quest for the American League Rookie of the Year award, Tolentino overheard Jackson talking with Canseco near the batting cage before the game. While Canseco blistered baseballs to all parts of the field, Jackson bragged about him to a group of reporters. He predicted on six pitches, Canseco would synchronically smash two home runs to right, two home runs to left, two home runs to center field, and then step out of the cage. Six thunderous cracks later Canseco strutted out of the cage. "He did it," confirmed Tolentino. "Jackson really took him under his wing." Said former teammate Dave Wilder, "José was the only player Reggie Jackson ever sat and watched hit during BP and be in awe."

The season also included a farewell tour scheduled for Jackson in each city the A's played. This way, fans could pay homage to the electrifying star and he, in return, could salute them. Aside from planning his heartfelt departure from the game, Jackson also felt he could strengthen the lineup and help the team contend. Mustering only eighteen home runs for the Angels the previous season, he wanted his return to Oakland to produce glimpses of the past. "He still wanted to be the old Reggie," remembered former A's hitting coach Bob Watson, who also teamed with him on the Yankees from 1980 to '81. "But for him to do that, he had to work twice as hard, and he did."

Watson believed Jackson's determination to stay in shape and his strenuous conditioning program prompted younger A's players to follow suit. "He was definitely a positive influence and role model for them," said Watson. "When the kids saw him doing all of the extra stuff, there was no problem asking them to do it." Rookie catcher Terry Steinbach relished the opportunity to play with Jackson. For Steinbach, growing up in Minnesota, watching Jackson thrill millions, and reading about his legend in newspapers made Jackson's arrival in spring training mind-blowing. "We were in awe of Reggie," confirmed Steinbach. "We were like sponges, trying to pick on anything that he could give us. He had tremendous credentials."

Those credentials couldn't help Jackson tame Canseco, however. "He grew frustrated with José," recalled Bud Geracie, the former A's beat writer for the *San Jose Mercury News* in 1987. "Jose didn't know the game, its history, and probably didn't respect Reggie's place in the game. I can recall Jackson expressing frustration with the guy."

Strength coach Dave McKay doesn't remember much of an impact Jackson had on Canseco, but did notice an annoyed Jackson shake his head in frustration on several occasions. "When José was doing something that he shouldn't have, Tony [La Russa] told Reggie, 'Hey, Reggie, that's why I brought you over here—to keep this guy in place,' and Reggie responded, 'He isn't going to listen to me—he won't listen to Babe Ruth,'" laughed McKay.

Several teammates, however, perceived their relationship differently: one egomaniac feeding the ego of another. Jackson, some say, convinced Canseco that he was the star of the team and he didn't have to work as hard as the others. That Jackson was too selfish to help anyone other than himself was another perception. Others felt Jackson was jealous of Canseco's budding stardom and how he drew hoards of attention, while some claim Canseco energized and pushed Jackson. During the season, Jackson explained for himself to the *Miami Herald*.

> I love him, he's like my son. People like to rip him. They say he's moody. When he came up last year, he was supposed to be Paul Bunyan. The media, even his peers, weren't fair to him. He hit thirty-three home runs. Led the league with 117 RBIs, and everybody said, "so what? That's what he was supposed to do."[2]

Hall of Fame closer Dennis Eckersley described Jackson as "mellow" that year, and recalled seeing him try to mentor Canseco as much as he could. Besides, Jackson had to prepare for each game, too, and his ego wouldn't allow his performance to dwindle. For Jackson, his reason for failure wouldn't be slacking. He tried to inject that mindset into Canseco. "He'd jack Canseco up, but he would also pump him up, in his own way," said Eckersley. "In José, he saw himself twenty years before, I think. He tried to help him, but at the same time I think he was envious. It's tough to see that when you're leaving the game. It's tough for anyone."

Former A's coach Rene Lachemann said Jackson's hard-nosed style of play and hustle rubbed off on Canseco and McGwire.

> One thing about Reggie Jackson was that you never saw him not run hard to first base. He played the game hard; the way it's supposed to be played. He respected the game and I think that's what they learned from him. Since he was a great power hitter himself, he was able to relate to the things those guys were going through, knowing that they were going to go through some tough times.

Right before Jackson's eyes emerged another up-and-coming bomber who captured the spotlight: Mark McGwire, who blasted thirty-three home runs by the All-Star break, a féat approaching Jackson's record of thirty-seven in 1969. At age twenty-three, McGwire and his record-breaking power didn't shock Jackson. In 1984, while McGwire played for Team USA and visited Boston's Fenway Park, he blasted a tape-measure home run that crashed off the back wall of the center-field bleachers. After the game, Jackson, who happened to be in town with the Angels, pulled him aside and said, "Son, when you hit one like that, you've got to watch it."[3]

Jackson watched plenty of McGwire's home runs in 1987. Jackson also overcame what could have hampered his season: a pulled hamstring, off-the-field issues, and frustration over being benched against left-handed pitchers. When McGwire clubbed three home runs in a game at Cleveland Stadium in July, Jackson waited to congratulate the rookie at the top step of the dugout. "It was a special effort, and I thought it deserved a special handshake, some recognition," Jackson told the media after the game. "I've played twenty years and only had three days like that one."

When McGwire blasted his league-leading thirty-third home run at the Oakland-Alameda Coliseum a week later, the crowd erupted and showered him with a standing ovation. As McGwire returned to the dugout in a business-as-usual manner, Jackson pushed him to leap out of the dugout and acknowledge the fans—which he did. "I've never done that my whole life," the unassuming McGwire admitted to reporters after the game. "I really don't know how to react to that. Reggie said, 'Tip your hat.' Reggie knows all about those curtain calls because he's had many of them."

Jackson tried to inject confidence and swagger into McGwire's game. He challenged McGwire to slow down his fast-paced home-run trot and savor the moment. "He's too fast," Jackson told reporters in 1987. "But he's a nice guy. . . . I'm going to leave him alone. The only thing I'll say is, 'Stay hungry.'" When asked about his relationship with McGwire in 1987, Jackson told the *Miami Herald*, "Big Mac and I talk every day. He's my friend and teammate. Great guy. Good man. Good upbringing. Nice family. Nice wife. He married his college sweetheart. Works hard. Doesn't take anything for granted. He's just glad to be here."[4]

Imparting his wisdom to two up-and-coming touted power hitters seemed sentimentally fitting. Jackson, whose brashness and unrivaled power owned the decade of the 1970s and early '80s, passed his mantle to Canseco and McGwire, a breed of future sluggers. Susan Fornoff, the A's former beat writer for the *Sacramento Bee*, 1985–91, described Jackson's enthusiasm. "He was eager to mentor both of them and at the outset referred to them as 'my sons,'" emailed Fornoff, who's also the author of the book *Lady in the Locker Room*. "And he did put in extra time with them."

Despite McGwire's surging success, though, Jackson gravitated to Canseco, according to teammates. Holding long-winded conversations with him in the clubhouse and dining with him on road trips, Jackson candidly offered him advice. "When Mark was hitting all those home runs, he used to still say that our season was going to be dictated by what José did—not on what Mark did," said former team captain Carney Lansford. "He talked to Jose a lot. He was a slugger and he liked sluggers. He loved watching him hit." In fact, Jackson viewed that, even though McGwire hammered homer after homer during the season, Canseco remained the centerpiece of the franchise. "No matter what he does, he'll still be in the shadow of Canseco," Jackson said in 1987. "That's absolutely to his advantage."[5]

In July, Jackson told Glenn Dickey of the *San Francisco Chronicle* that because Canseco garnered advanced praise and sparked comparisons with such greats as Mickey Mantle and Willie Mays in 1985, pitchers pitched him carefully. Not so with McGwire, who surprised everyone, according to Jackson. "Mark snuck up on people this year, but José never had a chance to sneak up on anybody."[6]

But watching two ripe, powerful bashers muscle their way into fame and grab attention from Jackson's farewell tour couldn't have been easy for him, according to former A's television analyst Ted Robinson, who broadcasted games from 1985 to 1987. "I don't think he ever expected that he was going to get overshadowed by these two guys," said Robinson. "He publicly handled it pretty well; but privately, I'm sure it couldn't have been easy for him, knowing he was going to the Hall of Fame and coming back to the place where he started, and having everything revolving around the two young guys."

Tipping his hat and saying goodbye to fans around the country was the easy part for Jackson. Staying healthy and playing at the level he expected was harder. In the final season of his colorful career, Jackson departed with a batting average of .220 and fifteen home runs while collecting forty-nine RBIs. He became so frustrated that by late May he had declined most interview requests. "I'm not up to it," Jackson told a reporter. "I'm sorry, man. I really am. Just write that I'm going bad."[7]

With flame-throwing pitchers like Boston Red Sox's Roger Clemens and Seattle Mariners' Mark Langston bursting into the league, Jackson admitted his difficulty catching up with a ninety-mile-per-hour fastball. After the season, he retired. That Jackson, McGwire, and Canseco accrued 1,609 career home runs spanning 54 seasons made the trio's season together one for the ages.

NOTES

[1]   Dan Shaughnessy, "Canseco Makes Powerful First Impression," *Boston Globe*, May 3, 1986.

2   Herald Wire Services, "McGwire, Canseco, Please Reggie," *Miami Herald*, July 3, 1987.
3   Hank Hersch, "Baseball's Young Lions," *Sports Illustrated*, July 13, 1987.
4   Herald Wire Services, "McGwire, Canseco, Please Reggie."
5   John Strege, "Big Mac's Secret Attack," *Orange County Register*, June 12, 1987.
6   Glenn Dickey, "Canseco More Fruitful as a Banana," *San Francisco Chronicle*, July 30, 1987.
7   Bud Geracie, "Jackson Isn't Producing, But A's Aren't Panicking," *San Jose Mercury News*, May 27, 1987.

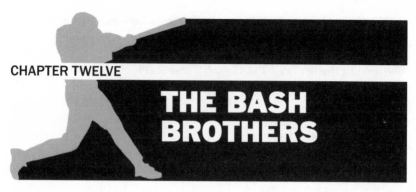

CHAPTER TWELVE

THE BASH BROTHERS

"It was a very different-looking McGwire who addressed reporters after the game. He looked dangerous, ready to explode. His responses were tight-lipped and abrupt, and his eyes were ablaze."

—Bruce Jenkins, *San Francisco Chronicle*
April 9, 1988

Nineteen eighty-eight. McGwire pumped iron all winter. Besides adding bulk to his burgeoning six-foot-five frame, McGwire saw that much had transpired after his remarkable rookie season. Although nurturing his newborn son, Matthew, commanded most of McGwire's time, he also profited from the exploding sports card collectors market. At times, McGwire earned $5,000 per three-hour session to scribble his autograph on baseball memorabilia. This booming business compelled him to travel the country and capitalize on the autograph craze, a market that saw his rookie card's worth rocket from fifty cents to fifteen dollars in 1988. Those monies helped Kathy and him purchase a three-bedroom home in Huntington Beach, California.

McGwire's early arrival in Scottsdale for spring training had taken a back seat to business matters. As a rookie, McGwire had a season for the ages. His record-setting forty-nine home runs had tied Chicago Cub Andre Dawson for the major league lead. McGwire and his agent, Bob Cohen, eyed an increase from the major league minimum of $62,500 he earned as a rookie. McGwire still showed up and entrusted his business dealings to Cohen, the Beverly Hills agent he had had since signing with the Athletics. Cohen reportedly hoped for a one-year contract worth $325,000 for his client, matching the contract the Los Angeles Dodgers bestowed upon second-year hurler Fernando Valenzuela in 1982. But the A's offer hovered around $225,000. As both parties postured and exchanged figures during the spring, they agreed during spring training to a base salary of $250,000 plus $50,000 worth of incentives. Being rewarded for his record-breaking season thrilled McGwire. "It turned out to be a very good contract," McGwire told reporters after he signed the contract. "I think both sides are very happy with it. I think I was fairly rewarded for what I did last year."

Former *San Francisco Chronicle* beat writer David Bush, who covered the A's from 1987 to 1994, sensed McGwire's enthusiasm after landing the contract, the largest of any second-year player in 1988. "When he signed his contract, and the A's had a press conference in Jay Alves, the public relations director's hotel room, he was so happy," recalled Bush. "He was so friendly and happy."

Complementing McGwire's enthusiasm was the ever-inflating muscular physique he attained through workouts. McGwire loved weight lifting. For two years, McGwire had religiously pumped iron year-round and admitted during spring training he was "addicted" to lifting weights. Some felt he dropped weight and lost strength and stamina toward the final months of his rookie season, mustering only sixteen homers after the All-Star break. This time, though, his chest and arms were noticeably larger. "I don't measure myself, but I know I'm bigger," McGwire said during spring training in 1988. "I hit the gym from day one at the end of the season last year. It's what keeps me going. . . . I want to be even bigger than I am now."[1]

Included in his workout regimen was an assortment of muscle-building and dietary supplements. McGwire hoped those additions would help him maintain his size and weight for the entire season. When Bush interviewed McGwire near his locker at the A's complex in Scottsdale, he noted the supplements in a *San Francisco Chronicle* article describing McGwire's bulked-up physique during spring training. "The top of his locker resembles a health food store, with jars of vitamins, amino acids, and something called 'Sudden Impact.' That isn't McGwire hitting the ball, but rather a drink of anabolic ingredients similar to steroids without the nasty side effects," wrote Bush.[2]

McGwire, however, was one of the many brawny figures on the A's. During the off-season the A's general manager, Sandy Alderson, acquired six-foot-five, 230-pound Dave Parker, a take-charge left-handed slugger from the Cincinnati Reds. Alderson also signed veteran Don Baylor, a right-handed hitter released by the Minnesota Twins in 1987, and stingy-gloved and powerfully built center fielder, Dave Henderson, who was a free agent. Catcher Ron Hassey and second baseman Glenn Hubbard were also lured via free agency. Those offensive additions comforted recently acquired starting pitchers Bob Welch and Storm Davis, who were guaranteed plenty of run support. With a strong nucleus of homegrown talent such as Canseco, McGwire, Luis Polonia, Terry Steinbach, and Walt Weiss, all of whom were groomed in the farm system, merging with the savvy veterans, the A's seemed built for a championship. Through Alderson's shrewd trades, calculated additions, and revolutionary emphasis on statistical analysis, he revived the A's from the ashes of the Finley regime. Former A's third baseman Carney Lansford recalls:

> He and Tony [La Russa] began acquiring great veteran players who still wanted to win. I remember walking out of the clubhouse to the field for the first day of spring training in 1988, and looking at the players and saying, "we definitely have a chance this year." We had a lot of veterans that had a lot of confidence and they showed that just by the way they walked on the field and how they handled themselves. We had every piece of the puzzle.

The team's swagger rubbed off on McGwire. Parker and Baylor imparted confidence in the twenty-four-year-old. Perhaps nothing showed their influence on him more than a Friday evening game on April 8. With several teammates pushing McGwire to send a message to opposing pitchers who casually plunked him during his rookie season, he roared at the next opportunity. When California Angels' starting pitcher Kirk McCaskill unleashed a steaming fastball in the top of the fourth inning straight at McGwire's head, he never meant to awaken a giant. McGwire, who had slammed a home run off him two innings earlier, ducked his head and dropped his bat. But the ball still crashed into his helmet. And when McGwire, still rattled from the jolt, finally regained his composure, he marched toward the mound, violently flung both arms in the air, and barked at McCaskill.

The confrontation turned into a mild bench-clearing verbal spat near the pitchers mound. Though McGwire never tackled McCaskill, his surprising response was enough to send a fierce warning to pitchers around the league who planned on throwing a similar pitch at him. "I wanted to know what the fuck was going on," McGwire told reporters after the game. "Excuse my French, but that's what I said." Asked to predict his actions if another pitcher threw at him during the season, McGwire promised, "I'll be thrown out of a lot of games and be fined a lot of money." To many, however, his sudden episodes of aggression unveiled a different version of McGwire, hot-tempered and harboring an edge. As *San Francisco Chronicle* columnist Bruce Jenkins explained after the game: "It was a very different-looking McGwire who addressed reporters after the game. He looked dangerous, ready to explode. His responses were tight-lipped and abrupt, and his eyes were ablaze." Jenkins later wrote, "Make no mistake, though, this incident marked a significant change in McGwire's on-field demeanor . . ."[3]

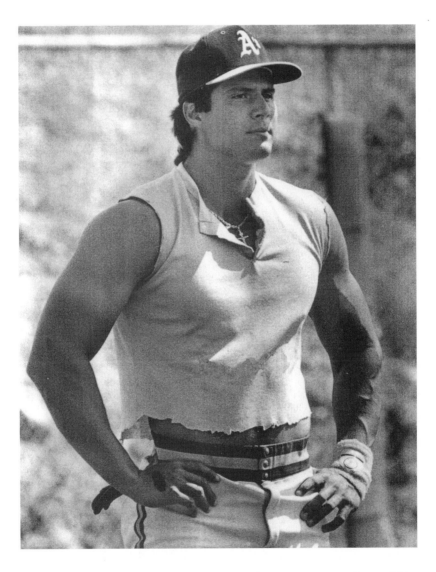

Poised for his Rookie of the Year season in 1986, Jose Canseco flaunted his ripped physique during spring training in Scottsdale, Arizona. Ron Riesterer/Oakland Tribune

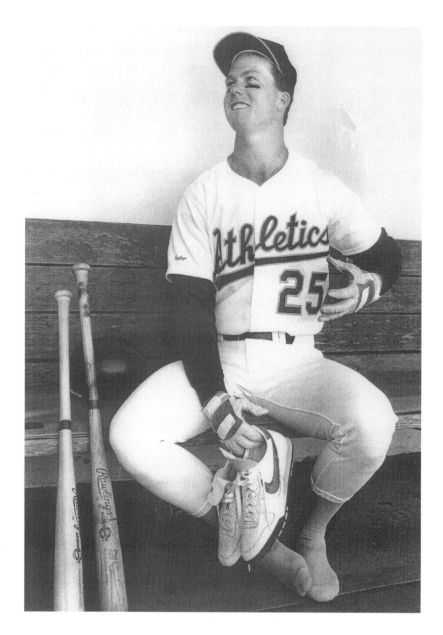

All smiles, a fresh-faced McGwire relished his Rookie of the Year season in 1987 when he exploded with 49 home runs, shattering the rookie record.
Ron Riesterer/Oakland Tribune

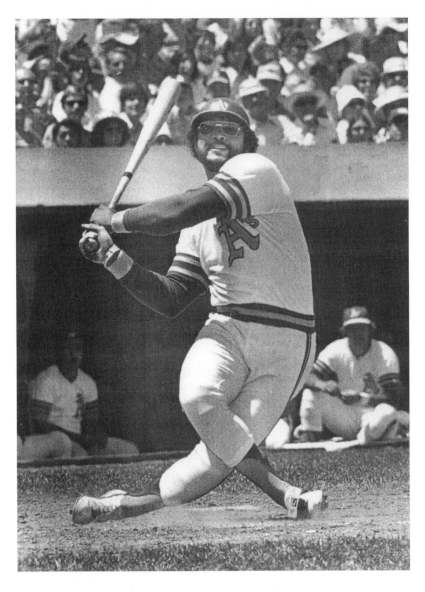

During the final season of his legendary career with the Oakland Athletics in 1987, Reggie Jackson passed his torch of elite power to up and coming sluggers Mark McGwire and Jose Canseco.
Ron Riesterer/Oakland Tribune

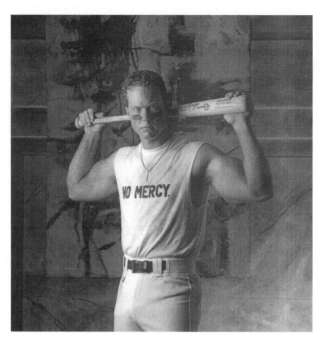

With his muscled-up frame, Mark McGwire added an edge to his game after his rookie season in 1987. Michael Zagaris

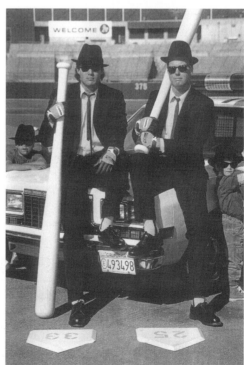

Posing for the hot-selling Bash Brothers poster in 1988, Canseco and McGwire embodied the Oakland Athletics' swagger and dominance of the late 1980s. Brad Mangin

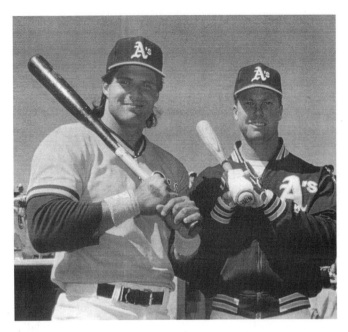

By 1989, Jose Canseco and Mark McGwire had ushered in the bodybuilding explosion in baseball and became the most thunderous power-hitting duo in baseball. Ron Riesterer/Oakland Tribune

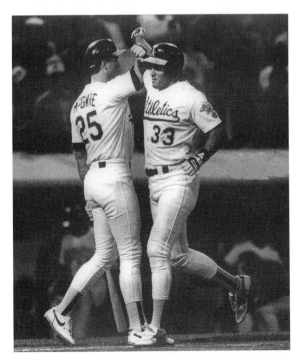

After belting a mammoth home run in 1989, Canseco slams his concrete forearm into McGwire's at home plate. Ron Riesterer/Oakland Tribune

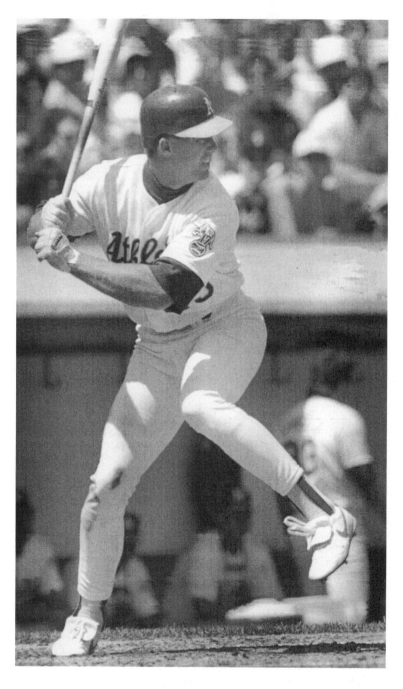

Despite his dismal season in 1991, when he batted .201, he still was the only player at that time to hit 30 home runs in each of his first four seasons. Ron Riesterer/Oakland Tribune

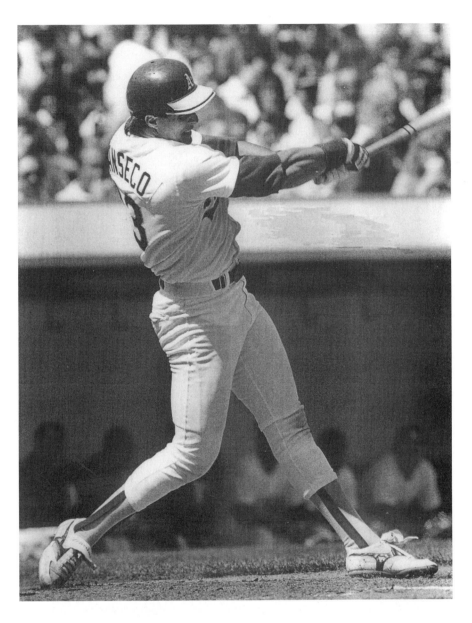

Even Canseco's vicious swing couldn't stop the A's from trading him to the Texas Rangers on August 31, 1992, which marked an end of an era in Oakland. Ron Riesterer/Oakland Tribune

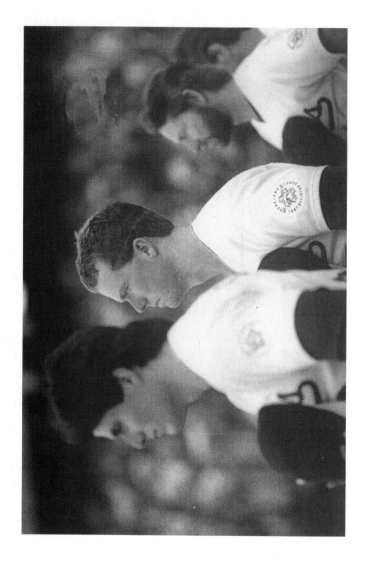

Paying homage to the American flag during the national anthem in 1987, no one could have guessed that eighteen years later Canseco and McGwire would face U.S. lawmakers in Congress on March 17, 2005. Ron Riesterer/Oakland Tribune

It was a change that was necessary, according to former teammate Dave Parker. After his arrival, Parker noticed pitchers trying to bully and intimidate the redhead by brushing him back. Parker advised McGwire that only he could eliminate those threatening pitches.

Pitchers were drilling him so much when I got there. I told him, "you're the only one who could stop that . . . you want to stop getting hit? The next time someone hits you, you need to go out there and shake him like a leaf. You should respect everyone but fear no one. Go out there and throw him around that mound, and you won't get hit the rest of the year." And he did against McCaskill.

McGwire refused to be bullied out of the league. Consequently, each time a pitcher brushed him back, he fearlessly inched closer to home plate. "He needed to make a statement," said former teammate Greg Cadaret. "He got a little more of an edge, but he was also maturing as a star." Releasing his anger toward pitchers represented only one of many changes in McGwire. On the road, his stardom and popularity along with all its accessories began taking its toll on his marriage. Women, intrigued by his celebrity, took notice. That was enough for Kathy, who filed for divorce in 1988 after three years of marriage. "There were too many things calling Mark's name," Kathy told *Sports Illustrated* in 1998. "Women, fame, glamour."[4]

It was 7:00 A.M. at Racquetball World in Fountain Valley, California, and Curt Wenzlaff carved time from his schedule to train McGwire. That McGwire was one of the premiere players in baseball didn't seem to matter to Wenzlaff. Bodybuilding was Wenzlaff's domain, and he harshly welcomed McGwire into it. "He was getting his ass kicked and it was good for him," said Wenzlaff.

McGwire grunted, sweated, and slowly pushed the dumbbells over his head, an exercise designed to tax the shoulders. McGwire had regularly pumped iron for over two years, but training with Wenzlaff was different, excruciating. Apart from being a connoisseur in muscle growth, Wenzlaff was an expert in human growth hormone and steroids. Merging those chemicals with weight lifting helped him chisel some of the finest physiques and transform athletes into superstardom. He didn't peddle steroids; he sold his expertise, a menu endorsing specific chemicals, foods, and workouts.

Wenzlaff's credentials intrigued McGwire, who delved into his mind. Not that McGwire was a steroid novice; he had already been exposed to the chemicals, its effects, and dangers. He asked Wenzlaff calculated questions, ones that clearly displayed his familiarity with the drugs. "He wasn't asking me, 'Gee…what are steroids?'" Wenzlaff said. "They weren't '101' college level questions; he was asking me '400' level questions, if you will, so he had already been exposed to it." Wenzlaff's, answers, however, didn't help soften McGwire's workouts. "You mother fucking bastard," McGwire roared at him, after completing another repetition. Although McGwire had had enough, Wenzlaff pushed him further. "He was pissed off at me, but I told him, 'I know you're a superstar, but you're working out with me, dude.' I pushed him to a different level and he was mad," recalled Wenzlaff. When Wenzlaff's friend marched in and heard the screaming, he thought both were prepared to scuffle.

Offering advice and expertise to McGwire, Wenzlaff began watching him metamorphose. "He truly changed in front of my eyes," Wenzlaff wrote in an email in November 2007. "Slowly and methodically, I witnessed an awakening of a selfish introvert, no one else mattered, almost an 'I'm in a different league' attitude. . . . I don't think anyone could convince me otherwise of the fact that steroids played a significant role in his self-imposed attitude adjustment."

Wenzlaff arrived in Oakland after stumbling into Reggie Jackson in a gym. His sculpted physique intrigued Jackson. They hit it off and Jackson eventually hired Wenzlaff to work in public relations for his recently purchased auto dealerships in Berkeley and Palo Alto. "When I met Reggie, I was scheduled to move to Hawaii," Wenzlaff wrote in an email. "There, I wanted to become a personal trainer in that climate. He also impressed me, especially by his athleticism and God-given talent for his age. So when the opportunity arose to work for him, I passed on paradise. All Reggie knew about my past was that I was an expert in working out and nutrition.

"Occasionally, we would share battle stories. He seemed equally intrigued with my past with regard to sleeping in deprivation tanks before each workout, my old regimens that involved being strapped to a machine, wearing an oxygen mask, breathing oxygen from a tank, and being zapped with a cattle prod when I felt I didn't have anything left. I spent many evenings in a gym (after it closed to the general public) crying because I just had my own ass served to me on a platter."

Wenzlaff soon moved into Jackson's home in the Oakland Hills. During his stay, he frequented the Oakland-Alameda Coliseum and met McGwire and Canseco. Wenzlaff insisted Jackson didn't know about his past or steroid use. "Reggie was a workout partner. Period. That was it," stressed Wenzlaff, who claimed steroid use in baseball was in its infant stages in the late 1980s when he became acquainted with McGwire. "He had a brother [J.J.] who was heavily into it [steroids], so he had already been exposed to it," said Wenzlaff. "Let's just say that I communicated with José and Big Mac. José opened the door for himself by writing his book [*Juiced*] but as far as Big Mac, all I'll ever say is, 'I trained with him a few times.'"

McGwire's attire, his interests, his personality, and his lifestyle shifted, according to teammates. While some claimed his off-the-field issues, including his divorce, caused the changes, others felt he was searching for his identity. Being a warm-hearted man surrounded by the rugged, strong-willed personalities on his team may have prompted a new image. Regardless of the reasons, teammates, media, and friends spotted the transformation. "I never saw a guy go from white bread to burnt toast faster. Within a year, he was a dark character," said Bud Geracie, the A's beat writer for the *San Jose Mercury News*, in 1988. "And it was almost a ridiculously clichéd morality play on how success can go to someone's head and change them. He really became prickly and grumpy; it was all quite mysterious. And now looking back, I certainly wonder if it wasn't something else: the classic symptoms of steroid use."

Former teammate Doug Jennings attributed McGwire's changes to seeing the glamour chasing Canseco, whose swagger and flamboyance commanded attention everywhere they traveled. "Mark saw the bad boy image in Jose and how much fan fare he got through it, and he wanted that attention," said Jennings. "But he was trying to be somebody he wasn't and couldn't fill that image because it wasn't his nature. That wasn't his personality. He was a very soft-spoken, easy going, and really good-hearted person."

The A's former director of scouting, Grady Fuson, witnessed him pass through several phases in his life: from the way McGwire acted, to the style in which he dressed and groomed his hair.

Something happened . . . and he took a turn into a different person. I saw him go through a couple of different changes in his life and he changed as a person. I never thought it would happen to him. When we drafted him, I thought he was really grounded . . . he came from a great, educated, happy and fun-loving family; I never once felt he didn't have his act together as a human being. He was your typical All-American kid. He wore nice collared shirts with jeans and a clean pair of tennis shoes. That was always his look. But I just saw this change. He was getting into the pimp look, the satin pants, and the pretty Italian shoes and, I remember saying, "that's not the McGwire I remember."

Fuson reiterated, though, that McGwire came full circle later in his career.

Hall of Fame closer Dennis Eckersley, who teamed with McGwire from 1987 to 1995 and later with the St. Louis Cardinals in 1997, said McGwire couldn't find himself. He said he didn't sense the changes turned McGwire into a bad person, but that they became more and more exaggerated with each passing year. "He really couldn't find who he was," observed Eckersley, who also claimed McGwire became much sharper over the years. "Each year he was something different. He was all over the map. One year he's a cowboy and the next year, depending on what girl he's with, he had the GQ look."

The changes trickled into his lifestyle and hobbies. While former A's coach Rene Lachemann points to McGwire's divorce and personal matters taking its toll on him, Lachemann, too, noticed his focus sway. "He kind of changed with certain things," said Lachemann. "This guy was a laid-back beach guy and all of a sudden he changed and was into fine art, which was way above his head. That wasn't him." Vice president of marketing Andy Dolich remembered, "When he first came in, he was extremely open, very friendly, and then became much more guarded in everything he did. As he became more successful and a bigger story, he went into a shell."

One shouldn't place too much emphasis on those changes, said former catcher Terry Steinbach, who roomed with McGwire during his rookie season. He believed the changes were a natural progression that reflected the circumstances surrounding his life. "Everybody changes," stressed Steinbach. "At that time, he had some personal issues and got divorced. A person might act a certain way if he's married with a child as compared to single and living a dream. He just did different things. I definitely don't think it was awkward or weird." Teammate Greg Cadaret said his new edge stemmed from teammates pushing him in that direction. ""It wasn't like he was becoming more belligerent or anything. People were just trying to teach him how to handle himself."

What certainly changed was the A's success. Fueled by a thunderous and physically imposing batting lineup and a stingy starting pitching staff, the club dominated the American League. Blazing a fourteen-game winning streak in May, the club barged into first place in the American League West and captured the national spotlight. The ingredients of brute strength, muscle-bound physiques, and unwavering confidence branded the A's as the sexiest show in baseball, one that many compared to an offensive line in the National Football League. "We were a traveling road show," said A's traveling secretary Mickey Morabito. "It was like the Rolling Stones were coming to town . . . it was incredible. With the big names we had, we were probably the first really high-profile team of this era. We almost had a superstar at every position."

Nothing exuded their swagger more than "the Bash." With fore-arm strength associated directly with power and home runs, several A's hitters acknowledged that by conjuring up a flashy alternative to the traditional high-five or handshake celebration. When A's hitters crossed home plate after belting a home run, instead of slapping hands together, they balled their first and pounded their forearms together. It was birthed during spring training when McGwire, who prized the added muscle he acquired during the winter, sat in the dugout and compared his enormous forearms with Canseco's. Shortly af-ter, when McGwire clobbered a home run, he strutted to home plate, raised his right arm, clenched his fist, and slammed his forearms into those of Canseco, Parker, and Baylor. The A's marketing depart-ment jumped on the phenomenon, and the craze whirled through the country.

"I thought with all the big guys we've got, why not change all the way over from high fives?" McGwire told reporters in 1988. "We've got a big team, so we bump forearms. I like it. It's unique."[5] That McGwire was at the forefront of such a snazzy trend offered more insight into the new side of him. Performance-enhancing drugs were instrumental in changing McGwire in 1988, Canseco claimed. He al-leged he and McGwire casually discussed steroids throughout the season and discreetly injected each other several times in the bath-room stalls at the Oakland-Alameda Coliseum. "It was only through using steroids and giving himself a new body that Mark really be-came more comfortable with himself, and stopped being so awkward around other people," Canseco explained in his book, *Juiced*.[6]

While McGwire, Canseco, Henderson, Parker, and Baylor were originally dubbed The Bash Brothers upon its inception, the name was soon solely lavished upon Canseco and McGwire. The two muscle-bound, twenty-something bashers from the Bay Area drew comparisons with other legendary duos such as Willie Mays and Willie McCovey, Mickey Mantle and Roger Maris, and Babe Ruth and Lou Gehrig. Canseco and McGwire merged into one phrase like Proctor & Gamble and Smith & Wesson. "They were a flashy, West Coast, hip duo that played in the World Series and attracted a lot of fans . . . it was a cult following," said Greg Cadaret.

With their explosive batting practice sessions, tape-measure home runs, popularity, and especially their weight-lifting sessions, both embodied a unique brand of player in the sport. Dolich reminisced on the duo.

Those two guys just started bashing forearms. We're talking about two of the biggest forearm bashers that ever existed and we were getting a fair amount of national publicity and television coverage. Plus, the gargantuan shots both hit. Those guys were hitting, you know, 80-90 home runs between them each season. That's a lot of forearm bashing. Winning teams generate enthusiasm. Their pure power rekindled the wackiness the A's had under Finley and the colorful names and the great teams that they had.

Glamour and fame chased the two. While many teammates claimed Canseco craved the spotlight, others also admitted McGwire, at the time, sought it, too. "They both got caught up in that bash shit," said Dennis Eckersley. Equipment manager Steve Vucinich said the Bash Brothers sparked a higher level of popularity for the franchise across the nation. "They were the beginning of that autograph craze," said Vucinich. "There were so many autograph hunters chasing us down and they tried to stay in the same hotel as us. It got to be sort of like the New York Yankees are now: A traveling rock show."

The surging popularity of Canseco and McGwire attracted companies hoping to ride their success. One of those companies, Costacos Brothers Inc., a Seattle-based business famed for its innovative sports posters, pounced on the opportunity. The operation began generating posters in 1985, after owner John Costacos, who had been selling t-shirts in a sporting goods store, asked a female employee for customers' most requested item. She replied that it was a poster of Seattle Seahawks strong safety Kenny Easley. John then contacted Easley's agent, Jeff Moorad, who introduced him to Easley. Soon after, John produced a poster of Easley called "The Enforcer." The successful project compelled John to search for other popular athletes who boasted a strong fan base. That's when he thought of Canseco and McGwire. "They were huge, and the A's were having a great season and were all over the news," said Costacos. "Originally we had come up with this concept called 'The Blast Brothers,' and then they started doing that forearm bash."

John contacted their agents, set up a photo shoot at the Oakland-Alameda Coliseum, and dressed them up as *The Blues Brothers*, after the 1980 film featuring Dan Akroyd and John Belushi. For the shoot, they wore black suits, black shoes, fedora hats, slim ties, and sunglasses, along with yellow socks. Leaning on the hood of an Oakland Police patrol car, they posed with oversized baseball bats. "Doing the poster with Mark is an exciting thing," Canseco told the Associated Press during the shoot in 1988. "I kind of can't wait to see how it turns out."[7]

Within two months of its release, Costacos sold 50,000 posters. "It was as popular as any poster we had done and it got a ton of press coverage," said Costacos. "Because they were such a big deal, had we had the distribution we had in our later years, it would have easily sold more than any poster, other than Michael Jordan. It was still one of the best sellers we had."

The bash became such a vogue that the A's marketing department and a Bay Area television station teamed up to produce a music video. Borrowed from Bill Pickett's 1962 song, "Monster Mash," "The Monster Bash" featured several A's players clubbing home runs, circling the bases, and smashing forearms together as they passed home plate. The video depicted the team's cockiness and the intimidating style of play in Oakland. The song's lyrics also encouraged fans to participate in the phenomenon: "If you're a fan of the Oakland A's/ You too can do the latest ballpark craze/When the A's big bats really come alive/don't waste your time with the boring high-five." Besides bashing, the A's did plenty of winning. Boasting a record of 54–34 by the All-Star break, catcher Terry Steinbach, third baseman Carney Lansford, closer Dennis Eckersley, Canseco, and McGwire were selected to the American League squad.

Nineteen eighty-eight. Tony La Russa was pissed off. It was February 24, and Canseco still hadn't reported to spring training, missing the club's first week of workouts in Scottsdale. What really annoyed him was the reason why: Canseco scheduled two autograph sessions at card collectors' shows in Philadelphia and New York, which delayed his arrival. "He needs to get his priorities straight," fumed La Russa, who hoped to experiment with Canseco in center field. But with exhibition games already looming, his tardiness smothered that idea. His absence didn't bode well with teammates, either. The previous season, he arrived late because of a financially driven contract dispute. His pattern became a tired act. Even though, technically speaking, under Major League Baseball's labor agreement, players aren't mandated to report to camp until March 2, his teammates voluntarily arrived early.

When Canseco, who had been picked up by McGwire and driven to Scottsdale Community College, had finally arrived, La Russa showed his displeasure. In a show of friendly badgering, his staff assembled a table, a large photo of Canseco, and a tarp on the field to welcome him. A sign read, "Welcome to Jose Canseco Autograph Day," and another one said, "Appearing for the first time: Jose (Card Show) Canseco from 10:00 a.m. to 2:00 p.m." The final one claimed Canseco would be lecturing on "Concepts of Team Play." Though it was a sarcastic gesture, La Russa clearly grew frustrated with his antics. "Who is giving Jose advice? I'd love to know who he listens to, so I can kick him over the goal post over there," La Russa told reporters during spring training in 1988. "He's signed. He's in his third year and he should be here. Whoever's telling him anything different is doing him a disservice."

On his team, however, one player offered him motivation. After watching Canseco take his cuts and dash around the bases during spring workouts, Dave Parker shook his head. A year before, Parker had teamed with another multi-talented player, Eric Davis, who boasted electric speed and explosive power, a rare combination. After observing Canseco on a daily basis, Parker challenged Canseco that he had the talent to become baseball's first player to hit forty home runs and steal forty bases.

"I made him believe he could be the first forty-forty guy," recalled Parker. "I told him, 'I played with Eric Davis, one of the best young players in the game, but after watching your foot speed, they should be talking about you being the first forty-forty guy.' After that, you could see a light go on in his head."

Canseco, who averaged thirty-one home runs and fifteen stolen bases each of his first two seasons, had participated in extensive leg trainings during the winter. Canseco figured four or five players had already reached the milestone, but after mentioning his goal to a group of reporters, they informed him that no other players had accomplished it. The closest, Bobby Bonds, while playing for the San Francisco Giants in 1973, was one home run shy of the mark. The twenty-seven-year-old outfielder snatched forty-three stolen bases and hit thirty-nine home runs.

Though no one doubted Canseco's uncanny talent, many questioned his drive and motivation. His suspect work ethic frustrated teammates and coaches. To accomplish such a feat meant Canseco would have to dedicate himself and remain focused, which meant spending more time at the ballpark and avoiding distractions. That was a daunting task for such an electrifying and self-absorbed figure. Many also felt that his size, six foot four and 230 pounds, would weigh him down over the long season and prevent him from swiping forty bases. Canseco remained confident. "I knew something that the reporters didn't. I knew that all my hard work, and the right combination of steroids, had already made me a much better athlete than I had been before. . . . Also, I knew that steroids would improve my stamina and keep me healthy and explosive throughout the long baseball season," wrote Canseco in *Juiced*.[8]

As the season progressed, teammates noticed Canseco's focus shifting. He spent extra time in the batting cage and sprinted early into the outfield to shag fly balls off the bat of La Russa. "Tony really took initiative with him," said Doug Jennings. "He took him under his wing and made sure he got his defensive stuff done every day. Everyone knew that José was pretty much an offensive player, but Tony went out there and hit him his fly balls and ground balls during batting practice before the game."

At the plate, Canseco also developed a two-strike batting stance, an approach endorsed by hitting coach Bob Watson and teammate Dave Parker. When Canseco faced a two-strike count, he closed his open stance and focused on making contact. That approach helped him pound fourteen home runs with two strikes. Besides accolades, financial incentives also motivated him. Earning $325,000 in 1988, he would be eligible for arbitration the next season. With agent Jeff Borris of the Dennis Gilbert Agency representing him, a monstrous season would guarantee a hefty pay increase the following year. Canseco had more than enough reason to concentrate on the feat. Former teammate Steve Ontiveros recalled:

> I saw him apply himself and he was a man on a mission. What a difference . . . it was night and day. You could see by the numbers he generated that something happened, something changed. And it was basically his work ethic and attitude. We could see the glimpses of greatness he had, when for one season, he decided to go all out. He was a force.

Curbing his off-the-field entertainment also helped him focus on the field. Though he never smoked cigarettes and rarely drank alcohol, he enjoyed a vibrant social life littered with beautiful women. Instead, Canseco secluded himself by staying in his hotel room and watching movies into the early morning hours. "He didn't go out a lot that year," said Jennings. "He spent a lot of time in his room, ordering room service and staying away from the media hype, so he could focus on his goal—to become the first forty-forty player."

Meeting Esther Haddad, a twenty-year-old beauty queen from Miami, also calmed him. Canseco first bumped into her at one of Miami's lavish fitness centers, the Scandinavian Health Club, in 1986. They locked eyes. But since it happened during the final weeks before Canseco headed to Arizona for spring training, nothing materialized. Her beauty mesmerized Canseco, though, so after the season he hunted her down and, through a friend, reconnected with her and they began courting. There was nothing drab about the couple: Canseco was the hunk of professional baseball and Esther had recently been crowned Miss Miami.

Canseco popped the question, and they were scheduled to marry after the season on November 5. The thought of Canseco finally settling down with one woman was strange for teammates, though.

Starting pitcher Dave Stewart didn't believe it. In fact, he was so convinced Canseco wouldn't get married by that date, he bet him $10,000. In turn, if Canseco didn't follow through with the wedding, he promised to pay $5,000 to Stewart. When Esther accompanied Canseco on most road trips during the season, it became apparent he felt the urge to settle down. While Esther calmed Canseco, American League pitchers couldn't silence his bat and popularity. Canseco clubbed twenty-four home runs and swiped twenty-two bases by the All-Star break, pushing toward his goal. With a batting average hovering around .300, his league-leading sixty-seven runs batted in and seventy-two runs also made him the leading candidate for the American League's Most Valuable Player. Focus, hard work, and steroids made Canseco a force. "He was the best player in baseball," said former A's radio play-by-play broadcaster Lon Simmons. "They talked about Kirby Puckett and he was good, but he wasn't as good as Jose Canseco."

Fans around the country noticed him, too. They voted him to start the All-Star Game at Cincinnati's Riverfront Stadium. Leading the American League players with 1,765,499 votes, he became the first outfielder since Fred Lynn to lead the league in voting. His performance, stardom, and muscle behind a dominating team lifted him on top of the baseball world. "He was the perfect crossover matinee idol," said Dolich. "Little boys wanted to be him; women wanted to date him; and guys wanted to hang out with him."

Aside from his offensive dominance, his dependable glove and range in right field garnered more praise. Working on his outfield defense with La Russa before games had paid off. "He was as talented a player as I've ever seen play the game," said former A's pitcher Bob Welch. "When I first got there, he played solid defense and ran the bases well." In fact, Canseco's outfield skills had improved so much that team captain Carney Lansford hailed him as one of the best right fielders in the league. His long strides and accurate angles toward the baseball impressed him. "I thought he should have won a Gold Glove in right field that year," recalled Lansford. "He was an outstanding outfielder."

His popularity reached its peak by September. His movie star looks and chiseled physique captured the hearts of adoring women across the country. Teenage girls taped posters of him in their school lockers and begged for his attention from the stands. When Canseco trotted to right field, girls screamed his name. When he walked into a card collector's show to sign autographs in July, observers compared the crowd's anticipation of Canseco to that of Elvis Presley. Companies stalked him for multi-million dollar endorsement deals. One of those corporations, American Express, paid him to swing a bat and pose nude from the waist up for a magazine advertisement in its "Portraits" series. *People* magazine also sent a reporter to Oakland to interview him. The article ran in October and featured Canseco and his fianceé, Esther. Canseco soon exploded into a national celebrity.

As Bob Rubin of the *Miami Herald* observed:

> With his dark, Latin good looks, a 6-foot-3, 230-pound body that's so perfect it makes me sick, and a public persona that has blossomed from shy (which used to be mistaken for moody and/or aloof) to relaxed and charming. Canseco will become a monster. Josemania will be upon us.[9]

Being lavished with such praise and fanfare was a platform he craved, according to teammates. Whether hearing a handful of screaming fans in a hotel lobby or clawing his way through autograph seekers and into the team bus, Canseco armed himself for the spotlight. "He didn't shy away from the limelight," said Jennings. "His bad-boy image was very attractive to a lot of people. He performed it to a T. He seemed to find his way into the media all the time. And he drew a lot of attention to himself, which he enjoyed." A's traveling secretary Mickey Morabito witnessed the onslaught and how Canseco handled the adoration. "He really liked the attention," said Morabito. "He probably enjoyed it more than anyone else."

Even as he absorbed the worship that accompanied his stardom, though, Canseco became a task to associate with, according to Jennings. That stemmed from his obsession to be the center of attention in a crowd, a desire that distanced even his closest friends. Jennings explained:

> One on one, José was great. He was very personable and easy to talk with, and extremely intelligent in baseball, but in a crowd he was very difficult to be around. It didn't matter who you were, he had to be the center of attention. Even if you were his good friend, you kind of got distanced from the crowd, because he had to be the focus of attention.

That attention, even from hoards of screaming, beautiful women, didn't seem to bother Esther, who traveled with Canseco on the road most of the season. In Oakland, she sat behind the A's dugout with other players' wives. Amid his rock-star appeal, she weathered the whistles and sexual innuendos shoved at her fiancé. "They can do all the screaming they want; they can write all the love letters they want; they can do whatever they want," Haddad told Michalene Busico of the *San Jose Mercury News* in 1988. "It doesn't matter. The wedding is still on, and they're just low. And José feels that way, too."[10]

On the field, Canseco made it clear that chasing his personal exploits would be secondary to his team's pursuit of a division title. What made his efforts more impressive was that his home runs and stolen bases came during crucial moments in games, pushing the A's to victory. And on September 19, the A's clinched the American League Western Division for the first time since 1981, edging the defending world champion Minnesota Twins by a score of 3-2. With the A's securing a play-off berth and Canseco having already hit his fortieth home run, this meant he could concentrate on swiping three more bases to reach his goal.

Four days later, in Milwaukee's County Stadium, Canseco entered the game needing two stolen bases to barge into history. Canseco swiped number thirty-nine in the top of the first. In the top of the fifth, he reached first base on a bunt single. With McGwire at the plate, Canseco took his lead, sprinted toward second base, and slid ahead of catcher B.J. Surhoff's throw. He was safe. "I wasn't taking a big lead, not giving any indication that I was going, and they weren't paying much attention to me," Canseco told reporters after the game. "So on the second pitch, I went." After stealing the base, he triumphantly grabbed the bag and lifted it over his shoulders.

The crowd cheered, and his teammates climbed to the top step of the dugout and applauded Canseco for becoming the first player to hit forty homers and steal forty bases in a season. But Canseco wasn't finished. Three innings later, he slammed his forty-first home run, a three-run shot that pushed his RBI totals to 120, establishing a new Oakland A's record. After his trail-blazing evening, Canseco shared his enthusiasm with reporters. "It's probably my biggest night," Canseco said. "I did break the Oakland A's RBI record, which I don't know if many people noticed. So I got the base and the ball. That's quite an achievement for one night."

Whether he could carry his season's success into the play-offs in October was another story, especially while engulfed in a scandal. A week later, while the A's were set to play the Boston Red Sox in the American League Championship Series, Thomas Boswell, a *Washington Post* columnist, appeared on CBS's *Newswatch* hosted by Charlie Rose. During the interview, Boswell claimed Canseco was "the most conspicuous example of a player who has made himself great with steroids."[11] Boswell said his statements stemmed from a conversation he had with La Russa, who admitted that Canseco had made "some mistakes" early in his career. It was clear, Boswell said, La Russa was pointing to Canseco's past steroid use. Boswell also noted that other players around the league refer to steroids as a "José Canseco Milkshake."

The buzz of steroids had been burning through media outlets, because a week earlier Canadian Olympic sprinter Ben Johnson, christened "the world's fastest human," tested positive for the banned substance Stanozolol, a water-based steroid. The Olympic Committee subsequently stripped Johnson of his gold medal in the 100 meters. While it was clear anabolic steroids had saturated the bodybuilding, professional football, and track and field communities, it became more apparent the drug had seduced its way into other competitive sports, including baseball. Boswell alleged steroids already infected professional sports, and baseball's best player, José Canseco, was the poster boy for its success. Said Jennings:

> You heard the rumors, but we didn't really know for sure; I never saw it. But you could see that his body type was so much different than the other players. At the time, he was in spring training strength. He was getting stronger as the season went along. That fueled the ability that he already had.

When Canseco learned of the accusations in Minnesota, he vehemently denied using the drugs and hinted at taking legal action against Boswell for his "slanderous" statements. "If I had used steroids," Canseco told the *Sacramento Bee*'s Susan Fornoff in Minneapolis in 1988, "it would have shown up in the urinalysis and blood samples we have done every year for our physicals. There's nothing there—and I don't see how he could have done that without looking at the samples."[12]

Boswell's claims rippled throughout the country and streamed into the playoffs. On October 5, the A's, who boasted 104 wins during the season, stormed into game one of a best of seven series with the Red Sox. With crafty left-handed starter and eighteen-game winner Bruce Hurst on the mound, the A's lineup braced themselves for a battle. In the booth, Reggie Jackson, known for his game-swaying home runs during the postseason, broadcasted the game on television for ABC. His presence in the ballpark prompted arguments over whether Canseco could capture his magic and muscle his team to the World Series, and become the new "Mr. October." Asked if Canseco could perform under the pressures of October, Jackson voiced his confidence to the *Miami Herald* before the game.

> Experience is a factor, but I make an exception with this guy. He has been in the national spotlight since his first week in the majors, when he hit five titanic home runs. After that everybody expected him to be a dominant player, so there has been pressure on him all along. Yes, there's more in October, but it won't be a great jump for him.[13]

During the game, meanwhile, as Canseco trotted out to right field, Red Sox fans taunted him with a loud chorus of "Sterrrr-oids . . . Sterrrr-oids." The jeering continued inning after inning and echoed throughout Fenway Park and over television airwaves. Canseco, who played along with the harassing fans, finally turned around and addressed the crowd seated behind the right field fence: he raised his right arm, rolled up his sleeve, and flexed his bicep for them. "He handled it well," said teammate Dave Parker. "He said things back sometimes. But most of the time, he was killing the baseball. That's how you beat that." Facing the needling fans, Canseco made his presence felt at the plate. In the top of the fourth, he muscled a Hurst 3-2 pitch over the Green Monster and into the net, producing the A's first run of the series. He clobbered two more home runs in the series, as the A's completed a four-game sweep of the Red Sox to capture the American League pennant.

"Jose Canseco is God," McGwire told reporters after the series.[14]

Canseco and the dominant A's barged into the eighty-fifth World Series, for the first time since 1974. Heavily favored against the scrappy Los Angeles Dodgers, who were coming off an emotionally charged seven-game series against the New York Mets, the A's were forecasted to maul the Dodgers in a swift four-game sweep. The Dodgers pitchers were considered unable to contain the A's muscle-bound bashers. Before the series, Canseco downplayed the momentum the Dodgers carried into the series. He told the media:

> An emotional edge is not going to get you anywhere. You can fight Mike Tyson against a midget and the midget might have an emotional edge, but I don't think he's going to hang in there for a long time. I think an emotional edge is overrated. I don't think anyone can shut us down for four or five games. I doubt it very much. Not with the power we have. It just won't happen. No way.[15]

It looked that way in the top of the second, when the A's loaded the bases and Canseco strutted to the plate. On the mound, Tim Belcher, a flame-throwing right-hander who played with Canseco and watched him electrify the Southern League in Huntsville in 1985, hurled a 1-0 slider. Canseco scorched a line drive that cleared the center-field fence and ricocheted off of the NBC television camera. As he circled the bases, Canseco smirked and raised both arms, an arrogant expression conveying he had left his mark on baseball's grandest stage. The grand slam seemingly capped a remarkable season for Canseco and the A's, who seemed poised to roll over the Dodgers.

The momentum, however, dramatically shifted in the bottom of the ninth inning, as Kirk Gibson, a pinch hitter who had carried the

Dodgers throughout the season, limped out of the dugout and hobbled to plate. With the A's clinging to a 4-3 lead and their unstoppable closer, Dennis Eckersley, on the mound, the match-up mirrored the series: a well-oiled juggernaut stalking a bunch that barely tripped into the World Series. And when Eckersley grooved a 3-2, two-out slider to Gibson, the pinch hitter stroked a game-winning, two-run home run to right to edge out the A's 5-4, snatching the first game of the series. Those dramatics set the tone for the series, as the Dodgers overwhelmed the A's in five games to capture the world championship.

The A's struggles in the series echoed that of Canseco and McGwire, who went 2-for-36, despite each hitting a home run. After Canseco smacked the grand slam in game one, he went hitless the remainder of the series. McGwire's game-winning home run in game three was his only hit of the series. Despite the disappointment from the shocking upset, 1988 propelled the duo into national prominence. The Oakland A's were a dynasty in the making.

After the series, Canseco prepared for another significant moment: tying the knot with Esther. Back in Florida, on October 25, 1988, they married in a brief civil ceremony on the second floor of Coral Gables police station.[16] Following through on his marriage meant that Canseco won the wager with teammate Dave Stewart, who owed him $10,000. Those monies would help pay the expenses of the formal wedding ceremony on November 5, held at Miami's Signature Gardens, an extravagant ballroom specializing in weddings. With more than 400 family and friends on hand, twenty-four-year-old Canseco, who donned a white tuxedo, married Esther in a Catholic ceremony.[17] After the wedding, the couple flew to Hawaii for their honeymoon. During the honeymoon, Canseco learned of more thrilling news: he was unanimously crowned the American League's Most Valuable Player, receiving all twenty-eight first-place votes by the Baseball Writers Association of America. The award cemented his place as baseball's most exciting player. After hearing the news, Canseco claimed his best seasons were still to come. On a conference call from Hawaii, Canseco told reporters, "I want to cut down on my strikeouts, I know I can hit for higher average, steal more bases. I am just twenty-four and I'm not going to stop improving."

NOTES

[1]   David Bush, "McGwire Bulks Up," *San Francisco Chronicle*, February 27, 1988.

[2]   Ibid.

[3]   Bruce Jenkins, "The Gentlemen Responds," *San Francisco Chronicle*, April 9, 1988.

[4] Rick Reilly, "The Good Father," *Sports Illustrated*, September 7, 1998.

[5] Gary Richards, "Hands Off: The Bash Is Here," *San Jose Mercury News*, April 11, 1988.

[6] Jose Canseco, *Juiced* (New York: HarperCollins, 2005), 75.

[7] Mercury News Wire Services, "Poster may mean cash in a flash for the bash brothers," *San Jose Mercury News*, June 18, 1988.

[8] Canseco, *Juiced*, 78.

[9] Bob Rubin, "Will Canseco Become New Mr. October?" *Miami Herald*, October 5, 1988.

[10] Michalene Busico, "McGwire seems like the kind of guy who'd give you the shirt off his back," *San Jose Mercury News*, October 2, 1988.

[11] Associated Press, "Canseco Denies Use of Steroids," September 30, 1988.

[12] Susan Fornoff, "Canseco Denies Use of Steroids," *Sacramento Bee*, September 30, 1988.

[13] Rubin, "Will Canseco Become New Mr. October?"

[14] Joe Goddard, "A's Totally Awesome," *Chicago Sun-Times*, October 10, 1988.

[15] Kevin Kernan, "A's Canseco Just Says No To Critics," *San Diego Union Tribune*, October 15, 1988

[16] Steve Rothaus, "Jose Makes His Biggest Catch," *Miami Herald*, October 27, 1988.

[17] David Hancock, "A Grand-slam Night for Canseco," *Miami Herald*, November 6, 1988.

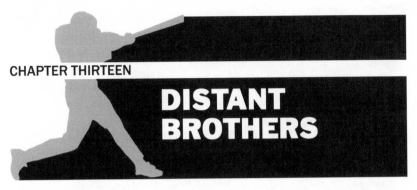

CHAPTER THIRTEEN

DISTANT BROTHERS

"They weren't the first [steroid users] in baseball, but they certainly were the most visible, and they alone certainly got a lot of other players on the bandwagon. They were young and up and coming and had a feeling of invincibility and it showed itself on the field."

—Curt Wenzlaff, one-time friend
July 2007

Nineteen eighty-nine. When McGwire strolled into San Diego's Bahia Hotel that winter for an autograph show, his stock had slightly dipped. Although he had been scheduled to sign one thousand autographs at nine dollars a scribble, as the event concluded, he was two hundred short of the mark. To justify his appearance fee, he signed the rest for the promoter, and the memorabilia would be distributed through mail orders. If it had been during his rookie season in 1987, when he had stormed the country and obliterated the rookie single-season home-run record, no sweat: the lobby would have been swarmed with autograph seekers, and within hours, he would have whipped through a thousand signatures. His popularity, though, had cooled from a fierce boil to a slight simmer. Not that batting .260, clubbing thirty-two home runs with ninety-nine RBIs, and lacing a game-winning home run in the World Series as he did in 1988 could be tagged a sophomore slump. But his teammate and accomplice in victimizing opposing pitchers, Canseco, overshadowed him and became an international star, hacking his way into the sphere of headlines and paparazzi. According to the *San Diego Tribune*'s Kirk Kenney, as McGwire sat at the table and welcomed each fan, a boy approached and asked him how José was doing. McGwire reluctantly answered that he was fine, he guessed.[1]

When fans yoked McGwire and Canseco and figured they were inseparable, both tolerated the perception. That they were teammates in their early twenties, who carried swelled physiques, valued weight lifting, and smashed prodigious home runs didn't forge a sacred friendship. Strength and conditioning coach Dave McKay remarked:

> They were two different people and hung out with two different crowds. They didn't have a lot in common, other than playing on the same team and being big and strong. They weren't very close or tight. I didn't really sense they didn't like each other, I just think they're two different types of individuals. You wouldn't see Mark and José hanging around a lot together. Mark had his group and José had his. They certainly weren't partners in the weight room. Absolutely not. There wasn't anything there.

Although media and fans chained the duo for their home runs on the field, Terry Steinbach didn't observe their relationship as teammates carry outside the clubhouse. Steinbach confirmed that, other than being acquaintances, both went their separate ways.

> They were cordial friends. But I don't think they were chomping at the bit to hang out after every game. They definitely weren't chomping at the bit to go work out together. Their time frames when one was sleeping and one was up weren't the same. . . . I didn't perceive them to be buddies for any extended period of time, at least to my knowledge.

Team photographer Michael Zagaris shared that opinion, too. While media wondered if a friendly rivalry had brewed, he didn't see one.

> They coexisted. They were never good friends, they never hung out together; they were very different people. They got along better in 1987–88, but in 1989, strain began to show. Because they were the Bash Brothers, a lot of people probably thought they hung out together. I don't think they disliked each other, although toward the end, there was nothing in common.

In addition to forearm smashing and home runs, their relationship featured friendly ragging and humor. Because Canseco's steroid use was obvious, McGwire often times referred to him as "No Nuts." And because of McGwire's glistening orange hair, Canseco called him, "Lightbulb Head." "They got along pretty good, though I wouldn't say they were social buddies," recalled former A's reliever Greg Cadaret. "They coexisted as superstars, but I don't think they went to dinner together. They were thrown together because of the Bash Brothers, but the way they lived their lives were opposite."

So were their personalities, claimed former A's captain Carney Lansford. "Mark had a completely opposite personality than José," said Lansford. "As brash as José was, that's how shy and quiet Mark was." Former A's marketing executive Andy Dolich felt that, besides thrilling fans with gargantuan home runs, what increased their appeal was how different they really were.

> Their personalities were so diametrically opposed. Mark was generally quiet, somewhat introspective, well-behaved, and very workmanlike, while José: Madonna, 200 miles-per-hour, Ferraris, a looker, an Hispanic background, when that sector was growing in the game, and total unpredictability. Both of them had really good senses of humor, but José's just didn't play well . . . José always surrounded himself with a posse before there were posses and Mark didn't.

Though former San Diego State baseball coach Jim Dietz never skippered Canseco, he was impressed enough with McGwire to determine who would be more suited to handle the distractions of success. Dietz, who coached McGwire during the Alaskan Summer League in 1982, claimed his upbringing would help carry him through obstacles. "He's very much a family-oriented person. Those types of persons, in my experience, can deal with it," Jim Dietz told the *San Diego Tribune* in 1989. "So he would handle that better than Canseco because Canseco is a very flamboyant, off-the-wall kind of kid. He probably did some things to enhance his body along the way. He took some shortcuts where I don't think McGwire would."

One-time friend Curt Wenzlaff spotted the differences, too, and said both bashers were integral to the game's shift into an offensive-driven style of play.

> They weren't the first [steroid users] in baseball, but they certainly were the most visible, and they alone certainly got a lot of other players on the bandwagon. They were young and up and coming and had a feeling of invincibility and it showed itself on the field. By their physical appearance, they were awesome specimens. With José at six-foot-four and Mark six-foot-five, those are large human beings to begin with. Then others began saying, "Well, hell, I might as well, too; I'm getting left behind."

Their contrasting personalities also attracted their own fan bases. Canseco, for example, received thousands of love letters and propositions from female fans, while McGwire opened his share of mail from admiring boys and autograph seekers. Canseco grabbed provocative lingerie and phone numbers from the hood of his car, while McGwire received homemade blankets.[2] Canseco was a rebellious, flamboyant sex symbol forced to fend off worshipping fans, and McGwire embodied a gentleman, a role model, a person whom parents hoped would play catch with their son or date their daughter.

"José and I don't compete against each other," McGwire told Tim Liotta of the Associated Press in 1988. "If he hits one out or I can, it helps the ball club. There's no competition between us. We're good friends."[3] Dave Parker downplayed any whispers of tension. "There was no animosity there," said Parker. "In fact, they used to joke with each other all the time. There was a friendly competition between those two guys."

NOTES

[1]   Kirk Kenney, "Oakland's Bash Brothers Have Earned A's," *San Diego Tribune*, March 4, 1989.

[2]   Michalene Busico, "McGwire seems like the kind of guy who'd give you the shirt off his back," *San Jose Mercury News*, October 2, 1988.

[3]   Tim Liotta, "Bash Club—For Heavy Hitters Only," Associated Press, May 17, 1988.

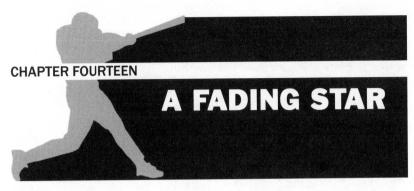

CHAPTER FOURTEEN

A FADING STAR

"He was the American League's most valuable player, the game's drop-dead handsome new superstar with a trademark neck twitch and sculpted body. He had the Bay Area in his pocket and baseball at his feet. But somebody tossed Jose Canseco the keys to the American Dream and forgot to tell him the rules. He might play baseball by A's Manager Tony La Russa's rules, but Jose Canseco has always played life by his own rules."

—Former A's beat writer Kim Boatman, *San Jose Mercury News*
May 7, 1989

January 22, 1989. David Valdez forgot to shove the gun and steroids into his luggage. Instead, they sat in his briefcase as he and Canseco passed through the metal detector at Detroit Metro Airport in the early morning hours. Canseco had been in Southfield, Michigan, to sign autographs at a sports memorabilia show and was scheduled to board a plane bound for Washington.[1] Much had transpired for Canseco during the winter: He had married Miami diva Esther Haddad, jammed several autograph shows into his calendar, signed a one-year $1.6 million contract with the A's, overhauled his three-car garage into a state-of-the-art gym, and endured the grumblings from his hometown fans in Miami for missing a parade honoring his record-breaking season.

His turbulent off-season continued on into that morning, when airport security stopped and probed Canseco and Valdez, along with three other men traveling with them. Pistols and steroids were a common accessory for Canseco, who claimed he needed protection because he carried wads of money from his card show earnings. Valdez and Canseco even carried a Florida sanctioned license to have a concealed weapon. That didn't mean much to airport security guards, who spotted the gun and arrested Valdez for illegally carrying a loaded semiautomatic firearm. After combing through his briefcase further, they also confiscated twenty-six pills, later identified as steroids.[2]

Valdez, who claimed he was Canseco's cousin and served as his personal attendant, had sped his way into legal troubles before. That previous September, a day after the A's clinched the American League West, he and Canseco visited a shopping mall in San Francisco. After the visit, they hopped on the freeway and headed back to the Oakland-Alameda Coliseum, where the A's were scheduled to play. As they rushed toward the East Bay, with Valdez at the helm, they encountered a traffic jam. At Canseco's request, Valdez veered onto the shoulder, hoping to land him at the Coliseum in time for batting practice. But a cop pulled them over and ticketed him. Because Valdez didn't have his driver's license with him, the stop lasted over thirty minutes, as police researched whether he was licensed in Florida. By the time the citation was complete and they headed toward Oakland, Canseco arrived in the A's clubhouse at 6:45 P.M., two hours after mandated.

It had been a chaotic winter for Canseco, one that began weeks after he belted his grand slam during the first game of the World Series. The off-season stained his image from baseball's bionic superhero to a troubled and self-centered egomaniac. In November, Canseco missed two appearances in Miami, one of which was a parade honoring him for his spectacular season. Because he had just married and was honeymooning in Hawaii, Canseco said he hadn't been informed of the parade. Canseco was also scheduled to throw out the first pitch before the University of Miami's opening game. With hundreds awaiting his presence, he didn't show up. Those incidents saddened and angered many of his supporters in Miami.

"Those other incidents aren't ignored, but I think the thing that most hurt the Hispanic community was when José didn't show up to a parade in his honor," Raul Striker, Sr., the former sports director for Miami's top-rated Hispanic TV station WLTV-TV, told the *Miami Herald* in 1989. "We're not talking about New York or Oakland or some other city having a parade for him but rather his own community, where he grew up and was loved. Many people became disenchanted when he didn't show up."[3]

Explaining his absence at the parade, Canseco told a reporter in 1989:

> They scheduled it for November 6 and my wedding was on November 5. They notified me of this parade two days before I was getting married. This was my wedding and honeymoon and you only get to do this once. I wanted some time to go on my honeymoon. So they rip me in the press and everyone thinks I'm a bad guy.[4]

Canseco didn't make friends with card show promoters, either. In February, he failed to show up at an autograph session in Rochester, New York, where he would have been paid $20,000 for a three-hour period. Thousands of fans were angered when promoter Jim Kelly notified the crowd that Canseco was a no-show. Canseco allegedly missed the flight to Rochester because Valdez was sleeping when Federal Express attempted to drop off the plane tickets at his apartment. For one reason or another, Canseco also skipped several other ceremonies, including award banquets in Baltimore and Miami. Canseco, who acknowledged his image problem, admitted he overextended himself. During spring training in 1989, he vented to a handful of reporters.

> I have not enjoyed my winters, period, because I've been doing so many autograph sessions. Next year I probably won't do any, because I'd like to stay home with my family on Fridays, Saturdays, Sundays. It's so consuming, its ridiculous—almost every weekend. People wouldn't understand. It was really hectic for me this year, between getting married, buying a house, fixing up the house, the card shows. You have no time for yourself.

Canseco could have taken advantage of the time off, especially blazing in his recently purchased 1989 customized metallic candy-apple-red Jaguar XJS V12, worth $75,000. The front of the license plate read, "Mr. 40-40," for his groundbreaking feat of hitting forty homers and stealing forty bases the previous season. His toy rocketed him from destination to destination throughout the winter. In February, Canseco was clocked and ticketed for allegedly speeding 125 miles per hour on Interstate 95 near Miami. "One day I'll take you for a ride in my car," Canseco once told a journalist. "You'll see; it's the weirdest illusion. You can be going 100 and it seems like you're going 50." [5]

The infamously magnetic vehicle also attracted loads of unwarranted attention. During spring workouts in Scottsdale, Arizona, he had his Jaguar shipped from Florida. Cruising back to the team's headquarters at the Double Tree Hotel around midnight one night, Canseco was pulled over by the Phoenix police. He initially received a ticket for allegedly failing to stop at a red light. Police, however, tacked on a cocktail of citations: driving without a license; driving with a fictitious license plate; and failing to provide proof of insurance. The next day an angry Canseco, who felt the police unfairly zeroed in on him because of his celebrity status, voiced his displeasure: "The thing about not showing leniency toward professionals or role models or whatever, that's kind of ridiculous. Who do they show leniency toward, the criminals?"

Canseco's image didn't get any better when, for the third straight season, he arrived late for spring training. His tardiness, though, seemed harmless compared to the set backs that loomed: during the first week of exhibition games, after fouling off a pitch, he felt a sharp pain in his left wrist. Diagnosed as a stress fracture in the hamate bone, the injury required a cast and haunted him and the club for the remainder of camp. It further prevented him from playing on opening night. He was also scheduled to miss April and most of May.

On April 21, Canseco arrived at the University of California San Francisco Medical Center for additional examinations on his injured wrist. When he and Esther showed up, they parked their Jaguar in a campus parking lot outside the university's Laurel Heights building on California Street. After they had stepped inside the hospital, a curious passerby, intrigued by the flair of the Jaguar, scoped the car and noticed a gun stored on the driver's side floor. The sight of the 9 mm semiautomatic Italian Army pistol, fully loaded with fifteen rounds according to the *Sacramento Bee*, compelled the passerby to alert campus police. [6]

After the police arrived, they ran the license plate and determined Canseco as the registered owner. When the couple returned, police arrested Canseco for possessing a loaded firearm without a permit on state property. He later pleaded no contest to the charges. "This is all bullshit," barked Esther, after posting $2,500 in bail to release her husband from San Francisco County Jail, according to the *San Francisco Chronicle* in 1989.

Veteran Bay Area sports radio host Ron Barr had first met Canseco in 1985. Barr hosted the show *A's Talk* on the team's radio affiliate, KSFO, and developed a healthy rapport with him over the years. Barr had no qualms asking Canseco about his need to carry a firearm. "He told me, 'Carrying a gun in my culture is like you carrying a wallet,'" remembered Barr, who currently hosts the nationally syndicated show *Sports Byline USA* based in San Francisco. "And he was absolutely right about that, I mean, he didn't think it was any 'big thing.' He was a typical Latin kid who was very talented, good-looking and acted that way."

Canseco, though, felt targeted by his newfound celebrity. Others blamed the Jaguar for his troubles, saying it elicited the wrong attention. One thing was for sure: Canseco's frequent run-ins with the law had clearly disturbed the A's front office. Even with his absence from the lineup, he was generating front-page headlines. "I am embarrassed for the organization, but I am not totally unsympathetic to the needs of José," Alderson said in a press conference before a game that evening. "We're not happy with the events that have taken place the past three or four months. We don't think it sends the right message to our fans."

By early May, Canseco's wrist had healed enough to convince the A's he could swing a bat and return to the field. But that field wasn't the Oakland-Alameda Coliseum. It was Joe Davis Stadium, in Huntsville, Alabama, where he obliterated the Southern League four years before. The A's hoped the rehabilitation assignment at Double-A Huntsville, scheduled for a week to ten days, would draw him closer to their lineup. After two painless batting practice sessions in Oakland during the week, Canseco was optimistic, though he had yet to make his season debut. Even without his presence in the lineup, the A's remained competitive, boasting an 18–8 record, one game behind the first-place Texas Rangers.

In Huntsville, Canseco faced live pitching for the first time in months. The likelihood, however, of him returning to the lineup anytime soon was stifled when he reaggravated his wrist after lacing a single to left field in his second game in Huntsville. This meant surgery to remove the small hook on top of the hamate bone was imminent, which sidelined him for two more months. "I'm twenty-four years old and have a long career ahead of me," Canseco said, after deciding on the surgery. "It's important to get these things out of the way early."

That Canseco missed the first three months of the season didn't sway his following from stuffing All-Star ballots. After he remarkably received the third most votes among American League outfielders for the sixtieth All-Star Game at Anaheim Stadium, fans voted him to start the game. Canseco, always welcoming the spotlight, hinted at making his season debut in the All-Star Game, which coincided with his scheduled return. Taking his hacks in the Midsummer Classic before debuting for his own team, however, didn't bode well with A's management. Starting him also didn't represent the club's best interest. The team had too much invested in his rehabilitation to carelessly allow him to face baseball's premiere arms while still recovering from surgery. After discussing the possibilities, the club agreed that Canseco wouldn't play in the game.

Though Canseco remained one of the most intriguing figures in baseball, his public image had taken a beating and slowly succumbed to less than favorable media coverage. In the May issue of *Gentlemen's Quarterly*, journalist Bruce Buschel penned a cover story on Canseco entitled, "The Battle Is With Himself." The article painted Canseco as a ridiculously talented, self-centered, irresponsible, and muscle-bound narcissist who recklessly marched to his own orders.

"Twins don't have much need for other people," Buschel wrote of José and identical twin, Ozzie. "Certainly not for this intruder, who had two strikes against him before arriving, being a reporter and an Anglo, two species of humanity José Canseco can usually duck here in Miami."

Referring to Canseco's record-setting 1988 season, Buschel wrote: "Some would bask in the afterglow of that for a lifetime; it doesn't seem to take José through an off-season. Dysphoria is his constant companion. You wish he were happier, as happy as you imagine you would be having lived every boy's fantasy."

"A nasty narcissism may serve a slugger more than serenity. After all, Canseco won Most Valuable Player, not Mr. Congeniality."

Speaking with Canseco on his freedom to steal bases and respect for A's coaches, Buschel wrote, "It is suggested that the coaches will not permit José to steal bases so regularly next season.

"'Coaches? They couldn't stop me last year and they tried everything,' Canseco responded.

'He means the Oakland coaches,' Ozzie corrects his brother. 'Not your opponents.'

'My own coaches?' José is flustered by the audacity of the thought. 'No one tells me what to do.'"

The issue arrived on newsstands in April and the article infuriated Canseco. His agent, Dennis Gilbert, immediately contacted *USA Today* to set up an interview with his client to curb the bad publicity.

Buschel felt, though, that his piece was factually balanced and exuded the edge intended for the magazine's demographics. Besides, as an avid baseball fan, he loved watching Canseco and even selected him for his fantasy rotisserie league in 1987, an acquisition that propelled his team. Combining his profession with his love for the sport thrilled Buschel, who looked forward to meeting the slugger. However, when he showed up on Canseco's driveway, he was rudely welcomed. "I wanted to thank him, but he didn't let me," recalled Buschel. "He started off by being pissed off that I was even alive. He was not happy to see me in his driveway. He looked at me like, 'what are you doing here and why are you bothering me?'"

Addressing Canseco's anger after the article was published in an interview for this book, Buschel said:

> I don't know why he thought I was going to be nice to him. Why would he assume that someone he had never met before is going to portray him in a flattering light when I'm just there to portray the person I meet? Nobody ever promised him how the story would go. I don't blame him for being hurt. There were a lot things in there that weren't particularly flattering.

Meanwhile, Canseco's off-field discretions remained in the news. On July 11, California Highway Patrol flagged down and ticketed Canseco. This time he had been driving his white Porsche down Crow

Canyon Road, a twisting route connecting his home in Danville to Oakland, at 51 miles per hour in a 35-mile-per-hour zone. His frequent
encounters with CHP on that road became comical, as if both battled
for the road's supremacy. For him, a five-hundred-foot blast was no
match for being ticket-free on Crow Canyon Road. Despite how easily
ripping a home run and swiping a base came to him at the ballpark,
Canseco quickly learned the feat couldn't help him tackle life. As much
as he dominated the game and absorbed troves of fanfare, playing by
life's rules came much harder to the twenty-five- year-old. "He led his
career the way he wanted," said former A's broadcaster Lon Simmons.
"He was oblivious to a lot of things. He just lived and floated on the
surface, but he didn't realize there were sharks underneath."

While former A's team captain Carney Lansford appreciated his
talent and how it helped the club, he admitted that teammates grew
frustrated with the distractions that followed the team. Canseco's circus began interrupting the clubhouse. Because Canseco ruled the
headlines, though, Lansford felt the commotion took pressure off the
other players. "He was always going to be in the paper about something," explained Lansford. "He showed up late to the park and he was
doing a number of things. A lot of guys perceived him as being really
selfish. He didn't want to give a lot of credit to other guys."

Former A's hitting instructor Merv Rettenmund claimed that despite the legal squabbles haunting Canseco away from the field, when
he arrived at the ballpark, he turned a switch on and prepared to play.

Zero distractions. He'd show up late, but zero distractions. One day,
when he was walking in late, [Ron] Hassey said, "you know what,
who really cares, because when he's playing, he can take us to the
top." If he came late and he was going to play, he always went up
stairs in the furnace room to do a soft-toss and get ready. He was so
good, he was too valuable to keep and too valuable to trade.

Rettenmund, in fact, admired his intelligence as a hitter. When it
came to predicting pitches and analyzing his swing, Canseco was very
studious. One of his friends, José Tolentino, who played with him in
the minors, recalled his attitude toward the media.

"He didn't care what people thought," said Tolentino. "He
wouldn't talk to reporters if he didn't want. He felt like his job was to
play baseball, hustle and get after it. He didn't brown nose and wasn't
a guy that knew how to treat the media."

Dave Parker, who kept the A's clubhouse loose and focused, felt
Canseco was learning how to handle stardom and the scrutiny that accompanied it. Dealing with that chaos for a young adult, when every

step is magnified, can be overwhelming, Parker claimed. That's why he fostered Canseco like a big brother and tried to keep him on task, which at times was draining.

> José was misunderstood. He just wanted to come to the ballpark, play the game, go home, and play with his toys. But I also tried to tell him, "When you're accomplishing great stuff, people are going to want to be a part of it; read about it; and know what you're like. That just comes with the territory." He could never adapt to the fact that his stardom could bring him that kind of attention.

Former A's pitcher Storm Davis recalled traveling and sitting with Canseco on buses to and from airports. "He's a very genuine person," recalled Davis, who pitched for the A's from 1988 to 1989. "The years that I played with him, I felt there wasn't any false pretense about him. He was very honest about what kind of person he was and what kind of player he was striving to be."

After a successful rehabilitation stint in Huntsville, Canseco returned to the A's lineup; his wrist had fully recovered. On July 13, in his season debut, Canseco clubbed a solo home run and drove in three runs against the Toronto Blue Jays at the SkyDome, a venue he always craved to hit in. "He walked into the clubhouse in Toronto, and I doubt he knew we were in first place," recalled Rettenmund. "He asked, 'hey, who leads the club in homers?' and Dave Parker said, 'I do, with nineteen.' Canseco then told him, 'oh, I'll catch you.' He wasn't joking; he really thought he would."

Despite the promising start, Canseco still claimed he was in spring training mode, since he had missed regular at-bats for six months. Still, he smacked five home runs in his first eleven games. "He came back cold turkey and hit a home run in his first game back, but it wasn't very pretty; his swing still wasn't very good," said Rettenmund.

Rettenmund remembered Canseco's unorthodox approach toward scouting opposing pitchers.

> You talk about a guy who had confidence. As a hitting coach, you were never sure if he really knew the pitcher, especially his name. If you said, "Roger Clemens," he just knew he threw hard and was going to throw him inside. I remember having a conversation with A's trainer Barry Weinberg, and we were betting that if he could ever stay healthy, he could hit eighty to ninety homers in a season. But he never could stay healthy.

When Canseco returned, fans flocked to stadiums to watch him take his cuts in the cage.

"When Canseco hit, we had to pull the batting cage back, because he'd hit the front pipe," said Rettenmund, who currently serves as the San Diego Padres' hitting instructor. "Everything he hit the trajectory was straight up. And then he would hit baseballs further than anyone I had ever seen. The distance was never impressive, but the height was."

On and off the field, his popularity skyrocketed. "When I go out to the mall with him, its like going out with Elvis Presley," former A's shortstop Walt Weiss told the *Boston Globe* in 1989. But not even Elvis had his own personal hot line. In September, Canseco, marred by bad publicity, started a phone line where his fans could call and receive daily updates about his life on and off the field. The concept had been fueled by fan interest and his desire to explain his side of the story on controversial media coverage.

The number, 1-900-234-JOSE, charged callers two dollars for the first minute and one dollar for each additional minute. Callers pushed buttons to navigate through different topics. From his day at a shopping mall, what he ate for lunch, to his experience at the ballpark, Canseco recorded a new message daily. Airing on local and national networks, the commercial for the hotline featured a white-clad Canseco leaning on his Porsche at Malibu Grand Prix, an arcade and track that neighbored the Oakland-Alameda Coliseum. "Hi, I'm José Canseco," he told viewers. "I want to speak with you, so call 1-900-234-JOSE and I'll give you the latest scoop on baseball and what's happening in my personal life. If you want to know if I take steroids, how fast I drive, or why I was carrying that gun, call me."

The idea signaled the first time a professional athlete had ever started a hotline and charged callers. While fans initially swarmed the line, it was later criticized for being boring and self-serving. Canseco had much more success on the field. In only sixty-five games and accumulating 227 at-bats during his injury-shortened season, he blasted seventeen home runs and collected fifty-seven RBIs. That's a home run every 13.3 at-bats. The A's, meanwhile, dominated the American League and barged into the American League Championship Series for the second consecutive season. And during game five of the series, Canseco left his mark.

Facing Toronto Blue Jay veteran left-handed starter Mike Flanagan, Canseco awed a packed SkyDome and millions across the world. In the top of the third, he clobbered a roof-scraping blast that climbed the air and reached the fifth deck in left field. The blast, conservatively estimated at 480 feet, landed in Section 540, Row 4, Seat 5. At the time, no player had ever conquered that territory of the venue. As he trotted around the bases, a silent reaction of astonishment and wonder swept through the crowd. After the game, teammates digested Canseco's home run.

"That wasn't just a home run. That was a home run of Biblical proportions," marveled Billy Beane in 1989.[7]

"The longest I've ever seen," Dave Parker claimed after the game.[8]

"The last time I saw one hit that far was Greg Norman on the first tee," said Mark McGwire, who was in the on-deck circle during the home run. "But I really didn't think he got it all because he hit it up so high."[9]

"It was a cut-fastball and it was a tough pitch to hit, but when he hit it, it never had the sound of a crack of a bat. It was a dead sound. He hit it straight up and at first, I thought it was going to hit the roof," recalled Rettenmund. "I was sitting by the walkway leading up to the clubhouse and when it landed, there was no cheering; no one said anything in our dugout; no one said anything on the field. Then [Dave] Parker, who was seated next to me told me, 'The man is illegal.'"

More perplexing was when Canseco claimed he didn't get all of it, a frequent response to many of his home runs. The home-run's trajectory prompted one to wonder if he ever fully squared and connected with a pitch, the distance the ball would travel. "He crushed it and hit it so hard and so far that I didn't even know where it went," spoke an amazed team photographer Michael Zagaris. "So after the game, when we're all in the shower, I told him, 'You hit the fucking shit out of that ball . . . you fucking crushed it,' but he said, 'No, I didn't, man, he jammed me.'"

In 1985, shortly after his brief call-up in September, Canseco crushed a home run off Floyd Bannister at the Oakland-Alameda Coliseum. The ball flew over the left-field bleachers and crashed off the back wall beneath the ivy. But after seeing where the ball had landed in the SkyDome five years later, one found it hard to believe he could hit one farther. Canseco told reporters after the game:

> I just missed it. I've got to get a hold of one tomorrow. I put a good follow-through on it but I really didn't hit it that well. . . . I mean, it's 328 [feet] down the line and this was only a few feet fair and very high. The ball travels well here. It may have gone farther than 480 and it may have been shorter. I don't think it was as far as you think. It was very deceiving.

His home run for the ages was one of the A's many highlights. They overwhelmed the Blue Jays in five games and carried their swagger into the World Series. Facing Bay Area rivals the San Francisco Giants, the heavily favored A's eyed a world championship. After snatching the first two games of the series, the A's were preparing to play game three at Candlestick Park on October 17, 1989. At 5:04 P.M.,

however, Mother Nature postponed game three, and the World Series, with an earthquake. Measured at 6.9, it rattled the Bay Area, killing
hundreds. The devastation put life in perspective for many players,
including Canseco. "When something like this happens, you realize
how small a part of life baseball is," explained Canseco shortly after
the earthquake in 1989.[10] After play resumed ten days later, the A's
steamrolled over the Giants for a four-game sweep and became baseball's
world champions.

Nineteen ninety. Swimming and playing volleyball on the beach
all winter in Miami, Canseco had managed to elude the radar guns of
local police that off-season. A furious Canseco, though, marched into
Phoenix for spring training in March. His anger, aimed at general
manager Sandy Alderson, stemmed from Alderson's comments before a scheduled arbitration hearing between the A's and him. Though
both parties avoided arbitration by settling on a one-year, $2 million
contract, Alderson viewed Canseco's off-the-field troubles as evidence
to sway the arbitrator. Feeling violated, Canseco seethed at Alderson's
stance. Canseco vented to reporters in 1990:

> That was a cheap shot. The A's have become a very classy organiza-
> tion, but Sandy didn't have to use those tactics. If he wanted to air my
> dirty laundry, he could have come to me privately with it—not bring
> it up to the media. There's so much I've done for this organization. I
> started the weight lifting on the club, I started the dieting, and I started
> the exercising. When I came to camp in '85, it was a mess. I don't think
> Sandy realizes that . . . if the A's don't respect José Canseco, then José
> Canseco has no reason to stay with the A's.[11]

Canseco hinted at filing for free agency and signing with another
club after his contract expired in 1991. Some speculated Canseco
wanted out of Oakland and lusted after a more hitter-friendly park.
The Oakland-Alameda Coliseum, he claimed, slashed his offensive
statistics, robbing him of ten to fifteen home runs a season. "His numbers were down because of his injuries, but also because of the
ballpark," said Rettenmund. "He used to keep track of the balls he hit
that would have gone out in other parks. Playing in Oakland at that
time, people wouldn't understand, was as tough as Petco Park to hit
home runs: Big yard, cold weather at night, long grass, and we had the
only ballplayers, the Bash Brothers, who could really challenge that
ballpark at night."

Canseco again battled injuries during the season. A sore right wrist
and a bulging disk in his back sporadically sidelined him. Canseco's
vicious swing had apparently taxed his back. For the second year in a

row, it appeared that injuries would hamper his season. That was frustrating news to Canseco, especially since the following year he would be eligible to file for free agency. "I was not getting around on even average fastballs and getting pitches right down the middle and fouling them off," Canseco told David Bush of the *San Francisco Chronicle* in 1991, regarding his back injury. "The bat head wasn't where it was supposed to be. My whole body was extremely weak, and I lost a lot of sleep because of the pain."

When he did manage to play, though, he contributed. By late June, Canseco already had twenty home runs and fifty RBIs. Fans voted him to start the All-Star Game for the third consecutive season, which was held at Chicago's iconic Wrigley Field on July 10. His peers also acknowledged his abilities. In a recent poll among players, Canseco was voted the best player in the game.

Whether Canseco cranked an enormous home run, ditched a scheduled appearance, or flaunted his Adonis physique, he certainly was tapped to be the player of the 1990s. Apart from his talent, he understood he attracted millions of fans. He also ushered in an unprecedented increase in players' salaries. Canseco's turbulent relationship with Sandy Alderson calmed when on June 27, 1990, Canseco signed a five-year contract with the Oakland A's for a reported $23.5 million. Included in the trailblazing contract was a signing bonus of $3.5 million, making him the highest-paid baseball player in history. With the A's recent run of post-season appearances, Alderson hoped he would retain most of his players and ink them to long-term deals. Canseco headlined his list. "The popularity I have, whether it's controversial or positive, people want to come out and see José Canseco play," Canseco said during the press conference to announce the contract in 1990.

Signing the contract and encountering such hefty luxuries marked a turning point for him. Canseco soon purchased a four-bedroom, 6,500-square-foot home, worth $1.3 million, in the affluent and gated Blackhawk community in Danville, California. Becoming baseball's first $5 million player, though, steered Canseco's focus away from baseball, according to teammates. They were bothered by his late arrivals to the stadium, sub-par work ethic, and comfort with becoming a one-dimensional designated hitter.

Canseco stopped working, and it showed in games. Canseco morphed into a bulked-up power hitter who depended on his fame and past accomplishments to justify his presence in the lineup. "When he started to be a designated hitter, a lot of guys had a problem with that," said teammate Carney Lansford. "Because he didn't want to apply himself in the outfield; all he wanted to do was hit. I don't think the organization was paying him $5 million a year to just hit. When he wouldn't go out to right field day in and day out, it hurt our team."

Former beat writer David Bush recalled, "He always said he wanted to be a complete player, then he signed his first big contract and after that it became, 'I'm a power hitter; I don't have to do anything else.' His total attitude changed; he stopped working on defense, and all he did was hit home runs."

Lon Simmons, who teamed with Bill King to broadcast A's games on the radio from 1981 to 1995, also noticed the sudden decline in Canseco's performance. "He had everything going for him. He had all the abilities that anybody could possibly have and they diminished overnight," said Simmons. "It wasn't a thing where they gradually went; suddenly he wasn't the player he was. He wasn't applying himself and that was his choice."

Simmons believed Canseco's priorities shifted due in part to his million-dollar income so early in life. He said the distractions and temptations attached to million dollar contracts could overwhelm anyone, including himself. "Hell, if I had $5 million at twenty-one, I'd probably be dead at twenty-two," chuckled Simmons. "That's why you can't fault all these young guys who are getting a lot money. It puts them into a spot that they're not mature enough to handle. It's amazing that some are capable of doing it."

His star in Oakland began to fade, too. Growing frustrated with his injuries that prevented him from playing, fans noticed he wasn't a five-tool player anymore. When he strolled to the plate, his hometown fans soon showered him with boos. When he muscled a monstrous home run, they cheered. Either way, Canseco elicited a strong reaction. "They saw that José was sort of moving away from his craft," said Andy Dolich. "Here was a guy that had all of the tools. Then it just became, 'well the heck with defense; I'm just hitting the ball to San Leandro.' But fans are really smart; they go: 'Hey, we want to see it all, not just a bit.'"

Former A's third base coach Rene Lachemann witnessed Canseco's enthusiasm for the game dwindle. His lackluster attitude toward the game prevented him from putting in the extra work to polish his outfield skills.

I got a feeling that sometimes he really didn't enjoy the game that much. He didn't enjoy playing the game of baseball. You have to have some fun in this thing, and I think he ended up getting a chip on his shoulder about people, he felt, were against him. He didn't give me a feeling that he was enjoying what he was doing, and when you're not enjoying what you're doing, it's hard to go out and work everyday.

Former A's hitting coach Bob Watson believed Canseco never reached his potential. For Watson, who tutored Canseco in the minor leagues and coached him in the majors, he, apart from the distractions, he could have slugged his way straight to Cooperstown. "He just scratched the surface," recalled Watson. "He allowed his off-the-field antics and exploits to cross over into the field and it really robbed him of what could have been a Hall-of-Fame career. I bet if you asked him if he would do it all over again, he would say he would probably change his focus."

Because Canseco figured he earned millions strictly to hit home runs, other elements of his game suffered and his focus shifted. Mickey Morabito observed:

All he wanted to do was hit home runs. And it was frustrating for Tony [La Russa], the coaches and teammates . . . he didn't want to work. He didn't want to work on his outfield. He was fascinated with hitting home runs. He realized that's what people talked about and he figured that was going to make him the most money. He slowly stopped being this five-tool player he once was when he first came up. He was an amazing talent, but got to be very lazy in the outfield. Why did it happen? I don't know.

Former A's reliever Rick Honeycutt, who currently serves as the pitching coach for the Los Angeles Dodgers, noticed Canseco slowly veering into another direction—away from the current pulling the A's. "He was making too many of his own calls, even in playing and how much energy he brought to the field," said Honeycutt. "He sort of separated himself from the team and almost became an individual about certain things."

That didn't stop the Oakland A's from muscling their way into the World Series for the third straight season. This time, the A's faced the Cincinnati Reds, a team featuring their own force, The Nasty Boys, a flame-throwing trio of relievers, Rob Dibble, Norm Charlton, and Randy Myers. While most experts predicted the heavy hitting A's to bury the scrappy Reds and capture their fifth world championship, the series took a shocking twist. After Canseco misplayed a crucial triple off the bat of Billy Hatcher in the bottom of the eighth in game two, leaving the A's in a 0-2 hole, La Russa and teammate Dave Stewart questioned Canseco's focus. "His concentration level is just shot," Stewart told the *San Francisco Examiner* after the game.

Losing game three in Oakland didn't help Canseco's cause. The next game, La Russa benched him. Canseco complained that he was being blamed for the team's collapse in the series, a meltdown capitalized on by the Reds. They completed a four-game sweep to win the World Series. Before game four, Canseco's wife, Esther, called La Russa a "punk" for benching her husband. "Let them sweep us. I should have worn a red dress," Esther told the *Miami Herald* in 1990. "Tony's going too far. He's putting all the blame on José when it's the whole team."

Nineteen ninety-one. The twenty-six-year-old Canseco filed for divorce from Esther in January. In the divorce papers, filed in Florida, Canseco claimed their marriage had been "irrevocably broken." But Esther, whom her lawyers claimed, "still loved José," attempted to move the divorce proceeding to California, a jurisdiction that splits assets. By April, both abandoned their petitions and reconciled. [12]

A month later, on May 11, Canseco was observed leaving pop sensation Madonna's apartment near New York's Central Park. The A's had been playing a four-game series against the Yankees in New York, when paparazzi spotted him walking from her apartment and into a cab in the early morning hours. The next morning, the front page of the *New York Post* featured a photo of him leaving her apartment. The headline shouted, "Madonna's Batboy? Did Baseball Star Reach First Base With Madonna?"

The story sparked rumors across the country, and many wondered if they were an item or had a brief rendezvous in her apartment, a fling between baseball's handsome superstar and the music industry's sexy material girl. "She had invited him to the debut of her documentary, *Truth or Dare*," remembered Zagaris, who was asked to fly early with Canseco for the New York visit. "He told me he went to the premiere and stood at her place and left around 4:00 A.M."

That same morning, Mickey Morabito observed a sleep-deprived Canseco climb onto the team bus bound for Yankee Stadium.

> In the photo on the tabloid, he had on these jeans and a white shredded jacket. When the guys were on the bus and reading the newspaper, here comes José from the hotel lobby and he was wearing the same outfit as he did in the newspaper. Guys are looking at the newspaper and then looking back at José. It was so funny. What he did with her in that apartment no one knows.

Canseco did finally gain favorable press coverage three months later, in Arlington, Texas, on July 4. In the Sheraton Centre Park, he treated thirty-three kids, who happened to be staying at the hotel, for an afternoon of hamburgers, french fries, and ice cream before he departed to play the Rangers that evening. [13]

He hoped for the same generous treatment from his hometown

fans in Oakland. By the middle of September, Canseco had clubbed forty-one home runs with 110 RBIs and twenty-four stolen bases, but he sensed fans didn't appreciate his performance. He also became frustrated when fans taunted Esther about his stay in Madonna's apartment. Because he was the highest paid player on the team and fans recognized his uncanny abilities, expectations were daunting for Canseco. In fact, he believed fans held his talent and salary against him. "I am being treated better by fans on the road than I am by the fans at home," Canseco told ESPN in 1991. "I have asked my agent to sit down with Sandy Alderson at the end of the season and explore playing elsewhere."

While Canseco claimed he didn't want to leave Oakland, he also wanted to feel welcomed. The following day, the *San Jose Mercury News* polled its readers on whether the A's should grant Canseco's request for a trade: 480 fans voted to trade him, 1,020 to keep him. "No matter what I do, the fans won't let me forget my past. I work with kids. I do charity work, and none of that matters except my past, which isn't really that bad," Canseco explained in 1991.

Canseco was also baffled by fans' reactions to McGwire. Earning only $700,000 less than Canseco and mustering a batting average hovering around .200, McGwire was lavished with cheers.

"But Canseco hasn't outgrown his resentment—not toward McGwire, but toward McGwire's image," wrote Kim Boatman of the *San Jose Mercury News* on September 22, 1991. "It galls him that McGwire is perceived as the All-American, red-haired boy, while Canseco is routinely portrayed as a bad guy because of his speeding tickets, fast cars, and occasionally fast company he keeps. Canseco can't understand why McGwire's matters remain private, while his are thrashed out in public."

Nineteen ninety-two. Days before spring training and on Valentine's Day eve, Canseco and Esther argued at 4:30 A.M. at a twenty-four-hour gas station on Kendall Street in suburban Miami. The argument escalated. Canseco allegedly grabbed her purse and pager. After he returned the purse, she hopped in her 1991 white BMW 850I and drove off. Canseco climbed into his 1985 Porsche and followed. The quarrel culminated when, blocks away, Canseco rammed his Porsche into the vehicle's passenger's side and rear. He slid out of his car and spit on her windshield. Minutes later, the Dade County sheriff arrested Canseco on aggravated battery charges.[14] Hours later, he was released on a $5,000 bond. In March, because the court had found no evidence of physical harm during the quarrel, the court spanked Canseco with twenty-six one-hour counseling sessions.

"I'm not a battered wife," Esther confirmed with Mirta Ojito of the *Miami Herald* in March 1992. "I'd never put myself in that kind of situation." Esther downplayed the episode: "We obviously have had our quarrels, but we've never had any violence. I think our quarrels are more publicized than anybody else's. I think this past incident could be interpreted as violence, but it's not."

Former teammate Doug Jennings, who also resided in South Florida and had spent time with the couple, recalled her unwavering devotion toward her husband. Jennings remembers:

> She truly loved him. They were both Cuban, so that was one of the things they had in common. She came from a well-to-do family, so it wasn't like she married him for the money. There were a lot of true feelings there on her part. But I'm sure, because of all of the things that were going on with him off the field, it led to a lot of distractions.

NOTES

1 "Police Arrest Man with Canseco," Associated Press, January 24, 1989.
2 David Bush, "Steroids Found on Canseco's Friend," *San Francisco Chronicle*, March 22, 1989.
3 Armando Salguero, "Fans Worry Canseco Is a Hero Gone Astray," *Miami Herald*, April 29, 1989.
4 Jeff Savage, "Going 40-40," *San Diego Tribune*, August 17, 1989.
5 *Miami Herald*, "Canseco Adjusting to Life—In the Very Fast Lane," March 10, 1989.
6 S. L. Price and Stephen G. Bloom, "Canseco Arrested For Carrying a Gun," *Sacramento Bee*, April 22, 1989.
7 Bob Rubin, "A's Close In," *Miami Herald*, October 8, 1989.
8 Thomas Boswell, "Follow That Ball And, Like Canseco's A's, It's More Than Halfway To Heaven," *Washington Post*, October 8, 1989.
9 Gerry Fraley, "A's Canseco Says He Didn't Hit Mammoth Homer Squarely," *Dallas Morning News*, October 8, 1989.
10 Bob Verdi, "In Candlestick Park, 60,000 Survive Scare," *Chicago Tribune*, October 18, 1989.
11 Bruce Jenkins, "Canseco Furious with Alderson," *San Francisco Chronicle*, March 28, 1990.
12 *San Jose Mercury News*, "Canseco's Giving Marriage a Second Swing," April 6, 1991.
13 *Lexington Herald-Leader*, "Canseco Turns Down Autograph Requests, But Treats on Him," July 1991.
14 *Wichita Eagle*, "Canseco Arrested after Fight with Wife," February 14, 1992.

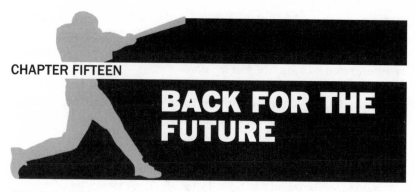

CHAPTER FIFTEEN

BACK FOR THE FUTURE

"McGwire's just a nothing these days, a non-factor. You don't worry about pitching to him. I don't know what's happened, but for some reason he just looks like a guy who will never get his swing back."[1]

— American League executive
1991

Nineteen ninety-one. Rick Burleson sensed he was on the hot seat. When Sandy Alderson and Tony La Russa pulled him aside and asked him this burning question, he recalled feeling uncomfortable and awkward. "They called me in and asked, 'We can trade McGwire for Wally Joyner straight up; right now, what would you do?'"

Burleson could have taken the easy way out. After all, La Russa had hired him as the hitting coach to help McGwire hit for a higher average. Batting .260, .231, and .235 from 1988 to 1990, respectively, McGwire had witnessed his average wither each year. Many felt that he was capable of better. Only his home-run totals made his offensive output acceptable. During his first four seasons he averaged a home run every 13.9 at-bats, a frequency second only to Babe Ruth. Despite that ratio, McGwire was clearly victimized by his past success, which triggered gaudy expectations for him every season. Any home-run total short of his astonishing rookie campaign when he blasted forty-nine home runs would label him an underachiever.

Some began dropping McGwire's name in the same sentence with former major leaguer Dave Kingman, a one-dimensional designated hitter with lethal power whose lifetime batting average dwelled in the low .200s. McGwire's hitting woes didn't affect his defense, however. Committing only five errors in 1,429 chances at first base awarded him the American League Gold Glove in 1990.[2]

Over time, McGwire had become obsessed with home runs, although that hadn't been his approach four years earlier. Going with the outside pitch and driving home runs toward the opposite field had been McGwire's trademark swing in college and the minor leagues. But now he tried to pull every pitch, which resulted in lazy pop-ups and groundouts, according to Burleson.

Burleson, who's currently a hitting coach in the Arizona Diamondbacks organization, hoped to steer him back to his elementary success. Before the season, he conceded that if he couldn't get McGwire to bat .250 and hit forty home runs, then he had failed. Four months into the season, however, McGwire had mustered only fifteen home runs and his average dipped to .196. That prompted La Russa to drop him to seventh in the lineup for the first time since 1987. Blaming McGwire and shipping him to the California Angels could have rid Burleson of the headaches and acquitted him of all McGwire's failures. Coaching highly paid and strong-willed A's superstars, such as José Canseco and Rickey Henderson, had been draining enough, but trying to harness McGwire puzzled him the most. McGwire was stubborn, in his own gentlemanly way.

Not that Burleson offered hollow instruction. A feisty infielder for the Boston Red Sox, California Angels, and Baltimore Orioles, he had batted .273 and slapped fifty home runs amid his thirteen-season career. On the field, his heart and hustle energized his team. McGwire admired that intensity and on several occasions invited him to his Alamo, California, home. McGwire, though, would stubbornly avoid talking hitting with him, his hitting coach, which frustrated Burleson. Still, Burleson, a scout for the A's the previous season, brooded over the trade and leaned toward keeping McGwire.

> It would have been easy for me to say, "Get Joyner because McGwire stinks." But did we want a guy who could hit for average, pick it at first and knock in some runs or did we want a guy who could maybe break records? They were two different guys: Joyner may hit you 20 homers and hit .300, but McGwire could hit 50 homers and if we got an average of .250 or .260 out of it, that was plenty.

There was plenty of anxiety for twenty-seven-year-old McGwire during his fifth full season. He battled back spasms during spring training, which sidelined him on opening night. He also endured the longest homerless drought of his career, a stretch spanning forty-one games that had begun the previous season. Hearing whispers of disapproval from several players' wives after his divorce from Kathy, a favorite, also took its toll. But nothing compared to the pain he endured while breaking up with his live-in girlfriend, Ame Blackshear, whom several players' wives had initially shunned from their inner circle. An emotionally taxed McGwire was seeing stars. Burleson alleges that the harsh breakup interrupted his life, taxed his emotions, and blurred his focus on the field.

> He had some personal things going on that year that I didn't even know about. What he went through shows that if your mind isn't where it's supposed to be, as far as games are concerned, playing baseball can be difficult. He struggled and mentally wasn't there day in and day out during the season. Because he had so many good seasons after that, only he knows how those issues off the field affected him.

After watching him struggle during the season, strength and conditioning coach Dave McKay, too, wondered if McGwire could rebound from his emotional and physical set backs. After all, players mired in such distractions often abort their entire careers and never recover. "He went through a lot," admitted McKay. "Being a young guy, we really didn't know what to expect from him. Sometimes players go through things and suddenly disappear and you wonder what happened. We were still wondering if he was going to be okay."

Former teammate Vance Law worked out with McGwire on the road during the season. Law, who played in Japan the season before, also heard rumors of those distractions overwhelming McGwire.

> I had heard there had been some girlfriend issues, but he never brought it to the ballpark. He played hurt an awful lot, but sometimes you have those kind of years, where you can't seem to get off the mark. It was tough to watch Mark, who had such great power numbers throughout his career, struggle. He struck out an inordinate amount.

Those off-field issues weighed heavily on his performance. McGwire endured several slumps and went hitless for long stretches of the season. By mid-July, he was mired in a 7-for-66 funk and hadn't homered in 100 at-bats. Others took notice of McGwire's decline. Despite being the only player to boast thirty—plus home runs in each of his first four seasons, he was no longer considered a threat and one of baseball's most feared sluggers. Instead, as one American League executive explained in 1991: "McGwire's just a nothing these days, a non-factor. You don't worry about pitching to him. I don't know what's happened, but for some reason he just looks like a guy who will never get his swing back."

Fueling that speculation was McGwire's rumored fear of the ball in the batter's box, which subconsciously tamed his aggressiveness at the plate. Some blamed his long swing and troubled vision, traced from his childhood, for his slumps. Others criticized his approach, claiming he had abandoned the middle and outer half of the plate. Still others credited opposing pitchers, who had finally adjusted and learned how to pitch to him. McGwire needed to make adjustments, coaches stressed. As the recommendations, opinions, and tips to regain his stroke bombarded him, he became more guarded about discussing his hitting troubles. "He stays away; he doesn't want to talk," Burleson told Lowell Cohn of the *San Francisco Chronicle* in 1991. "He's elected to stay with what he has. He talks the least to me about hitting out of all of them." [3]

McGwire soon lost his passion for pumping iron, an obsession since college. Beefing up his body through lifting weights had been his therapeutic fortress, a channel to release his slumps and frustrations. Now it had suddenly become a task and burden. Though he physically showed up in the gym, he lacked intensity, physically and mentally. The muscle-loss had curbed his power. "It probably had something to do with my performance," McGwire confirmed in 1992. "It sort of screwed me up mentally, too. I didn't feel good about myself." [4]

Even while McGwire had lost his touch at the plate, he remained in the hearts of his fans scattered across the country. Playing for a highly publicized franchise that powered its way into the World Series for three straight seasons maintained his popularity. On July 9, fans voted him as the American League's starting first baseman in the All-Star Game in Toronto's SkyDome. That marked the fourth consecutive season McGwire was elected to start the Midsummer Classic. However, after an ear infection sidelined him and would worsen if he flew, the A's medical staff recommended McGwire skip the trip to Toronto. Replacing him on the roster was an emerging first baseman for the Texas Rangers, Rafael Palmeiro. "This is probably one of the toughest decisions I've ever made," McGwire said of his decision to miss the All-Star Game in 1991. "My heart and gut instinct is to go. I do thank the fans from the bottom of my heart . . . but that extra 7 1/2-hour flight could have hurt me. When you get right down to it, I could have easily hurt myself for the last half of the season."

McGwire never stopped battling to crawl out of his slump, though his mental state and relentless feedback had clearly drained him and contributed to his disappointing season. Even so, after each game, McGwire faced the media and addressed his slump. "I've talked to too many people. There was a time when I was getting really upset with it," McGwire said in 1991. "It's to the point where if you want to be humorous about it, just to keep you sane, yeah, I have to be. I have to have a good attitude toward it." [5]

McGwire's positive attitude during his dismal season couldn't stave off management from pondering options. In late August, the A's promoted first baseman Ron Witmeyer, a twenty-four-year-old left-handed prospect who had batted .258 with thirteen home runs while playing with Triple-A Tacoma. Prior to Tacoma, Witmeyer had been a seventh-round draft pick from Stanford University in 1988. Many speculated that Witmeyer's call-up had been a decoy to motivate McGwire. La Russa downplayed the rumors, though. He claimed Witmeyer's offensive production warranted the call-up, not McGwire's struggles. But some perceived the call-up too coincidental. "It was almost like it was a scare tactic for Mark," recalled A's former director of scouting Grady Fuson. "He struggled so much, we didn't know what the big club was going to do." Coincidentally or not, Witmeyer's presence awakened McGwire's bat. With Witmeyer looming, McGwire cracked a home run in three consecutive games. "I'm not sure Witmeyer got five at-bats," said Fuson. "It was a matter of days before McGwire kicked back in and the rest was history."

By the final series of the season, however, McGwire would require assistance in salvaging his dented pride and massaging his failures into respectability. When McGwire tagged his twenty-second home run of the season on October 1, at Kansas City's Royals Stadium, it would be his final hit of the season. Clinging to a .204 batting average with four games remaining, he went 0-for-8 in consecutive games. That meant another hitless game would drop his average below .200, a bankruptcy for hitters. Trying to rescue him of the embarrassment, La Russa mercifully benched him for the final two games at Texas's Arlington Stadium. When the season ended, he sat on a .201 batting average. "All the coaches and players felt bad with the way the season went for him," recalled Burleson, who coached for the Boston Red Sox the following season. "Tony did the right thing by sitting him out the last couple of days. I felt it was the professional thing to do for the player."

That didn't prevent skeptics from bashing McGwire and claiming his best years were behind him. "People were down on him," said former A's third base coach Rene Lachemann. "Everybody thought he was done and couldn't hit anymore. They also thought he had fear at the plate." After the season, McGwire admitted that his season-long offensive collapse stemmed from several non-baseball-related matters. Nagging injuries also compounded those effects. "I was messed up mentally, messed up physically, and I never got back on track," he told the Associated Press in 1992.[6]

In November, a long trek back home to his roots, in Claremont, California, enlightened McGwire. For him, he needed to retreat to his old self and early successes. During the drive, he battled himself, brooded over his life, and searched for answers. "During the entire five hours down, I just thought," McGwire told Pedro Gomez of the *San Jose Mercury News* in 1994. "I never played the radio or stopped. I just thought the whole time. I knew what I needed to do but it wasn't easy. There's a stigma that goes along with getting the kind of help I needed."[7]

Help emerged during the off-season. First, he began meeting with a Bay Area psychologist, which rejuvenated McGwire. In his baseball life, McGwire began working with A's new hitting coach, Doug Rader, who had been recently fired as the California Angels' manager. They instantly connected, and Rader stretched his confidence and tweaked his approach. "That was a huge turning point in his career as a hitter," said Lachemann of Rader's influence. "When Rader got a hold of him, it was an entirely different thing."

Seeking advice from a familiar face and respected friend, A's farm director Karl Kuehl, also capped a life-changing winter. Kuehl had watched McGwire rocket through the farm system and had been familiar with his swing. McGwire needed honesty, and Kuehl could provide it. In Scottsdale, Kuehl critiqued his hitting mechanics, guiding him through the same hitting drills he practiced when he first arrived in the minors. After taking several hacks, McGwire asked Kuehl about his swing. "I told him, 'There's nothing wrong with your swing, Mark. It's the same one you've always had,'" remembered Kuehl. "Then he said, 'Well, that's what I've been telling everybody, and they're all telling me my swing is screwed up.'"

But Kuehl did notice a change: McGwire had moved closer to the plate. McGwire said the change started after opposing pitchers brushed him back several times. A rumor floated around the league, claiming that pitchers who pounded him with inside fastballs could disable his bat. McGwire had had enough and refused to be bullied out of baseball. "To prove he wasn't afraid of the ball, he got even closer to the plate," said Dave McKay. "And that wasn't the place for him to be, because he couldn't extend his arms."

Moving closer, however, didn't stop pitchers from exploiting his weakness. Kuehl offered McGwire two alternatives: back off the plate or learn how to handle the inside fastball. McGwire chose the latter. "Within ten minutes, he was real consistent and worked on it during spring training and into the season," said Kuehl. "All of a sudden he had that short, quick swing [that] made him the player he became."

Nineteen ninety-two. Doug Rader set the record straight. He grew tired of fielding countless questions about McGwire's decline and ever-dwindling batting average. Though McGwire had impressively averaged thirty-five home runs over the last five seasons, a hint of discontent arose among fans and management. Becoming the fifth A's hitting coach in six years, Rader inherited those worries. Poised for the challenge, Rader marched into spring training and stifled any doubts, insisting McGwire would rebound. He assured everyone that McGwire had worked out his kinks and predicted he would have a tremendous season. Dave McKay recalled how Rader infused confidence in McGwire and silenced any whispers that contributed to his lackluster performance.

> Rader came into spring training and said, "This guy's going to be fine." If someone talked about him having this problem or that problem, Rader made it clear that he didn't want to hear it. It got to the point where he became angry. He really stood up for Mark and brought a lot of confidence to him. He played a big part in helping him.

So did packing on twenty pounds of muscle. During the winter, after a seven-month layoff from serious weight lifting, McGwire returned to the gym, gaining noticeable strength and size. Pushed by his younger brother J.J., a bodybuilder, McGwire acquired more muscle. J.J. moved into McGwire's recently constructed home in Alamo, California, and briefly returned to play football at Hayward's Chabot College, a Bay Area junior college. At six foot three, 250 pounds, J.J. possessed an explosive strength that awed teammates in the college's weight room. That he acquired that strength through juicing was whispered about by many of them. His return to the football field was cut short, however. During the opening kickoff in the first game of the season, J.J. was blind-sided and leveled on the field. The injury threatened his season, so he dropped out and disappeared from campus. He soon pursued competitive bodybuilding.

Former A's beat writer Bud Geracie remembered McGwire's muscle-popping entrance. "He showed up that spring and it was absurd how big he got," said Geracie. "I remember telling him he looked like a tight end for the Raiders. But he wasn't comfortable with us making any sort of fuss about how big he had gotten."

When he arrived in Scottsdale, he weighed 240 pounds. He credited his confidence at the plate with his increased muscle. "The ball's been jumping off my bat. My swing feels strong, really good," McGwire said during spring training.[8] Reestablishing himself among the league's premiere sluggers wasn't his only motivation. Before the season, he voluntarily took a pay cut of $150,000. McGwire not only wanted to prove that his previous season had been a fluke, he also wanted to play for a new contract and understood a productive season would guarantee a hefty one.

McGwire was poised for a comeback. He felt comfortable, not only because of his beefed-up build, but also because he was more secure in himself. That led to a new look: red curly hair bursting from the rear of his cap and a bushy goatee. Because he had portrayed the innocent, clean-shaven, all-American stereotypical image too long, he wanted to project a "mean" side of himself, one he seldomly exposed. Those changes signified a fresh start for McGwire. "A lot of people never see my mean side," McGwire said. "They think I have such a baby face that I never get mean."[9]

Pitchers encountered that fierce side of his bat during the season. McGwire ripped twenty-eight home runs and amassed sixty-nine RBIs by the All-Star break. For the sixth consecutive season, he earned a spot in the All-Star Game, held at San Diego's Jack Murphy Stadium. McGwire offered fans a firework's show the day before. During the All-Star Home Run Derby, he erupted by blasting twelve home runs, including seven on seven straight swings. McGwire's home-run output even shocked McGwire. "I was surprised to hit that many because I don't hit home runs in batting practice," McGwire explained to reporters after the derby.[10]

The Home Run Derby marked a significant change in the caliber of home-run hitter he had become and was perceived: besides hitting homers in bunches, he capped them with tape-measure distance. He muscled balls into uncharted territory in various American League ballparks. The monstrous blasts entertained fans and generated buzz when he stepped into the batting cage before the game. The bionic power Canseco had demonstrated upon exploding into the majors in 1985, McGwire was now flexing seven years later. McGwire suddenly overshadowed Canseco in the lineup and clubbed balls farther than him. His power helped the A's secure a commanding lead in the American League Western Division heading into September.

But the A's soon dismantled the power-hitting tandem of Canseco and McGwire. On August 31, in one of the most blockbuster trades of the era, the A's shipped Canseco to the Texas Rangers. The trade represented an end of an era for McGwire and the A's. José Canseco, the player who he had trailed by one year through the minor leagues and into Oakland, the player with whom he had teamed to revive the once fledgling, small-market franchise into national prominence and shoulder to a trio of World Series appearances, had departed. The Bash Brothers' era in Oakland was over. "It's hard," McGwire said after the trade. "This is the end of the one-two home-run punch. We were ranked in the top five all-time, and now it's broken up."[11]

By trading Canseco, the front office hoped McGwire would become the centerpiece of the franchise, though he faced free agency after the season. With a depleted farm system and several other A's players, including Terry Steinbach, Ron Darling, and Dave Stewart, embarking on free agency and eyeing a healthy raise after the season, the juggernaut Sandy Alderson had masterfully constructed appeared to be headed for the inevitable: a period of stocking the farm system and rebuilding, the same process that hatched prospects such as Canseco and McGwire. Though McGwire saw the writing on the wall, it didn't quench his spirits or his bat. He finished the season with forty-two home runs and 104 RBIs, while hitting an improved .268, despite missing twenty games with a pulled rib-cage muscle. Meanwhile, the A's boasted a record of 96–66 and snatched their fourth division title in five years. However, during the American League Championship Series, the A's ran into the sizzling Toronto Blue Jays who overcame them in six games to advance to the World Series.

The club's early exit from the play-offs stirred an emotional reaction from players. Those players who had witnessed the club crawl out of the ashes of the Charlie Finley-owned dynasty and dominate the late 1980s and early '90s sadly sensed the end of an era. With the economics of baseball, the A's ownership wanted to slash its payroll to $30 million, and some doubted if they could afford to secure the core superstars. That players would be enticed by sizable salaries and longer contracts from other teams was a reality. Players and Tony La Russa came to grips with it. The run of supremacy was over, they realized, and a new blueprint was eminent. "We had a feeling on the plane going home that this was the end," remembered Rene Lachemann, who departed and became the manager of the Florida Marlins after the season. "There were a lot of others that ended up leaving and things changed from then on. We played great baseball and it was the end of a great time."

Meanwhile, McGwire and agent Bob Cohen branched out and entertained offers from other clubs during the winter. The Atlanta Braves, Chicago White Sox, and Boston Red Sox all showed interest in McGwire. At one point, he appeared ready to sign with the Red Sox. With the seductive Green Monster in left field, playing eighty-one games at the cozy, power-hitter friendly Fenway Park, McGwire could accumulate torrid home-runs totals. But negotiations fizzled shortly after. After the A's re-signed pitcher Ron Darling, catcher Terry Steinbach, and outfielder Ruben Sierra (acquired in the Canseco trade) to long-term contracts, it became clear McGwire could end up staying in Oakland. He wished to play on a competitive club and didn't want to be a part of a rebuilding movement. By signing those players, the A's showed him their desire to remain in contention. On Christmas Eve, McGwire signed a five-year, $28 million contract with the A's, crowning him the highest-paid first baseman in baseball at the time. Included in the package was a $7 million signing bonus, which cemented the deal. "I wanted to make the right decision, and I know I did," McGwire confirmed after the deal had been announced.

Across the Bay Bridge, the San Francisco Giants, the A's cross-town rivals, had also landed a larger-than-life slugger, Barry Bonds. In December, Bonds signed a six-year deal worth a reported $43.75 million. With Bonds cranking moon shots at Candlestick Park and McGwire electrifying fans at the Oakland-Alameda Coliseum, the Bay Area hosted two of the most feared offensive weapons in baseball.

By 1993, baseball's culture had shifted, and a revolution had emerged. Many players spent the off-season lifting weights and showed up to spring training weighing heavier and carrying increased muscle. They recognized that owners had dished out long-term multi-million-dollar contracts to the game's elite offensive players such as Canseco and McGwire. Players such as speed burner Vince Coleman of the St. Louis Cardinals and Rickey Henderson of the A's, the all-time stolen base leader, had been left behind. The market dictated that owners placed more value on players who could hit forty home runs than on those who could swipe sixty bases. Home runs were the biggest attraction in baseball, and fans, owners, and players recognized it by the enormous salaries allotted to power hitters. More home runs equaled more money. So, players hopped on the bandwagon, grabbed dumbbells, and muscled up.

Players such as Barry Bonds of the Giants, Lenny Dykstra and Mickey Morandini of the Philadelphia Phillies, Brady Anderson of the Baltimore Orioles, Mike Greenwell of the Boston Red Sox, Mickey Tettleton of the Detroit Tigers, and Eric Davis of the Cincinnati Reds showed up to camp noticeably larger. Even pitchers hoping to increase their velocity pumped iron. The more seasoned weight lifter, McGwire, marched into Scottsdale carrying 250 pounds. Ruben Sierra had also gained twenty pounds of muscle during the winter and came in weighing 220. Teammates were taken aback by his dramatic transformation. "The game changed based upon what was being asked," explained former A's outfielder Doug Jennings. "The game became more about power and velocity than it did about strategy and finesse. Owners were looking for bigger and stronger players to hit home runs. That really pushed players to do things that might have compromised their health."

As *Oregonian* reporter Dwight Jaynes wrote in 1993: "Weight lifting has finally come out of baseball's closet and is a respected part of training. In fact, every major league clubhouse now has weight lifting equipment." [12] One of the movement's staunchest ambassadors, McGwire, soon became a beefed-up endorsement for weight lifting in baseball and encouraged other players to join the craze. "It's part of my game," confirmed the twenty-nine-year-old in 1993. "I not only do it, I tell others to do it."[13]

College and high school baseball players soon spotted how the landscape of the game had changed. They, too, flooded gyms around the country and hoped to muscle their way into the majors. Steve Friend, the head baseball coach at Chabot College in Hayward, California, noticed his players weaving weight training into their workouts. One of the most successful coaches in California Community College history, Friend has steered his powerhouse program to a record of 555–260 over his eighteen-year tenure. Over the years, he has watched players getting larger through a year-round workout program. "We experienced a great deal of success on the field that could be attributed to additional strength levels—players hitting balls further and the reduction of muscle-related injuries. As players experienced strength gains and subsequent bodily changes, they also became mentally tougher," Friend wrote in an email in 2007.

Bob Milano, University of California-Berkeley's former head baseball coach for twenty-two years, pointed to the late 1980s as the period when baseball players, at every level, began embracing weight lifting. In an email dated 2007, Milano wrote:

> Around the late 1980s, I noticed a large group of our players lifting above and beyond what was required. From the '90s on, it became a very important off-season routine for players. And during the season, they lifted two, three times a week to maintain their strength, while lifting lighter weight with more repetitions. That helped players with bat speed and also increased their power.

McGwire's increased weight, though, stressed the rest of his six-foot-five frame. Little by little, different parts of his frame ached and failed him. In early April, a strained muscle in his lower back forced him out of a game. A week later, he sustained another unrelated back injury, which sidelined him for six games. In May, after running the bases, McGwire, who was leading the club in homers and RBIs, left a game early in Texas with a strained bruised left heel and a strained arch. He was then placed on the fifteen-day disabled list. The nagging condition, plantar fasciitis, required a cast and robbed him of the remainder of the season, except for two at-bats in early September. The A's missed his presence in the lineup, and he grew frustrated for not contributing. "When he was hurt so much and barely played, he just got sick of us always asking him about his foot and his return," recalled former A's beat writer Ron Kroichick. "That created a lot of tension between him and the writers. The foot injury was a real flat point in his mood and his relationship with the media."

Pain haunted McGwire the following season, too. He re-aggravated his left heel, which prevented him from running and deprived him of the leverage to generate power at the plate. The pain had spread to another part of the heel. He visited several specialists around the country, but his condition hadn't improved. Though he tried to play through the pain, after playing forty-seven games, he opted for season-ending surgery. After signing his multi-year contract, he played only seventy-four games over the next two seasons.

It was a turbulent period for Major League Baseball as well. Although budget-conscious owners wanted a salary cap, the mighty Players' Union refused. So, August 11, 1994, brought on baseball's eighth work stoppage in twenty-four years. The strike swallowed the season and wiped out the World Series for the first time.

While owners and the Major League Baseball Players Association (MLBPA) were negotiating a new agreement during the off-season, McGwire shredded his body through an extensive cardiovascular program with recently hired strength and conditioning coach Bob Alejo. The goal of the workouts was to lose weight to lighten the load off his feet. He ran on the treadmill and rode on the stationary bike all winter. McGwire strolled into camp carrying a ripped, bodybuilder's physique, boasting only eight-percent body fat.[14]

After tension between owners and the MLBPA had temporarily softened and both parties finally reached an agreement during the spring of 1995, McGwire returned to the lineup and smacked several home runs. But a deep bone bruise on his left foot, a concussion, and strained back carved his season. Still, he cranked out a home run every 8.13 at-bats, leaving him with thirty-nine for the season. Fighting injuries for four consecutive seasons wore on McGwire and cast him in a fragile light. Some blamed weight lifting for his injuries. Many couldn't comprehend how a player so conditioned and powerfully built could be so delicate and vulnerable to injuries. As Bob Padecky of the *Santa Rosa Press Democrat* penned in 1995:

> Instead of chasing Ruth and Hank Aaron, McGwire is chasing doctors, trainers, and the latest hot opinion. This is the reality he has to face: McGwire didn't go on the disabled list until his sixth year of pro ball. Now in his 12th year, he's been on the DL in each of the last four seasons, with most of his stays lasting a significant amount of time.[15]

Besides missing chunks of the season, McGwire would also miss the Haas family, the family-based ownership that had purchased the

A's from controversial owner Charlie O. Finley in 1980. Principal owner and philanthropist Walter A. Haas, Jr., resurrected the once dilapidated franchise to keep the team in Oakland. He forged a bond with the community and paid competitive salaries to his players to continue the franchise's winning tradition. At times, while the team was losing money, he fulfilled payroll from his own wallet. The climate changed when the Haas estate sold the team to Steve Schott and Ken Hoffman, Bay Area real-estate developers, in 1995. Shortly thereafter, Tony La Russa, McGwire's only big league manager who steered the club's on-field success for parts of ten seasons, departed to manage the St. Louis Cardinals. To slash overhead, other staffers in the organization had been handed pink slips. The change of ownership tossed a brand new pitch to McGwire.

NOTES

[1]   Mark Maske, "Rickey Henderson, McGwire: Less Than Expected," *Washington Post*, September 8, 1991.

[2]   Steve Kornack, "McGwire Lets Bat Do His Talking," *Detroit Free Press*, April 28, 1991.

[3]   Lowell Cohn, "Burleson Not Always a Hit With A's," *San Francisco Chronicle*, July 2, 1991.

[4]   Ron Kroichick, "McGwire Ponders Move from Oakland," *Sacramento Bee*, March 29, 1992.

[5]   Kim Boatman, "McGwire Plans to Smile While Riding Out Slump," *San Jose Mercury News*, July 18, 1991.

[6]   Associated Press, "Bash Brother Back," April 18, 1992.

[7]   Pedro Gomez, "McGwire Says He Has Developed Mental Strength," *San Jose Mercury News*, February 21, 1994.

[8]   Kroichick, "McGwire Ponders Move from Oakland."

[9]   Ibid.

[10] Associated Press, "McGwire Turns on Power," July 1992.

[11] David Bush, "A's Kiss Jose Goodbye," *San Francisco Chronicle*, September 1, 1992.

[12] Dwight Jaynes, "Weightlifting Gave McGwire More Lift," *The Oregonian*, April 11, 1993.

[13] Ibid.

[14] Mark Maske, "The Bash Is Back in McGwire," *Washington Post*, June 13, 1995.

[15] Bob Padecky, "A's McGwire May Be on the Road to Ruin," *Santa Rosa Press Democrat*, August 6, 1995.

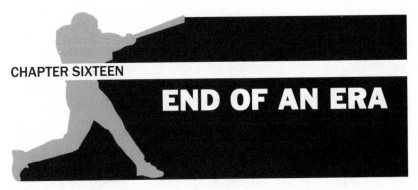

CHAPTER SIXTEEN

END OF AN ERA

"I guess it probably won't really hit me until later on. Right now, I'm just in a dream state, wondering if this really happened. I hope they will miss Jose Canseco the person and Jose Canseco the player here. I will miss the A's. . . . I've never known baseball anywhere else."

—José Canseco
August 31, 1992

Nineteen ninety-two. When Pamela Pitts walked into her office on Monday afternoon she sensed something brewing. Since it was August 31, the last of baseball's two trade deadlines, she figured she'd better show up. As an administrative assistant for the Oakland A's, she created, updated, and secured each player's personnel files. To Pitts, their privacy was important, and she was leery of anyone snooping near her filing cabinet. Addresses, medical reports, contracts, divorces, and every document chronicling a player's history with the organization had been tucked inside those folders. As she approached her desk, she noticed Canseco's folder sat on her cabinet. It had clearly been tampered with.

Canseco had been playing in his second season of a five-year contract and wasn't eligible for free agency until 1996. That his file was opened seemed strange. "I immediately said, 'What the hell is going on here?'" recalled Pitts, who learned that a press conference announcing a trade had been scheduled within minutes. Shocked, she rushed downstairs and crept into the press conference. Cameras flickered, and reporters buzzed and congregated. Canseco, still wearing his A's uniform, walked inside the room, sipping a Coke. Microphones, television cameras, and tape recorders surrounded him. Pitts reluctantly tied those events together and came up with the inevitable: Canseco had been traded.

"I was standing in the back of the room and caught eyes with José, and once I started to cry, I turned around and left," Pitts remembered, fighting tears. Pitts had forged a connection with Canseco; she had monitored his progress in the organization since the eighteen-year-old arrived in 1982, which included cheering on his marriage with Esther in 1988 and supporting the couple through their high-profile separation in 1992. "I didn't want to be standing there crying with all of the media there. I figured I would hear about it later." Pitts said.

It was a scene fit for theatre inside the Oakland-Alameda Coliseum that Monday evening, an appropriate farewell for José Canseco, the flamboyant and controversial muscle-bound Oakland A's icon. The A's traded Canseco to the Texas Rangers for switch-hitting superstar Ruben Sierra, twenty-six; starting pitcher Bobby Witt, twenty-eight; and reliever Jeff Russell, thirty-one; plus $500,000 in cash. The blockbuster trade, perhaps the biggest in A's history, was sparked on August 27 and gained momentum over the ensuing weekend. Tom Grieve, the Rangers' general manager at the time, phoned Sandy Alderson on Thursday afternoon.

To Alderson and Grieve, mulling over trades and comfortably tossing around prospects' names with each other wasn't foreign. They had developed a professional relationship and had swapped players before. "My relationship and rapport with Sandy was probably better than almost any other general manager," confirmed Grieve, who's now a television analyst for the Rangers. "When we talked, there wasn't any posturing, smoke screens, or gamesmanship; we pretty much both knew each other to the point where we could get to the bottom line; if we could do business, great, if not, we'd get on with it."

Grieve had several players embarking on free agency and doubted he could sign them to long-term contracts after the season. One of those players was Bobby Witt, a durable, flame-throwing starter who battled fits of wildness. Looking to bolster his rotation for the pennant drive and into the post-season, Alderson showed interest in Witt. Alderson also steered his focus on pitcher Jeff Russell, a veteran, hard-throwing, right-handed closer with twenty-eight saves under his belt. Alderson, though, showed the most interest in twelve-game winner José Guzman, a twenty-nine-year-old starter from Puerto Rico.

Alderson clearly lusted after pitching and figured dangling twenty-eight-year-old Canseco, with three more years on his contract, would seduce Grieve. Two days later, Alderson spruced up the discussions and included Canseco. "I'm sure Sandy started thinking he could add a bunch of players down the stretch for the pennant race that would give him depth," speculated Grieve. "It seemed to me that he was more than happy to include Canseco in any kind of trade discussion." Grieve offered Witt to Alderson for prospects. Alderson balked and conjured up another proposal: Guzman, Russell, Witt, Sierra, and a prospect for Canseco.

Alderson also eyed first baseman Rafael Palmeiro, a sweet-swinging slap hitter. Grieve refused. "Then I countered and asked him, 'How about Witt, Russell, and Sierra and cash considerations for Canseco?'" Grieve remembered. Alderson agreed and pulled the trigger. "It was a huge trade," said Grieve. "It happened very quickly and went very smoothly." Landing three players to bolster Alderson's team wasn't his only motivation for trading Canseco. He grew frustrated with Canseco's antics: "Whether it was an incident with his wife, his cars, and gun arrest, he had become a distraction."

There had also been speculation that Alderson peddled Canseco because of his alleged steroid abuse. It was believed that because Canseco had become so muscular, he had lost his athleticism, particularly his arm strength and flexibility. He had become a bodybuilder in a baseball player's uniform. Alderson denied that steroids played a part in the trade. "None of that was even a consideration. We didn't say, 'Geez, let's trade him because we suspect he's using steroids'; that didn't even enter into my mindset," confirmed Alderson. "You're talking about a guy who'd been with the organization for ten years, at that point, and there might have been two or three instances where the suspicions of him using steroids arose."

Keith Lieppman, the A's farm director at the time, had flown into Oakland the day of the trade and sat in a closed-door meeting with La Russa and Alderson to mull over the trade. While some members of the A's organization agreed that the A's could survive without Canseco, others felt he could still contribute to the club. "Alderson went around the room and asked for everyone's opinion and it wasn't a slam-dunk. We didn't have to do it," said Lieppman. "It was open and a lot of people had different comments and input. It was an interesting congregation of people and ideas. But there was a general consensus that for the betterment of the organization, there were too many distractions with José at the time. It had reached that point."

The distractions piled. Teammates fumed when Canseco exited the Oakland-Alameda Coliseum during the eighth inning of a game for personal reasons. Team leaders Carney Lansford and Terry Steinbach ripped Canseco in Bay Area newspapers. "To be honest, I don't really give a [expletive] about José," Steinbach told a Bay Area reporter. "Seriously, you're talking team. Team is twenty-five guys. We've got twenty-four guys on this team."[1]

The trade deadline was set for midnight Eastern Standard Time, which translated to 9:00 P.M. on the West Coast. For a club to add a player who would be eligible to play in the post-season, he must first clear waivers and the transaction must be completed by the deadline. Dave Henderson, the A's center fielder whose locker was adjacent to Canseco's, remembered talking with him before the game in the clubhouse. "He was bragging before the game he wasn't going to be traded," recalled Henderson.

By trading Canseco, Alderson hoped the trio of players could help his team plow deep into the playoffs; the A's already boasted a record of 79–51 and held a commanding seven-game lead in the American League Western Division. "We had a chance to get three guys who would have an immediate and positive impact on the team in three different areas: The starting rotation, the bullpen, and someone we thought would be a quality replacement for José."

Before the trade could be officially announced, Alderson and Grieve had to tie up loose ends and massage details. One of those details was the health of Sierra, who had been diagnosed with chicken pox and was quarantined back in Texas, sidelining him for a week to ten days. For the Rangers to obtain Canseco, he had to pass through the waiver wire unclaimed. Meanwhile, the A's were scheduled to play the Baltimore Orioles that evening at 7:05 P.M. As game-time approached, upstairs in the press box several beat writers, including John Hickey, Ron Kroichick, and David Bush, routinely combed through the starting lineups. Bush spotted a minor discrepancy in the A's pregame notes and brought it to the attention of the A's press-relations director Jay Alves. Alves smirked at Bush and prepared him for the news. "He told me, 'If what I think is going to happen, happens, you guys won't care about that.' He hinted that there was something big about to happen," Bush recalled.

Kroichick, who was then the A's beat writer for the *Sacramento Bee*, remembered sitting in the press box and readying himself for the game. "I don't recall there being rumors before the game and one of the amazing things about it was they kept it really quiet," said Kroichick. "There wasn't speculation in either Texas papers or Northern California papers. I recall it being very sudden." For A's television announcer Greg Papa, who along with Reggie Jackson broadcasted the game for former cable television network Sports Channel, the intriguing plot was the Bay Area return of twenty-three-year-old hurler Mike Mussina, a first-round draft pick from Palo Alto's prestigious Stanford University. "There had been some gossipy rumors, but it wasn't at the forefront of our minds," said Papa. "Mussina was the big story going into the game."

After A's pitcher Kelly Downs wiggled out of a jam in the top of the first, behind the scenes Canseco passed through the waiver wire unclaimed, which finalized the trade. Because no team, including the New York Yankees and Boston Red Sox, figured the first-place A's would trade their highest paid player, they passed. The Rangers then claimed him. Now taking Canseco off the field uninjured was the next step.

Canseco, who played right field to open the game, trotted into the dugout and was scheduled to bat third in the bottom of the first. Between innings, he fastened his helmet and grabbed a bat. Lead-off batter Rickey Henderson flied out, and utility third baseman Jerry Browne battled Mussina. Canseco headed to the on-deck circle to warm up, when he was summoned from the dugout. "He was literally in the on-deck circle," said David Bush, former A's beat writer for the *San Francisco Chronicle*. "Then he saw that finger from the dugout saying 'come here.' He turned around and went back into the dugout."

That finger belonged to A's bench coach Tommie Reynolds, who informed him that La Russa needed to speak with him. La Russa broke the news to Canseco and hugged him. Stunned, Canseco headed back to the clubhouse. Confusion and speculation had spread over the airwaves and hovered over the stadium. La Russa ordered utility infielder Lance Blankenship to grab a bat and hit for Canseco. As Blankenship rushed out of the dugout and dug his cleats into the batter's box, the television monitor featured Canseco's name and statistics underneath. Papa recalled the chaos:

> There were a million different things going through my mind. On the air, I'm telling the audience that Jose has a history of migraine headaches, which he did, and that might be the reason he was replaced. The entire time, I remember talking about why he wasn't in the lineup, which was not uncommon because he was doing that a lot. But at the same time, I knew it was August 31, the trade deadline. I was communicating with the truck a lot and we were scrambling to find out what was going on. I remember distinctly going to commercials and saying, "Well, today *is* the trade deadline—the A's didn't trade Canseco—did they?"

Thanks to A's statistician and historian David Feldman, Papa learned the Texas Rangers had scheduled a press conference to announce they had obtained Canseco. "It was the most surreal night I had ever had," said Papa. "It was fascinating theatre." Some criticized A's management for coldly yanking Canseco from the on-deck circle, claiming that the procedure was tacky and retaliatory for the headaches he caused the organization. However, Grieve and Alderson insisted there was absolutely no malicious intent and claimed that last-minute salary adjustments and medical opinions had dictated the timing of the trade. "When they called him back from the on-deck circle, that's when it happened to be finalized," recalled Grieve.

Shortly after, the A's also planned a news conference to announce the trade during the game. Sports Channel television producer Michael Ireland decided to remove a television camera from the field and plant it inside the interview room, where the press conference would be held. After streaming sound from the press conference, the network scaled the game camera down and simultaneously showed both. This way, viewers could watch the game and also see and listen to the press conference live. "I told José this was the end of an era for us," Alderson explained to reporters during the press conference. "In many ways he personified the A's the last few years. Rightly or wrongly, José represented this organization."[2]

Minutes later, Canseco entered the room and addressed the media about his shocking departure. "I guess it probably won't really hit me until later on," Canseco admitted to a swarm of buzzing reporters in the interview room. "Right now, I'm just in a dream state, wondering if this really happened. I hope they will miss José Canseco the person and José Canseco the player here. I will miss the A's. . . . I've never known baseball anywhere else." Former A's closer Dennis Eckersley, who teamed with Canseco from 1987 to 1992, observed him in the clubhouse after learning of the trade. "That was the first time I had ever seen him visually upset. He was shocked; there might have been a tear. He might have been emotional," stressed Eckersley. "I almost felt sorry for him. He represented the A's more than McGwire did, at that time. He was more of the figurehead than McGwire, even though they both went hand-in-hand with the bash shit."

On the field, the game certainly had less significance, as the trade ignited shockwaves throughout the rest of baseball. "It's surprising because you usually don't see a team that's seven games in front trade their best player," New York Mets' general manager Al Harazin told the *Daily News* of Los Angeles in 1992. "It's a little backward."[3] Former strength and conditioning coach Dave McKay, though, claimed other issues spurred the A's willingness to shop Canseco. "A lot of people wondered how we could trade a guy like that," explained McKay. "But we had trouble keeping him on the field. In the long run, we just thought he was breaking down and was going to keep breaking down. He physically looked good, but not for baseball. He was young and had tremendous talent, but it just didn't bother him not to be out there as much as it would most players." Added team photographer Michael Zagaris: "They probably felt it was a good chance to get rid of someone they felt was starting to go on the downside and starting to put celebrity over career. They also had a chance to get Ruben Sierra, a rising star."

Among the media covering the event, members of the A's staff, and teammates in the clubhouse, the reactions varied:

"Stunned," said beat writer David Bush.

"Surprised, but not shocked," recalled A's team photographer Michael Zagaris.

"Shocked, really surprised, and I didn't expect it," said Pamela Pitts.

"The fan inside me said, 'How can you trade José Canseco?' I didn't see it coming," A's traveling secretary Mickey Morabito remembered.

"It wasn't a great surprise," recalled former A's broadcaster Lon Simmons.

"I think he kind of wore his welcome out and Sandy took a lot of heat for it. He was the icon, the rock star — How can you trade the lead singer?" said Ted Polakowski, the A's director of minor league operations.

"Not at all surprised," Carney Lansford claimed.

"I knew there was a possibility," confirmed equipment manager Steve Vucinich.

"There had been rumors," said former A's reliever Rick Honeycutt.

"I wasn't too shocked," said former A's strength and conditioning coach Dave McKay.

But to many observers, the trade signified the end of a thrilling string of success and popularity for Oakland, highlighted by stellar pitching, stingy defense, and an intimidating crop of hitters. With several A's players, including McGwire, free to troll the free agent market after the season, many felt that the core of the teams' superstars would scatter. "It was a shame because it was the end of an era," reflected Bruce Jenkins, a columnist for the *San Francisco Chronicle*. "The A's peaked when they had Canseco, McGwire, and Parker in the lineup. They were a larger-than-life team; they were an amazing phenomenon. Trading Canseco obviously changed their image and everything else."

Broadcaster Greg Papa also sensed the close of an eclectic chapter for the storied franchise, a narrative steered by sheer dominance. "To me, it was a real changing of an era for A's baseball," confirmed Papa. "After they traded Canseco, they were not the same team for years and years, until the [Tim] Hudson, [Mark] Mulder, [Barry] Zito era of the A's."

Fans sniffed that, too. Over the next week, thousands of angry fans bombarded the phones lines at the A's executive offices. The love-hate relationship between Canseco and A's fans had been turbulent and forgiving over the years: When he carelessly struck out with the bases loaded, fans booed. When he blasted a three-run home run, they cheered for him. In either instance, they wanted to watch him hit, and weren't prepared for his abrupt departure. Fans demanded a piece of Alderson.

"People in the Bay Area were outraged, partly because it took them completely by surprise. They liked José," said Alderson, who's now the CEO for the San Diego Padres. Alderson's secretary, Suzi Davis, and administrator Pamela Pitts manned the phone lines and endured countless calls of outraged fans cursing and screaming, expressing their disapproval. Pitts remembered the outcry.

> If we could have been spit on over the phone, that's how it was. It was hell. She [Davis] and I felt like we were being beaten to death because of the outrage. Hundreds and hundreds of angry fans called in. We were screamed at, yelled at, and cursed at. After you've been yelled at so many times, you start to realize that you can't take all this abuse. I've never had that much venom thrown toward my direction. I was going home every night and crying. It was amazing how fans were so angry and upset. It was awful.

Back in Texas, managing general partner and future U.S. president, George W. Bush was thrilled to add Canseco to the lineup. "Obviously we're pleased with the deal. It's a big deal and we're impressed how Tom Grieve handled it,"[4] Bush told the *Dallas Morning News* shortly after the trade had been finalized. To Tom Grieve, landing Canseco meant unlimited possibilities. With a new state-of-the-art stadium, Rangers Ballpark in Arlington, scheduled to open in 1994, Canseco could pack the stadium and muscle his club back into the playoffs. Grieve shared his motivations:

> Canseco was a huge personality. We also viewed him as a frontline middle-of-the-order guy. Maybe not quite the same player he had been in his heyday, but a guy who could still be very productive and had a lot to offer. I'm not going to say that marketing had nothing to do with it. But the underlying reason for anything like that has to be the long-term success of your ball club, and we felt it would be improved with José.

Whether the A's could thrive and still draw fans without Canseco's bat and mystique remained to be seen. Teammate Mark McGwire pondered the future and paid homage to the A's Bash Brothers-fueled reign. "The Bash Brothers are done. José is gone. It's the end of an era,"[5] observed McGwire.

The A's captured the division title, but were knocked out of the playoffs by the Blue Jays. A seven-year postseason drought for the franchise followed.

NOTES

1. Associated Press, "Quotes of the Week," August 16, 1992.
2. Pedro Gomez, "A's Shocker: Canseco Traded," *San Jose Mercury News,* September 1, 1992.
3. Elizabeth M. Cosin, "Walk the Waiver Wire," *Los Angeles Daily News,* September 2, 1992.
4. Gerry Fraley, "Bush Praises Grieve But Defers His Decision on His Return," *Dallas Morning News,* September 2, 1992.
5. *San Jose Mercury News,* "José's Other Moments," September 1, 1992.

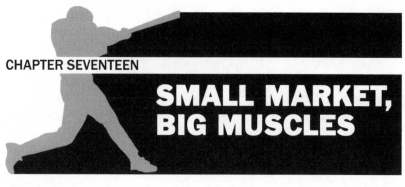

CHAPTER SEVENTEEN

SMALL MARKET, BIG MUSCLES

"Sandy felt it was important to bring Jose back, who was huge in Oakland, to help with the attendance and draw the interest of fans. At that point, we were struggling as a team and we didn't have the pitching to win, so we had to do other things to keep the interest of our fans. And having the Bash Brothers back together was a step that he felt was important."

—Former A's manager Art Howe
July 2007

By 1997, thirty-two-year-old Canseco had established a "reputation," according to one former major league manager. After playing for the Texas Rangers and Boston Red Sox for two years at each stop, Canseco was widely recognized among his peers as the most seasoned steroid user in baseball. As one former teammate confirmed, "In an era when everyone was doing it, he was the best at doing it." While back, hip, and arm injuries slashed his playing time, costing him 279 games during that period, Canseco still averaged a home run every fifteen at-bats. That he produced and remained a feared hitter in the game couldn't deny the fact that his skills had clearly diminished, however. Whispers started that his tireless steroid use had stiffened his frame and, over time, impaired his body from playing. Canseco had been labeled a run-down, bulked-up, one-dimensional designated hitter. Tom Grieve, the Rangers' former general manager, explained:

> The thing I was a little surprised at when I saw Canseco was how far his physical skills had diminished, even though he could still swing a bat. When we acquired him, I imagined him as a younger player and very athletic. But he was stiff; he couldn't run or throw; all he could do was swing a bat. He was incredibly strong, obviously through steroids. He was basically a bodybuilder who could still swing a bat but

couldn't play the game anymore. He looked more like Mr. America than a baseball player.

After two embarrassing moments during a four-game span in 1993, the fans and the media's perception of him as a bona fide superstar had started to fade. The first occurred at Cleveland Municipal Stadium on May 26, 1993. When Indians' first baseman Carlos Martinez drove a ball to the outfield, it bounced off Canseco's head and sailed over the right-field fence for a home run. Canseco subsequently became the subject of blooper shows and jokes around baseball. The next series, at Boston's Fenway Park on May 29, Canseco convinced his friend and rookie manager Kevin Kennedy to let him pitch during the bottom of the eighth; Canseco had always toyed with the prospect of pitching. With the Rangers trailing 12-1, Kennedy figured that planting Canseco on the mound would excuse him from taxing his bullpen amid the mauling. Canseco allowed two hits, three walks, and three earned runs during his one inning appearance. His statistics, though, were the least of his worries: after throwing his second pitch, he tore his ulnar collateral ligament in his right arm, which required season-ending surgery. [1] Grieve observed:

> He was more of a high-profile rock star than, say, a George Brett or Don Mattingly. I never viewed him as a ball player. Personally, I thought he was a good guy; he was prompt, bright, and clever, but he just couldn't play anymore. Steroids probably made him into a player he never would have been and then robbed him of it a lot sooner than he would have liked. You saw him rise so fast, and it was obvious he was going to take a fall.

Perhaps what Canseco provided off the field for the Rangers fueled Grieve's lineup. After Canseco arrived in Texas in 1992, it mysteriously coincided with the hitting revival of Rafael Palmeiro, a childhood friend from Miami. Before being traded from the Chicago Cubs to the Rangers, Palmeiro was considered a fledgling run producer with limited power.

The sweet-swinging first-round draft pick from Mississippi State, however, maintained a high batting average. His graceful ability to spray the ball to all fields and find holes convinced many that he could one day capture a batting title. Weeks after the Rangers acquired Canseco, Palmeiro immediately clobbered seven of his twenty-two home runs for the season. His batting average had also increased. During fifteen games of teaming with Canseco, Palmeiro batted .385. Asked to explain how Canseco's entrance had swelled his offensive numbers, he explained to a reporter in 1992, "I was down because I wasn't having the kind of season I should have. Having José is like a new life for me."[2]

The next season, in 1993, Palmeiro strolled into spring training carrying twenty pounds of added muscle. He claimed that pounding the weights, hiring a personal trainer, and tweaking his diet during the winter accounted for his transformation.[3] Besides trying to help his team knock the Oakland A's out of first place, generating a big season was an added incentive for Palmeiro: free agency loomed after the season. Already having inked a one-year contract worth $4.55 million in January, he eyed the blanket of a long-term and lucrative contract. That motivation elevated his play during the season.

He not only increased his batting average by twenty-seven points, from .268 the previous season to .295 in 1993, he also bolstered his home-run totals. Having hit a home run in every thirty-four at-bats during his first seven seasons, Palmeiro more than doubled his frequency with thirty-seven total, hitting one every sixteen at-bats. To justify his abrupt power surge, some people claimed Palmeiro had matured as a hitter. According to Canseco, he introduced, schooled, and injected Rafael Palmeiro, along with teammates Ivan Rodriguez and Juan Gonzales, the heart of the lineup, with anabolic steroids shortly after he landed in Texas. "Soon I was injecting all three of them," Canseco wrote in his book, *Juiced*. "I personally injected each of those three guys many times."[4]

The word soon spread around baseball that Canseco represented more than a player or an offensive threat in the lineup. His experience weaving steroids into his career, through trial and error since 1985, and also consulting others on how to use them, was acknowledged among players. Not that Canseco was an absolute authority on the complex world of performance-enhancing chemicals. Players had questioned his seemingly disproportionate and top-heavy body: his lanky legs hadn't caught up with his broad shoulders and wide chest. He had simply been a self-proclaimed guinea pig of a phenomenon enhancing player performance, ripping the soul out of hallowed records and altering the game. His decade of experience with the drug had intrigued several players. Above offering advice on hitting mechanics to teammates, Canseco helped them in other ways too. Adding Canseco to a team meant inviting the bodybuilding culture and its baggage into the clubhouse. One former teammate, who preferred anonymity, explained:

> He was the most publicized and recognizable guy, but players were doing that stuff in the minor leagues to get to the big leagues. He was

the more openly noticeable guy, but he wasn't the minority; there were a lot of guys doing it, but they got away with it, because they didn't want anyone else to know about it. And José, just by being so naïve, didn't think a whole lot of it as being wrong, so he didn't have a problem with letting people know he did it. But there were more than just him doing it, believe me. He definitely helped some people out that he knew about, but him being the "Godfather" of that stuff? They were doing that long before he got there, it just wasn't as publicized.

The A's reacquired him shortly before the 1997 season. In January, Canseco broke the news of his return to the A's to the *Boston Globe*. While the trade hadn't been officially announced, pending physical and salary allocations, Canseco had quarreled with Red Sox general manager Dan Duquette and desperately wanted out of Boston. "I don't think [Duquette] communicates with his players, if at all," Canseco told the *Boston Globe*. "He wants everything under his control. Any coach or other member of the staff that doesn't submit to that control is fired or demoted." [5]

On January 27, Sandy Alderson sent promising, young right-handed starter John Wasdin, the A's first-round draft pick in 1993, to the Red Sox for Canseco. On and off the field, Alderson needed a spark to inflame the rebuilding franchise. New owners Steve Schott and Ken Hoffman had slashed operating expenses, and team pillars, catcher Terry Steinbach and shortstop Mike Bordick, had fled via free agency. The only residue remaining from the A's supremacy of the late 1980s was Mark McGwire. The previous season, attendance had dropped to 1,148,380, which was the lowest in the American League. Victories didn't come any easier on the field, either: the A's went 78–84, twelve games behind the first-place Texas Rangers. Across the Bay, the San Francisco Giants had gained momentum.

Besides Barry Bonds ripping home runs and thrilling fans with his five-tool arsenal, the city's board of supervisors had also approved a privately financed, baseball-only, 40,000-seat stadium on the China Basin's industrial waterfront. The stadium, Pacific Bell Park, was scheduled to open in the year 2000. [6]

Alderson was also frustrated by being perceived and treated as second-class citizens to the Oakland Raiders. City officials had recently lured Al Davis and the silver and black back to Oakland by allocating $100 million for renovations on the Oakland-Alameda Coliseum. The construction efforts ripped out the bleachers and robbed fans of the tranquil scenery of the East Bay Hills. Instead, a bank of seats, named Mt. Davis, hovered over the outfield. In fact, the season-long renovations forced the A's to open the 1996 season at Las Vegas's Cashman

Field, which strained relations between the A's and stadium officials.

The stadium's makeover also dropped attendance and revenue. The club wanted a baseball-only stadium in Oakland, but Alameda County board of supervisors president Gail Steele claimed, "There's no way in hell it will happen here."[7] Because the A's had an escape clause in their contract after the 1998 season, it was speculated that the A's would exercise it and bolt to potentially lucrative markets, such as Sacramento, Las Vegas, or San Jose. Trading for Canseco would generate fan interest and provide a financial Band-Aid before the franchise's ensuing move. To Alderson, reuniting Canseco and McGwire could provide excitement back in Oakland. "The reuniting of the Bash Brothers was basically a marketing effort on our part," admitted Alderson.

A's manager Art Howe admitted his club, characterized by youth and zeal, lacked the pitching to become a contending one. While the A's were grooming young players and restocking their farm system, they relied on other ways to attract fans to the stadium. "Sandy felt it was important to bring José back, who was huge in Oakland, to help with the attendance and draw the interest of fans," recalled Howe, who's now the bench coach for the Texas Rangers. "At that point, we were struggling as a team and we didn't have the pitching to win, so we had to do other things to keep the interest of our fans. And having the Bash Brothers back together was a step that he felt was important."

The A's long-time equipment manager Steve Vucinich conceded that the duo's popularity a decade before could stir emotions and grab Bay Area headlines. "We needed a little kick-start because of [Barry] Bonds across the Bay," said Vucinich. "The Bash Brothers were back and I'm sure it sold some tickets. We knew it was the end of long-term contracts for both, so we knew it was probably a one-year deal."

But Alderson first wanted to run Canseco's return by McGwire. Before Alderson pulled the trigger on the trade, he posed the possibility to McGwire in December. McGwire, who was clearly the leader of the A's clubhouse at the time, supported the idea and welcomed Canseco's return. "I think it would be a great acquisition to have him back," McGwire said in a statement before the trade was announced. "We were considered one of the best one-two home run combinations. It would be exciting to get back together again. It would be good for the organization, and it would also help our attendance."

Thousands of Bay Area fans thought so, too. They crammed the A's ticket office and stormed the phone lines to purchase tickets. Roughly $45,000 worth of tickets was sold in one day.[8] The week-long ticket explosion boasted the highest number of ticket sales since 1992, the last season Canseco donned an A's uniform. Fans purchased eight times more season tickets than the previous season. As enthusiastic fans cruised into the parking lot at the Oakland-Alameda Coliseum to snatch tickets, a billboard outside the stadium read, "He's Back . . . Welcome Back, José." "This was a chance to acquire one of the most dominating sluggers in the last decade,"[9] assistant general manager Billy Beane said in 1997.

Eric Carrington, the A's media relations director from 1997 to 1999, came to Oakland after serving in media relations with the Las Vegas Stars, the Triple-A affiliate of the San Diego Padres. When he first arrived in the A's offices in January, he said phones wouldn't stop ringing. "A's fans are really loyal to players who wore that A on their hat," said Carrington. "That was neat. Even with all of the negative publicity José had, when he came back, it was like they all forgot and embraced him."

Long-time Bay Area columnists Glenn Dickey, Lowell Cohn, Bruce Jenkins, and Art Spander, who covered him when he broke in with the A's in 1985, were also intrigued by his return. And when Canseco reported to Papago Park, the A's spring-training headquarters in Phoenix, on a sunny Saturday morning in February, he didn't disappoint them. "José was great with the older writers and they always knew he wasn't going to shut them out," recalled Carrington. "They were all excited for him to come back and were waiting out front when he came in. Everybody wanted to interview him. When he showed up, the whole atmosphere was electric."

The interest in Canseco and McGwire's reunion had also carried over nationally. Media titans ESPN and *Sports Illustrated* flew to Phoenix for interviews, photo shoots, and to produce on-air segments. While reliving those thunderous years of their youth was something they tolerated during interviews, Canseco and McGwire insisted they were no longer the Bash Bothers. Now they were Mark and José, two very different and separate individuals. Plastered on the wall in Papago Park's weight room was the infamous Bash Brothers poster, produced by Costacos Brothers in 1988. The popular poster had reporters zooming in on the subject.

Several writers approached McGwire about the significance of the duo headlining the A's lineup again, but he downplayed it. "We really didn't know each other personally, and we never hung out," McGwire said. "People just associate us because of all the Bash Brothers stuff. That was a big thing for the A's at a time when the team was winning . . . but things have changed. We're older, we're wiser, we're the veterans—that's really the big difference."[10] Art Howe recalled McGwire distancing himself from the marketing ploy and Canseco. "Mark grew out of that," said Howe. "That was the old days. He wanted to be his own man."

The A's traveling secretary Mickey Morabito claimed that by 1997, after more than a four-year hiatus, the duo had nothing in common. Morabito, who had accompanied both on planes and to hotels at the peak of their popularity in the late 1980s, said their relationship had disintegrated. "When he came back, they didn't have the same camaraderie and rapport they once had," said Morabito. "They were never guys who would go and hang out together, but in the clubhouse they were a team. By that point, I didn't get the feel that there was any chemistry at all between those two guys."

Added Sandy Alderson: "When two guys create a reputation in their early twenties, and reunite ten years later, they're going to be two different people and the chemistry is going to be different. I didn't notice any unusual distance between them, but I also didn't notice that they were close, either."

According to Canseco, however, he and McGwire were the big brothers of steroid use for younger players in the clubhouse. "Before too long, it seemed like everybody was doing it," Canseco wrote in *Juiced*. "The bathroom stalls were the laboratory, and players would inject themselves right there. Everyone knew why you were going in there; they'd see two guys going into a stall together, and make cracks."

Canseco and McGwire had also embarked on different junctures in their careers: Canseco, a dangerous but injury-prone slugger, was riding on the residue of his past popularity and stardom. He hoped that coming back to Oakland would help thrust him back into an all-star caliber player. Canseco also claimed he had matured as a person. With five years having passed since he was traded to Texas, Canseco had calmed his once flamboyant lifestyle. After divorcing first wife, Esther, in 1992, he married Jessica Seikaly, a Hooters waitress he met in Cleveland in 1993.

But falling in love wasn't the only change that mellowed him. He also became a father. Josie, his newborn daughter, was born during the off-season in November. Fatherhood provided Canseco a new lens on life. "I have to say I have a lot of respect for José — he's come a long way," McGwire said in 1997. "We've really been nothing alike, but he's mellower now, more approachable. Seeing him coming from the person he was to the person he is now — well, I guess a lot of things have changed." [11]

Conversely, McGwire had elevated himself into baseball's elite power hitter. Pounding thirty-nine and fifty-two home runs in 1995 and 1996, respectively, McGwire rivaled Babe Ruth, incredibly averaging a home run every 8.13 at-bats.

Poised to test the free-agent market after the season, McGwire and his agent, Bob Cohen, eyed a lucrative contract, beyond what the A's

could afford. Life's challenges and baseball's slumps had also emotionally matured McGwire. He had tasted the glee of success and the
doldrums of failure, which shaped him into a seasoned veteran. That,
along with becoming comfortable at the plate, made him a resource
for younger players and arguably the most feared hitter in baseball.

He effortlessly muscled booming, tape-measure shots that drew
silent admiration from his peers near the batting cage. Though Canseco
had received similar reactions a decade earlier, this time, however, the
roles were reversed. "José was probably starting to decline as a player,"
said Art Howe, who inserted both of them in the same hitting group
during batting practice. "In the old days when they were together,
José was the man, the premiere power hitter in the game. He was the
guy who set the tone. But that year, he couldn't hit home runs like
Mac—not even close."

Former A's television announcer Greg Papa admired McGwire's
unprecedented displays of power during batting practice. Papa still
recalls him launching several astounding blasts before a game at
Boston's Fenway Park. "His batting practice was extraordinary there,"
marveled Papa. "It was much greater than Canseco's had ever been
earlier in the decade. Mac was just hitting towering, tape measure
shots."

The enormous attention McGwire received during batting practice pushed Canseco. He tried to keep up with McGwire and launch
his own skyscraping drives, but sadly fell short. Canseco was clearly
not on the same plane as McGwire. After a month into the season,
Canseco asked Howe if he could come out of McGwire's hitting group.

> He told me, "You better get me out of that group; I'm going to hurt
> myself trying to hit home runs like he's hitting." He recognized the
> fact that McGwire elevated himself to a new level. He wasn't at that
> level anymore, but I give him a lot credit for that. He recognized that
> himself and handled it well. His time had passed.

McGwire flexed his muscle in games, as well. Facing the Cleveland Indians at Jacobs Field on April 30, McGwire drilled a
mesmerizing home run off of 1988 World Series nemesis Orel Hershiser
that cleared the bleachers and crashed off the Budweiser sign in left
field, 485 feet from the plate. On June 24, he obliterated a ninety-seven-
mile-an-hour Randy Johnson fastball into the second deck in left-center
field at Seattle's Kingdome. The gargantuan missile estimated at 538
feet, was the longest in the venue's history. "It was absolutely incredible," said Eric Carrington. "When he hit it, the whole place went quiet."
McGwire soon left memories of his trademark colossal home runs at

each stadium he visited. Greg Papa, who broadcasted both games on the A's television network, observed, "He was as powerful a hitter as he's ever been, at that time."

Former A's infielder Mark Bellhorn admired the West Coast home-run duo, Canseco and McGwire, in their heyday while growing up in Florida. A second-round draft pick by the A's from Auburn University in 1995, Bellhorn was promoted after second baseman Scott Spiezio went on the disabled list in June. When he strode onto the field, it was surreal to be suddenly playing alongside the two. "I'd only been in pro-ball for a couple of years and suddenly I'm playing right beside McGwire," said Bellhorn, currently playing for the Cincinnati Reds organization. "To watch some of the balls he'd hit was amazing. He would take an easy swing and the ball would go a lot further than everybody else."

Canseco, though, also flashed glimpses of power. By mid-June, he smacked fifteen home runs. Despite the added muscle in the lineup, however, the team's starting pitching couldn't contain opposing batters and quickly fell out of contention. Still, Canseco and McGwire were a novelty on the road. And scheduling interviews and tackling endless media requests was Eric Carrington. Before the season, Carrington did his homework. Hoping to learn more about dealing with Canseco and McGwire, he elicited feedback from several members on the A's staff. Both could be difficult, they warned him. But Carrington soon discovered Canseco was the most cooperative.

> When I first met José, I had all these preconceived impressions as this prima donna, a jerk, and he turned out being the total opposite. He almost seemed contrite. He was an easygoing laid-back kind of guy. He was totally easy to deal with. He did pretty much everything I asked. You'd see him talking to younger guys on how to handle stuff. He gave time to pretty much everybody that wanted to talk with him.

Carrington couldn't say the same of McGwire. "I had heard that Mark McGwire would be hard to deal with and a lot of that came true," confirmed Carrington. "It wasn't easy to ask him to do stuff. He had a certain persona, probably because he was Mark McGwire."

Carrington blamed most of McGwire's standoffish and guarded demeanor on coming to grips with leaving Oakland and hearing his name constantly linked to trade rumors by June. Unlike the Canseco trade in 1992, Alderson had made it clear to media and fans during the season that McGwire's departure was inevitable.

Alderson said he recognized the financial challenges of the franchise and how trading McGwire's contract would benefit the budget. If

McGwire remained with the club, he would most certainly sign else-where after the season. That scenario would mean the A's would only receive compensation picks. Alderson judged that the A's were better off obtaining established players and prospects than draft compensations.

> We prepped everyone in the Bay Area that Mark was on his way. He bought into it; people bought into it. But in the final analysis, there weren't a lot of potential takers. He'd be a free agent after the season. Other than the St. Louis Cardinals, the only other team we seriously talked with was the Anaheim Angels.

In the trade discussions with the Angels, Alderson wanted Tim Salmon, a twenty-eight-year-old up-and-coming power hitter, as a foundation for the trade. "They weren't interested in parting with him [Salmon]," said Alderson. "Plus, I think they felt they were in the driver's seat in obtaining McGwire via free agency after the season."

To McGwire, the anxiety and uncertainty of his future began tak-ing its toll. As trade talks snowballed, McGwire became tightlipped with reporters and bottled his emotions. On separate occasions in May and June, McGwire, angered by a third strike call, uncharacteristically scoffed at plate umpires, Jim Joyce and Rich Garcia, prompting two ejections. At Detroit's Tiger Stadium on June 10, he erupted. Steve Kettman, the A's beat writer for the *San Francisco Chronicle*, detailed the incident for readers the next day.

> McGwire put on one of the most prodigious displays of anger in his career, and he did it with a schoolboy-in-a-snit insouciance. He grabbed two bats and his helmet and tossed them out of the dugout, then he grabbed two more and flung them, too. Finally, he reached for a couple more to make it an even half-dozen and heaved them, too.

Art Howe acknowledged that the trade rumors had drained McGwire. "He got pretty emotional. It was affecting him offensively, performance-wise," admitted Howe. "Two days before he got traded, he asked out of the lineup. That was the only time he asked out of the lineup—right before he was traded." By July, however, McGwire wasn't the only one on the trading block. Hoping to dump more payroll, the A's mulled over trading Canseco to the New York Yankees. In late July, Canseco, who had been recovering from off-season back surgery, ag-gravated his back again. The injury cost him a week of playing time and eventually landed him on the disabled list. "He only played about four months for us, but he still put up some decent power numbers," remembered Howe. "But his back was bothering him."

With McGwire's unavoidable departure looming and Canseco's absence from the lineup, the organization looked to the future by calling up touted prospects Ben Grieve and Miguel Tejada. While Alderson's marketing-driven plan to reunite the Bash Brothers had initially sparked enthusiasm, by August his plan had evaporated. "It wasn't the great reunion they were hoping for," said Greg Papa.

Meanwhile, trade discussions surrounding McGwire between Alderson and his former farm director Walk Jocketty, now the general manager of the Cardinals, had intensified. With McGwire's former manager Tony La Russa along with former A's coaches Dave Duncan and Dave McKay now on staff with the Cardinals, their familiar faces could help ease the adjustment of playing in the National League and switching organizations. Though McGwire figured he might one day finish his career back in Southern California and be close to his nine-year-old son, Matthew, the ten-year veteran understood the economics and business of baseball. He welcomed the opportunity to be reunited with his former manager and coaches in the Midwest.

Closure couldn't come any sooner for McGwire and several of his teammates. Steve Karsay, an A's former starting pitcher in 1997, grew tired of addressing trade rumors in the clubhouse. "Everybody in the clubhouse wants the situation to be over," Karsay told reporters shortly before the trade deadline. "It's got to take a toll on everyone, [wondering] if Mark is going to be traded. He doesn't know. We don't know. It's tough."[12]

Months of speculation finally culminated on Thursday afternoon, July 31, the trade deadline. After several days of deliberating and finalizing the deal, the A's sent McGwire to the Cardinals for twenty-seven-year-old reliever T.J. Matthews, who was 4–4 with a 2.15 earned run average, and right-handed pitching prospects Eric Ludwick and Blake Stein. McGwire was thrilled at the prospect of playing in St. Louis, a baseball-enamored city. He also anticipated the feeling of stalking a championship, an adrenaline rush he lacked during his final five years in Oakland.

Still, after thirteen years embedded in the same organization, leaving the A's was bittersweet. The organization crowned him the tenth pick in the country in 1984, and supported him through his agonizing slumps and nagging injuries. "I think Mark wanted to stay with Oakland, because that was the only organization he knew and he really loved it there," said Howe. "He got pretty emotional about being traded. It's always tough for a player who has been with an organization his whole life and suddenly be traded to another club. It hurts. We would've loved to keep him, but we couldn't afford him."

After learning of his departure, McGwire held a press conference in the bowels of the Oakland-Alameda Coliseum, shortly before the A's played the Baltimore Orioles at 7:05 P.M. During the press conference and amid emotional farewells in the clubhouse, McGwire showed a different side, according to Carrington. "He was crying in the clubhouse and during the press conference," said Carrington. "It was a sad and somber day, but I got the impression it was a weight lifted off his chest. He was sad to leave and wasn't guarded."

McGwire said his heartfelt goodbye to the Oakland A's and Bay Area fans. "I grew up with this organization. It was not an easy decision, but everyone comes to a crossroads in your life when change will be good for you," a choked up McGwire explained. "I came to that crossroads. They've [fans] been through thick and thin with me: My down year in '91. The '93 and '94 injury years. They saw someone turn his career around. For the fans that stuck with [me] through the years, thank you."

One of the saddest players in the ballpark, however, was teammate Jason Giambi, a twenty-six-year-old rising star. Growing up in Southern California, Giambi watched McGwire crack home runs with an aluminum bat at USC's Dedeaux Field in the early 1980s. Like McGwire, Giambi played in the Alaskan Summer League and starred for the United States Olympic club. Grabbed by the A's in the second round in 1992, Giambi smacked his way through minor league stops at Modesto, Huntsville, and Tacoma before arriving in Oakland in 1995. For over two years, McGwire took the rookie under his wing and groomed him to be the A's next leader and the franchise's superstar. Both became inseparable. "You could see how they were pretty close," said Mark Bellhorn. "He was his mentor and showed him how to do things. He obviously knew he was going to leave at some time and Jason would eventually take over."

Carrington said their relationship translated away from the field and clubhouse. "Giambi was like his little brother," recalled Carrington. "He did everything with Giambi. But when he left, it became Giambi's clubhouse."

Though Giambi embraced the role of clubhouse leader, seeing his best friend depart crushed him. "This is probably one of the saddest days of my career," Giambi told reporters in the clubhouse after learning of the trade. "We were best friends. He took me under his wing and taught me how to play the game at this level. I won't forget the things he taught me."[13]

With the final cog of the A's championship years headed to St. Louis, the club turned their attention to monitoring the progress of younger players. That meant Canseco, who had returned from the disabled list on August 20 and needed 122 at-bats to reach the 568 required to trigger a guaranteed $4.5 million contract for the following season, would be deprived of playing time. Additionally, without McGwire, Canseco had lost his marketing worth to the A's, it seemed. Canseco saw the writing on the wall and approached Art Howe. "Right after we traded Mark, he came back and asked me, 'Art, level with me: Am I going to get those at-bats to qualify for my option?'" Howe recalled. "I said, 'I'll be honest with you: No, you're not. I'm going to be playing these other kids, so you're not going to reach it.' He was going to play, but not get enough at-bats to qualify for his bonus."

With over a month remaining in the season, Canseco reaggravated his back on the base paths in a game. He packed his bags and returned to his home in Florida, where he would remain for the remainder of the season. Some wondered if Canseco would succumb to his back injuries and retire. But in an era of performance-enhancing drugs, one couldn't count on it.

NOTES

[1] Associated Press, "Injury Might End Canseco's Season," June 29, 1993.
[2] Dave Van Dyke, "Canseco Boon For Palmeiro," *Chicago Sun-Times*, September 20, 1992.
[3] T.R. Sullivan, "With Free Agency Looming, Palmeiro Knows a Big Year Means Bigger Payday," *Fort Worth Star-Telegram*, February 27, 1993.
[4] Jose Canseco, *Juiced* (New York: Harper Collins, 2005), 135.
[5] Gordon Edes, "Sox Deal Canseco Back to A's," *Boston Globe*, January 25, 1997.
[6] Jeordan Legon, "Giants Exec Takes Pitch for Ballpark," *San Jose Mercury News*, November 14, 1996.
[7] Susan Dowdney, "A's May Say Ciao If They Don't Get Stadium," *Contra Costa Times*, June 6, 1996.
[8] Glenn Dickey, "Rakish Canseco Restores A's Allure," *San Francisco Chronicle*, February 12, 1997.
[9] Mike Lefkow, "Canseco's Arrival Has A's Getting Ready for Big Bash," *Contra Costa Times*, January 28, 1997.
[10] Jennifer Frey, "Getting Together For Another Bash," *Washington Post*, March 20, 1997.
[11] Ibid.
[12] Steve Kettmann, "McGwire Deal Still Not Done," *San Francisco Chronicle*, July 31, 1997.
[13] Ricci R. Graham, "McGwire Trade Hits Giambi Hard," *Sacramento Bee*, August 1, 1997.

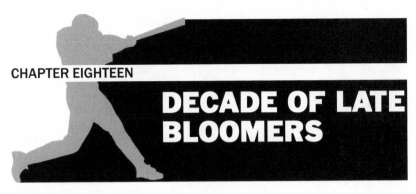

CHAPTER EIGHTEEN

DECADE OF LATE BLOOMERS

"I feel stupid for not realizing how rampant steroids were; I wasn't paying attention. Jose was pretty obvious, but you would have to say Mark was, too."

—Former A's closer Dennis Eckersley
May 2007

Nineteen ninety-seven. If McGwire and Canseco epitomized an unrivaled pedigree of millionaire, muscle-popping, and supplement-fueled power hitters in the 1980s and early '90s, Mike Piazza represented an advanced crop exploding into the game in the mid-1990s. By that time, designer steroids and personally hired trainers created a subculture in baseball. Players had prioritized their relationships with private trainers over hitting coaches. Sophistication had also soared. For example, players had figured out which chemicals caused particular effects, which ones chiseled fat, and which ones added bulk. Drugs that accelerated foot speed, healed joints, increased bat speed, bolstered stamina, and also temporarily provided a psychological edge, had revolutionized the game. To justify their freakish muscle growth, some players endorsed creatine monohydrate, a natural over-the-counter muscle-building supplement, to masquerade their steroid use. They praised creatine as the supplement of the 1990s.

Underground steroid education filtered through the game. It was common knowledge among players that oil-based testosterone dramatically increased strength and added weight. Oral forms of steroids such as Dianabol also packed on mass. Additionally, the chemicals Winstrol, otherwise known as Stanozolol, and Equipose had been favorites among bodybuilders to help shed fat before a competition. Human Growth Hormone, or HGH, contained properties to help players recover from bone and tissue-related injuries. Some players also included milk thistle in their cycles, an herb reportedly designed to help the liver survive the strain of toxic chemicals passing through the organ.

"It massages your liver," Ken Caminiti told the *San Diego Union-Tribune's* Tom Krasovic in February 1997. That year, Caminiti developed an abnormality in the enzyme levels of his liver. In the interview, Caminiti blamed his liver abnormality on the anti-inflammatory medication he ingested to help him play through his tendon and cartilage problems. "I take a lot of things for my liver because I had high enzymes when my blood was tested," he told Krasovic. "The doctors say the anti-inflammatories might have been bad for the liver. I was just trying to play." Caminiti failed to mention that months before he used steroids throughout the 1996 season. He died of a heart attack in 2004. He was forty-one.

Players acquired and used those chemicals for muscles and fame. By using, though, they also mortgaged their liver and increased their risk of heart attack. The bodybuilding culture had seductively, but dangerously, enveloped America's Pastime. To many players, steroid use wasn't about cheating or physically harmful effects. It was a matter of stretching their dream. "When I was faced with the decision, in my mind, of my career ending or keeping it going, I compromised my morality and beliefs," said F. P. Santangelo, a former major league player, and one of the eighty-four players linked to steroids in the Mitchell Report released in December 2007. "I did what I thought I had to do."

Taking banned performance-enhancing drugs wasn't only about gaining muscle and slamming tape-measure blasts; it was about enhancing performance and rebounding from injuries. The culture bred an unfair sport for those players who shunned steroids. Some players chose a drug-free weight-training regimen. But the immense pressure to survive and remain relevant in the sport pushed others to experiment. "Suddenly players got smarter than you," said former A's strength and conditioning coach Dave McKay, one of the first avid weight lifters in the game. "I was oblivious that there were that many players doing it. Obviously there was a lot going on."

Mike Piazza played in the thick of the movement. Piazza, the former Los Angeles Dodgers' All-Star catcher and Hollywood celebrity with soap-opera good looks, had been a sixty-second round draft afterthought in 1988. A heavy-footed first baseman for Pennsylvania's Phoenixville Area High School in 1986, Piazza had been ignored by scouts. Only after the urging of Dodger icon Tommy Lasorda, his father's confidante, did Piazza get a shot. The reasons behind the scouts' reluctance played out during Piazza's first two seasons, however.

As a struggling minor leaguer in 1990, he battled through adversity and wanted out of baseball. Teammates ridiculed him, and many figured he had been drafted as a favor. Piazza wanted to prove he deserved a professional contract and belonged. He worked harder. After two lackluster seasons in the minor leagues, Piazza exploded in 1991, placing himself among the top prospects in the organization. At Single-A Bakersfield, he batted .277 and smashed twenty-nine home runs, inching his way closer to the majors. The next season, Piazza ripped through other minor league stops at Double-A San Antonio and Triple-A Albuquerque. By 1992, Piazza strutted into Dodger Stadium. A year later, he batted .318 and clubbed thirty-five homers, grabbing the National League Rookie of the Year award.

Piazza defied the science of scouting. His was a feel-good story, a timeless tale that old-time scouts marvel about around the table. "That was damn great job of scouting," said legendary scout Dick Wiencek, praising the scout who signed Piazza. He embodied the hope for sixty-something round draft favors. Coinciding with Piazza's stardom and stellar work ethic was his dramatic strength gains. A poster boy for late-budding superstars, he packed on slabs of muscle through pumping iron during his first five years developing in the organization. That accelerated his bat speed and spawned him into a freak. "I know I've worked very hard to get better," Piazza told the *Long Beach Press-Telegram* in 1993. "And I've matured a lot physically. When the Dodgers signed me, I weighed 190 pounds. I've put on 25 pounds since then through an intensive weight lifting program. I've benched pressed 285 pounds and done full squats with 350." [1]

By 1997, twenty-eight-year-old Piazza was a five-time All-Star and one of the game's most dominating offensive juggernauts. He averaged thirty-three home runs a season and headlined every offensive category. Beyond his resume of statistics, though, Piazza was a marvel in the batting cage. His explosive strength and lightning bat speed helped him pepper balls onto Dodger Stadium's pavilion. The way the right-handed batter muscled home runs toward right-center field and the booming sound of the ball leaving his bat made his abilities seem bionic. To this day Piazza is recognized as arguably the game's greatest offensive catcher. One could ponder the whispers if he had invaded the game in the 1980s. But, in the decade of the 1990s, he was one of the myriad players who had scurried to weight rooms, got stronger, and helped turn baseball into a game of Wiffleball.

Though that doesn't mean Piazza used steroids, he certainly symbolized what baseball was about in the 1990s: a carnival of heavy-hitting figures monopolizing the game. While some stubbornly refused to find comfort in steroids, others, sucked by the current of the culture, succumbed to the temptations. Juiced players ran the show.

Hall of Fame closer Dennis Eckersley, who retired after the 1998 season, reflected on the era. "I feel stupid for not realizing how rampant steroids were; I wasn't paying attention. José was pretty obvious, but you would have to say Mark was, too," admitted Eckersley.

San Diego Padres' legendary hitting coach Merv Rettenmund wasn't so oblivious.

"I knew [Ken] Caminiti was taking them," said Rettenmund. "Because there he was with a blown-out arm, he's an MVP candidate if he can keep playing, and he's taking steroids, but so what. He would tell you: I'd ask him how his arm was today and he'd say, 'It's not good, but it will be better by the weekend.' And then he starts swinging better.

"At the time, I didn't even know if they were bad or illegal. I said, 'So what if he's taking them.' Everyone in baseball knew it. And now they want to bring all this stuff out. If someone's caught now, it should be a year suspension. But back then, everyone knew it; everyone in the New York office knew it; everyone knew it when they were going for the home run race."

Rettenmund said neither Senator George Mitchell nor his investigative team interviewed him for the Mitchell Report, but he wished they had. "Baseball should step out and some of these people should say, 'hey, we knew, and we're sorry and we're going to have to just put that time behind us and go on, man.'"

Home-run totals rocketed and traveled further than ever before. From 1996 to 1998, major league players amassed 14,666 round-trippers. That figure is 3,249 more than the previous three seasons, which included a strike-shortened one in 1994. Those torrid totals fueled several speculations. As Jeff Miller of the *Orange County Register* observed in 1998: "Baseball has become a buffet, an all-you-can-eat orgy of offense, and isn't it perfect that the action is centered on the plate? More players have puffy forearms and thick chests and pound high-octane protein shakes loaded with muscle food."[2]

While some claimed the baseball had been juiced, others felt that the cozy, hitter-friendly, state-of-the-art-ballparks were to blame for the home-run revival. Some even blamed expansion, more specifically the watered-down pitching of newly formed teams, such as the Colorado Rockies and Florida Marlins, both established in 1993.

The mid-1990s spit out the Blake Street Bombers, Andrés Galarraga, Vinny Castilla, Larry Walker, and Dante Bichette. They were the murderers' row of the Colorado Rockies' potent lineup. With booming blasts, they awed fans and took full advantage of the home-run-friendly climate at Denver's Coors Field.

On the East Coast, in Baltimore, thirty-two-year-old lead-off batter Brady Anderson, who mustered 103 home runs during his first eleven years of professional baseball, abruptly reached fifty in 1996. Those were enormous totals compared to the eighteen he hit in each of the next two seasons. "The huge alarm clock in baseball was Brady Anderson," said MSNBC.com baseball analyst Ted Robinson. "He was the seminal figure for that discussion. What he did that year was so shocking."

Anderson, another player who sculpted his frame through strength training, nutritional supplements, and a rigorous cardiovascular routine, had been a staple of the decade's surging "Late Bloomers." His teammate Rafael Palmeiro had also cracked his share of home runs. Beginning in 1995, he muscled 206 over the next five seasons. The weight-lifting revolution had even driven Orioles' iron man, Cal Ripken, to the bench press. Groomed by old-time baseball traditionalist Earl Weaver and his father, Cal, Sr., Ripken had avoided weights as a young player in the early 1980s. A notoriously sturdy and dependable shortstop with home-run power, he personified durability. He broke Lou Gehrig's consecutive games played streak of 2,130 in 1995. After the season, urged by Anderson, Ripken pounded the weights and muscled up, too. Anderson told Thomas Boswell of the *Washington Post* in July 1996:

> For years, I've told Cal, "when The Streak is over, come lift with me and I'll show you how much better you can be." Cal has enormous natural strength. Wrestling around in the clubhouse, he can throw you around like you're a little kid. But in the weight room, I'm lifting hundreds of pounds more than he is. As a home run hitter, he's never touched his potential. Watch what he does the next few years.[3]

Boswell wrote the following in the next paragraph: "Scouts already have noticed that he [Ripken] seems to have a 'new body.'"

Former Oakland A's backup catcher Mickey Tettleton, at twenty-eight, revitalized his career with the Baltimore Orioles in 1989. A former fifth-round draft pick, Tettleton, whose average hovered around .190 with the A's in 1987, was handed his unconditional release in 1988. The next season the powerfully built, six-foot-two, 215-pound slugger cranked twenty-six home runs, earning a spot on the American League All-Star team. From that point, Tettleton transformed himself from a light-hitting catcher, a blip in the lineup, to one of the league's most dangerous switch-hitting power hitters over the next eight seasons. Tettleton attributed strength training to his power surge.

Former pinch-hit specialist Matt Stairs surprisingly clobbered twenty-seven home runs for the A's in 1997. Before signing as a free agent with the A's in 1995, the Canadian had spent most of his seven seasons in the minor league affiliates of the Montreal Expos and Boston Red Sox. During that time, he played in a major league game only fifty-eight times. Stairs was considered a backup, light-hitting journeyman, a utility player. Stairs hit so poorly for the A's to start the season in 1996 that they placed him on waivers that April. After that season, however, he hit eighty-five homers over the next three seasons, landing him a two-year extension worth $5 million. Stairs attributed lifting weights, consuming energy drinks, and eating "sixteen egg whites per day" for his improved performance and weight loss off his once five-foot-nine, 225-pound frame. Said A's general manager Billy Beane, "Matt will be the centerpiece of this club for the next two or three years."[4]

Perhaps no player arched more eyebrows than former Arizona Diamondbacks star Luis Gonzales in 2001. Playing for Jefferson High in Tampa, Florida, in 1985, the lean six-foot-two standout weighed 150 pounds. Before breaking in with the Houston Astros, alongside Ken Caminiti, Craig Biggio, and Jeff Bagwell, Gonzales was a lukewarm prospect who had made up for his shortcomings by working hard. "Every young kid dreams of playing in the major leagues, and this is an opportunity for me to get in the door," Gonzales told the *Dallas Morning News* in 1991. "If they told me to pitch, I'd go pitch. I don't care what I have to do just so long as I get there."

Gonzales, a left-handed line-drive hitter, had averaged roughly thirteen home runs during his first seven seasons. In 1997, after signing with the Detroit Tigers, he bumped into Brad Andress, the team's strength and conditioning coach and former offensive lineman at Penn State. Andress had played a significant role in the physical development of former Tigers slugger Mickey Tettleton. Andress cast his spell on Gonzales. And beginning in 1998, thirty-year-old Gonzales elevated his home runs totals to twenty-three, twenty-six, and thirty-one, over the next three seasons, respectively. In 2001, he smashed an astonishing fifty-seven home runs, powering the Diamondbacks to a world championship. Gonzales claimed that strength training and working out with his newest personal trainer, Greg Bucher, a Phoenix-based bodybuilder, helped him produce such a season. "Yes, I'm surprised by his power," Bob Watson, Gonzales' former general manager with the Astros, told the *Arizona Republic* in 2001. "If he was honest, he'd tell you the same thing. He always had a sweet swing and hit balls to left-center. The added muscle and strength definitely helped him out and did not hurt his swing." The bodybuilding culture, along with all its supplements, had infected baseball.

That's what discouraged left-handed hitter Ben Grieve, a slender, smooth-swinging outfielder who was the A's first-round draft pick in 1994. At six foot four, 210 pounds, Grieve flashed power and gracefully sprayed balls to all fields, prompting many to hail him as one of the game's future superstars. Grieve first suspected steroid use when he spotted several A's players dramatically blow up. "It's safe to say that a player that's not using steroids would have to work three to five times harder than a user, just to keep up and that might not even guarantee the same results," Grieve wrote in a December 2007 email. Still, Grieve remained natural.

And it worked. After batting .288 with eighteen homers in 1998, he earned a spot on the All-Star team and eventually earned the 1998 American League Rookie of the Year award. In 1999, he slammed twenty-eight home runs; the next season he hit twenty-seven. For those efforts, the Oakland A's rewarded him a four-year, $13 million contract in 2000, which, to this day, Grieve gratefully says, "gave me enough money that I could retire at age thirty and never have to work a day in my life."

After the 2000 season, however, the A's traded Grieve to the Tampa Bay Devil Rays in a three-team swap that landed Kansas City Royals' star Johnny Damon and Devil Rays' reliever Jim Mecir in Oakland. Though Grieve hit nineteen home runs in 2002, his stroke faded shortly thereafter, he desperately tried to match his previous form. That never happened. After he briefly latched on with the Milwaukee Brewers and Chicago Cubs, he sadly found himself at Triple-A Iowa in 2005. Grieve had had enough. At age twenty-nine, he retired that year. If there were an ideal candidate who would have benefited from steroids it was Grieve. The drugs could have energized his sometimes-perceived lackadaisical body language. They could have helped the slow-footed outfielder blaze on the base paths, adding another weapon to his game. Increasing his power and bat speed by using the chemicals could have also inflated his home-run totals and morphed him into one of baseball's heavy hitting figures. "I never felt the pressure, but if there was ever a time for me to use steroids it would have been after my first year in Tampa, when I struggled," emailed Grieve. "But I had been successful before without using, so I felt I could do it again. It never happened."

For a steroid-free player in the 1990s and 2000s, trying to do it the right way and hustle into stardom was a long shot. Muscled-up players dominated the game. If Grieve would have been plucked out of the 1990s and dropped into the '80s, he would have certainly had a chance at enjoying a long, illustrious career. Instead, he happened to play during the movement's peak, and many of his steroid-fueled peers passed him by, making him a casualty for staying natural. Grieve wrote in a December 2007 email:

I compare it to stealing money. You are breaking the rules of baseball (as well as the law) in order to make money for yourself. At the same time, you are taking away money from someone who might have had a chance if it wasn't for you. To me, you could make the argument that it should be a crime . . . I'm happy every time a players is accused because it demeans their accomplishments.

That other players used steroids and robbed him of playing time and roster spots also angered him.

To see a player you know is taking steroids and producing is definitely frustrating. Especially knowing that on an even playing field, you're a better player. The knock on me was always my defense, and although I know steroids wouldn't have helped me in that aspect of my game, I do believe they would have given me a chance to stick around longer just based on the offensive benefits they would have given me. The amount of money I've seen players make, that I have a strong feeling took steroids, is astounding, not only in Oakland but also in Tampa Bay.

Grieve claimed "at least three to four" players were juicing in the A's line-up in 2000 and wouldn't be shocked if upwards of seven were also using. Canseco and McGwire, forefathers of baseball's bodybuilding craze that had players flexing their muscle as never before, rode the wave, too.

Thirty-three-year-old McGwire found a nest in St. Louis. He instantly made a mockery of the daunting adjustments players face when they switch leagues. To many players, hoping to flawlessly adapt to a different galaxy of baseball—new teammates, unfamiliar ballparks, unknown pitchers, and a different brand of play—can cause headaches. Those difficult elements didn't seem to bother him. McGwire's universal home-run swing spanned both leagues. When he was traded from Oakland to St. Louis in August 1997, he launched twenty-four home runs to wrap his final fifty-one games of the season. That's remarkably a home run every 7.25 at-bats, a thrilling finish that capped his fifty-eight home-run season.

Local fans and media embraced the Paul Bunyan-looking redhead. He thrived in the baseball-crazy atmosphere at Busch Stadium, entertaining fans by peppering tape-measure bombs in the left field's upper deck. Not that McGwire's moon shots were his sudden trademark in baseball; he had been on a headline-making home-run pace his final two-and-a-half years in Oakland. But to many St. Louis fans, McGwire, six foot five, muscles and all, had been veiled behind the small-market, under exposed rebuilding conditions in Oakland. Even while he consistently smacked blasts for over a decade in Oakland, he never received his due. Bay Area columnist Mark Purdy of the *San Jose Mercury News*, wrote on the eve of the trade:

> In spite of this, McGwire was never The Man around here. Meaning that, he was never the most dominant sports personality in the Bay Area. Not even close. Not even in his own sport. Do you remember one local McGwire endorsement deal? Or any television commercials, except the ones for the A's themselves? How did this happen? Think back to 1987, McGwire's rookie season. When he showed up here, all muscles and freckles from Orange County, the Athletics' commanding celebrity was José Canseco. And by the time José was traded in 1992, Rickey Henderson and Dennis Eckersley were more larger-than-life. After they left, Bonds was The Man, working on the other side of the water in San Francisco.

In the Midwest, however, Cupid couldn't have engineered a more fitting and timely marriage between McGwire and his bride, St. Louis. Arriving in the Gateway City, McGwire discovered that his long and self-evolving journey had taken him full circle. The fresh-faced, bright-eyed, all-American boy, who ended his interviews with "Thank you" in his years of innocence, had already tasted the sweetness of thriving and was ready to return to his roots. "To me, when he embraced that All-American boy image again in St. Louis, which America really needed, that took him to the highest level," observed former teammate Doug Jennings. "He found himself there and really took the hearts of America. That was the real rise of Mark McGwire and becoming who he really should have been from the very beginning."

Early arriving fans crammed the left-field seats to watch McGwire take his cuts in the batting cage. The affection fans lavished on him overwhelmed McGwire. "I've never had that feeling," McGwire said in 1997. "I almost was embarrassed because there were other guys that had to hit, too. The fans were roaring. Believe me, I will never forget this. . . . In Oakland, we'd only get a couple of hundred people watching batting practice."

After playing in St. Louis for a little over a month, McGwire relished the atmosphere and soon signed a three-year, $28 million deal on September 16. Included in the deal, which was worth less than market value, was a $1 million signing bonus and a fourth year option that would seal the pact of nearly $40 million. Since he also deferred a quarter of the monies until after he retired, the Cardinals could secure other players. McGwire, who could have garnered millions more as a free agent during the winter, proved that landing top dollars couldn't sway him from the peace he found in the city by the arch. "I tell you what, it makes me float every time I come to the ballpark, to play in this stadium and play in front of these fans," McGwire said during the press conference announcing the deal. "I've never been treated like this as a ballplayer. I'm overwhelmed. I'm going to say that probably for the rest of my career."

What choked McGwire up the most during the press conference was his announcement to donate $1 million a year to establish the Mark McGwire Charitable Foundation geared toward sexually and physically abused children. Because he had close friends that had been victims of such abuse, McGwire claimed that he felt compelled to launch his foundation. "Let's just say children have a special place in my heart," McGwire said.

If children had a special place in his heart, home runs had a special place on his bat. The relentless comparisons drawn between McGwire and legendary baseball icons Babe Ruth and Roger Maris had snowballed the following season. Coming into the 1998 season, McGwire accumulated a home run every 11.94 at-bats over his eleven-year career. With the recent home-run explosion in baseball, it seemed fitting that a player of McGwire's caliber could blast his way into baseball's hallowed record books. That he finally seemed at peace, injury-free, and energized by the adoring fans at Busch Stadium helped create a magical stage. Fans and reporters buzzed that this could be the season McGwire surpassed Roger Maris's thirty-seven-year-old single-season record of sixty-one home runs.

Up north, twenty-nine-year-old Sammy Sosa, a strapping, charming, Dominican-born right fielder for the Chicago Cubs, had established himself as one of the National League's dangerous sluggers. Averaging thirty-seven round-trippers each of his last three seasons, the six-foot, 220-pound, right-handed hitter exuded an unrivaled passion for the game. Sweating hard on the island of the Dominican Republic to make his way to the United States and play in the major leagues, Sosa took nothing for granted. After six sub-par seasons playing in the farm systems of the Texas Rangers and Chicago White Sox, Sosa muscled up and found his stroke in the Windy City.

McGwire and Sosa relentlessly assaulted opposing pitchers with a barrage of home runs, barging toward Maris's record. By June 17, McGwire had already smacked thirty-three, while Sosa had thirty. Though headlining different lineups, the tandem captured America's attention. People of all walks were mesmerized by the story. The stretch run and pennant races had all taken a back seat to the home-run chase. On August 11, Sosa cracked home run nos. forty-five and forty-six against the San Francisco Giants at 3Com Park, catching McGwire. Like two heavyweight boxers exchanging blows in the final round of a stomach-turning match, McGwire and Sosa rejuvenated fan interest.

The country's heart-pounding romance with Sosa and McGwire had also lured troves of reporters from around the globe. Steve Wilstein, an Associated Press feature writer, had been one of a dozen writers who waited patiently for McGwire near his locker after an August game. With pen and pad in hand, Wilstein hoped to gather McGwire's quotes to churn out a story. The delay granted Wilstein time to scope McGwire's cluttered locker. His eyes zoomed in on a small brown bottle. The label read, Androstenedione. Though he flew into St. Louis to chronicle McGwire's feats on the field, that name and that bottle reverberated through his mind. When the curious Wilstein returned home to California, he called a doctor friend and asked, "What's Androstenedione?" The doctor explained that the drug was a precursor to testosterone and could harm the heart.

Wilstein immediately expanded his research and soon discovered the National Football League, International Olympic Committee, and National Collegiate Athletic Association had banned the over-the-counter pills, which had anabolic qualities. And on August 21, he broke the story and revealed how America's fence-clearing savior—on the cusp of shattering one of baseball's most famed record—had been taking the pills for over a year. Wilstein wrote in his 1998 article:

> No one suggests that McGwire wouldn't be closing in on Roger Maris' home run record without the over-the-counter-drug. After all, he hit 49 homers without it as a rookie in 1987, and more than 50 each of the past two seasons. But the drugs' ability to raise levels of the male hormone, which builds lean muscle mass and promotes recovery after injury, is seen outside baseball as cheating and potentially dangerous.[5]

When McGwire heard about the article, he angrily responded and hoped to set the record straight. He also informed reporters that other players had used the supplement. "Everything I've done is natural," emphasized McGwire. "Everybody that I know in the game of baseball uses the same stuff I use." "Why would people fathom that I've done steroids?" McGwire later asked. "Because I lift? It's foolish. It's because I played with [José] Canseco and it came up one year with him."[6]

The controversy briefly placed a cloud over McGwire's record-breaking pace. As word that McGwire had used the supplement whirled around the country, the sales of Andro, the nickname to which the pills were commonly referred, skyrocketed. "We would have forecasted $30 million in andro sales this year," Grant Ferrier, editor of the *Nutrition Business Journal*, told the Associated Press in December 1998. "McGwire added $10 million."

While other players may have been using the supplement, McGwire was chasing greatness. Still, the distraction that questioned the legitimacy of his power couldn't calm the enthusiasm the country felt over watching him and Sosa hunt sixty one. Some, in denial, refused to accept or allow the speculation that McGwire cheated to hamper such a larger-than-life story, one steered by integrity, hope, and morals. Nor did the frenzy stifle McGwire's power. He belted no. fifty-three at Pittsburgh's Three Rivers Stadium on August 23. But that same afternoon in Chicago, Sosa had just blasted nos. fifty and fifty-one. With little over a month left, both were closing in on history.

The media was also zooming in on McGwire. Reporters stalked his every move, and camera crews waited for him as he emerged from the dugout before every game. Though becoming the center of attention had drained him, he recognized that flirting with the record would draw relentless coverage, an onslaught he faced as a rookie in 1987. That microscope had sapped Roger Maris when he approached Babe Ruth's cherished thirty-four-year-old record in 1961. Treated as a second-class citizen to teammate and media darling Mickey Mantle by the press, Maris received death threats and began losing hair from the stress.

McGwire showed his discomfort through his body language. He sighed. He rolled his eyes. He reluctantly answered. He never sought the spotlight, but his bat always seemed to drag it along.

The charisma McGwire lacked was what Sosa possessed. To Sosa, absorbing the showers of praise he received energized him. Since no one had expected him to pursue such a legendary mark, he played loose, as if he had nothing to lose. He smiled. He laughed. His signature dash toward right field and affectionate two-finger salute to fans at Wrigley Field had endeared himself to millions around the globe. But it wasn't just his personality that hailed him as baseball's modern-day Babe Ruth. After Sosa smacked no. fifty-four to match McGwire on August 30, McGwire erupted for his fifty-fifth later that evening, reclaiming the lead. A week later, on September 7, McGwire clubbed no. sixty-one off Cincinnati Reds' starter Mike Morgan, tying Maris's record. After McGwire circled the bases and stepped on home plate, he blew a kiss and pointed toward the sky to pay homage to Maris. "I admire everything that Roger went through," McGwire said after the game. "Because I've been through it, too, now."

Two days later, on September 8, Hollywood couldn't have scripted a more intriguing plot. With the Cubs and Sosa invading Busch Stadium that Tuesday evening, McGwire needed one homer to break the mark. With the Maris family in attendance; his son, ten-year-old Matthew, a batboy, in the dugout; and parents, John and Ginger also in the stadium; McGwire eyed a record-breaking moment. FOX network spruced up the scene by carrying the game and broadcasting it nationally. A anticipating crowd of 49,987 and hundreds of international media surrounded McGwire at every at-bat. In the bottom of the first, McGwire grounded out to short.

But in the bottom of the fourth, at 9:18 P.M. EST, McGwire drilled a low, searing line drive down the left-field line off Cubs' starter Steve Trachsel. Because the bullet wasn't one of McGwire's no-doubt-about-it, towering trademark blasts, fans traced the ball from its inception off the bat. Seconds later, the crowd erupted when they noticed that the ball had barely cleared the fence. The distance didn't matter: no. sxity-two did. McGwire trotted around the bases and muscled himself into baseball immortality. As FOX announcer Joe Buck described the home run for millions of television viewers: "It's down the left-field line. . . . Is it enough? . . . Gone," Buck roared. "Don't forget to touch first base, Mac. You are the new single-season home run champion."

The game paused. Sosa rushed in from right field and congratulated him. McGwire hugged him and triumphantly lifted him in the air. Then he jogged into the stands and embraced the family of Roger Maris. The tear-dropping moment capped a radiant season for baseball, filled with hair-rising plots that weaved the sport back into the fabric of American culture. In McGwire, Americans were reminded that heroes still existed.

McGwire completed his awe-inspiring season with an unprecedented seventy long balls. But he wasn't the only one to conquer sixty-one: Sosa ended his season with sixty-six. McGwire proudly savored his exploits. "I don't think I will ever let go of the moment," McGwire explained to reporters after breaking Maris's record. "I don't know if I will ever be here again, so how can you let it go? What I have done is fabulous. I'm going to enjoy it right now."

For McGwire, however, the proud feeling of holding a record that had twice survived almost four decades lasted only two seasons. On the West Coast, in San Francisco, Barry Bonds eclipsed his mark of seventy by smashing seventy-three in 2001. Bonds's season for the ages overshadowed McGwire's. Baseball traditionalist began to question those inflated numbers and sensed the game's equilibrium had clearly changed. On Friday, October 5, while ESPN aired a game between the Cardinals and Astros, while McGwire was at-bat, the network interrupted to provide coverage of Bonds's first at-bat of the game in San Francisco as he embarked on the record. Bonds smashed no. seventy-one.

"What he's done is absolutely phenomenal. It's in the stratosphere," McGwire said after Bonds broke his record. "I know when I was going through it and not seeing pitches to hit, and then getting a pitch to hit. He just hasn't missed them. And the amazing thing is, everything he's hit, he's hit over the fence. That's hard to do. It's almost like he's playing T-ball."

Players were juicing, the game had changed, and McGwire knew it. "He was certainly surprised that the record was broken so soon," admitted Dave McKay, the first base coach for the Cardinals. "You think about how many hits you get a year and for seventy of them to be home runs? I thought, 'Who in the world would ever break that record?'"

By 2001, patellar tendinitis, a nagging injury stemming from his surgically repaired right knee, had sidelined him for parts of two seasons. The injury had also altered his approach and robbed him of his foundation at the plate, which is crucial for power hitters. After hitting sixty-five home runs in 1999, McGwire's production sunk the next two seasons. At thirty-seven, McGwire wrestled with the harsh reality that his injuries wouldn't allow him to play at the level he and his fans were accustomed. And with the emergence of hot-hitting outfield prospect Albert Pujols, who replaced him at first while he was injured, he recognized the Cardinals were in good hands. After fifteen seasons, McGwire, pondered retirement. McKay recalled:

> I knew it was going to be his last year before anyone. I kept telling Tony [La Russa] he's not coming back next year. He [McGwire] was pretty emotional when we talked about it. He told me, "they [fans] expect fifty home runs or more; I can't do that. Because of this ankle, I can't do that. I feel like I'm cheating these people and I don't want to cheat anyone." He expected so much out of himself and didn't want to go through the frustration of knowing what he's capable of doing and not being able to do it.

McKay tried to convince McGwire to play longer, suggesting that former Cardinals' star Jack Clark, who belted thirty-five home runs in 1987, had been a fan favorite in St. Louis. But it was a different era of baseball, and while thirty-five home runs was widely considered exceptional in the 1980s, the total had lost its dignity in the 1990s. Any total short of fifty or sixty, McGwire thought, would be considered a disappointment. "He told me, 'you don't understand; I won't wear this uniform next year,'" McKay recalled.

After McGwire batted only .187 and collected twenty-nine home runs during another injury-hampered season, the thirty-eight-year-old announced his retirement on Sunday, November 11, 2001. By retiring, he walked away from a guaranteed $30 million extension that would have stretched his career until 2003; the agreement had been reached with the Cardinals during spring training, but was shelved and never signed. Known for his explosive ability to hit balls farther than most and reviving the country's love for baseball, McGwire softly exited the game. Without the ego-feeding frenzy of a packed press conference, he called ESPN, claimed he was "worn out," and informed them that for the first time in seventeen years, he would not be headed to spring training in February.

> After considerable discussion with those closest to me, I have decided not to sign the extension, as I am unable to perform at a level equal to the salary the organization would be paying me. I believe I owe it to the Cardinals and the fans of St. Louis to step aside, so a talented free agent can be brought in as the final piece of what I expect can be a world championship–caliber team. So I am walking away from the game that has provided me opportunities, experiences, memories and friendships to fill 10 lifetimes.

Departing the game with 583 homers and three World Series appearances (1988–1990), he departed as baseball's most habitual power hitter, clearing the fences every 10.6 at-bats. Not even Babe Ruth, who hit a home run every 11.8 at-bats, boasted such frequency. Seventeen home runs shy of six hundred, a class that, at the time, only Hank Aaron (755), Ruth (714) and Willie Mays (660) graced, McGwire ranked fifth on the all-time home-run list. Media outlets across the country praised McGwire for his seemingly unselfish and noble deed. "That's just how he was," recalled Mickey Morabito, the A's traveling secretary. "He was quiet. He withdrew away from things and didn't seek any publicity for himself. At the end of his career, that's the way he was going to be."

McGwire's decision to hang up his spikes seemed well timed. By the fall of 2001, hints that several major league players were using steroids to enhance their physique and performance had emerged. Though baseball's members-only, tight-lipped steroid culture was no longer a secret, many wondered just how widespread the chemicals were in the sport. Concerns that baseball's most famed superstars could be breaking the law by chemically forging their careers and manipulating the integrity of the institution's sacred records had surfaced.

Columnist around the country finally felt at liberty to explore the issue and question the sobriety of America's pastime. What reporters had overlooked for more than a decade, pointing to other reasons associated with baseball's booming offensive revival, had now begun to make sense. Years of off-the-record suspicions of rapid muscle growth and a mysteriously sudden jolt of performance of several aging players had now validated whispers: rampant illegal steroid use had jaded the game, an evolution, some say, was inevitable. Colorful columnist Skip Bayless of the *San Jose Mercury News* wrote in October 2001:

This is no longer your grandfather's baseball. Many of baseball's most talented players have discovered the wonders of nutrition, strength training, supplements and—in some cases—testosterone boosters such as steroids, combined with heavy lifting. . . . When did baseball finally get off the couch? It started in the late 1980s. In Oakland, McGwire and José Canseco began competing in the weight room and experimenting with supplements.

Head trainers and conditioning coaches speculated that the growing numbers of tendon and ligament injuries could be traced to steroid use. Team doctors had also expressed concern over growing numbers of steroidal athletes in baseball and the health hazards associated with the unsupervised use of the chemicals. Former Major League superstar Ken Caminiti admitted to *Sports Illustrated* in 2002 that he juiced during his Most Valuable Player season in 1996. He also claimed that he had been one of hundreds of steroid users in baseball. The public gradually became aware of baseball's dark secret.

"It's no secret what's going on in baseball," admitted Caminiti, who had been the first major leaguer to freely disclose his steroid use. "At least half the guys are using steroids. They talk about it. They joke about it with each other."[7]

That performance-enhancing drugs could have played a significant role in the economic boom of baseball starting in 1998, enhancing the billion-dollar industry, spurred a public relation's nightmare for Major League Baseball. In June, Congress warned baseball owners and the MLBPA to solidify an agreement on a steroid policy at the bargaining table or U.S. lawmakers would be forced to intervene. "Like it or not, professional athletes serve as role models," Republican Senator John McCain told the Senate Commerce Committee in 2002. "That's more important than whether a group of highly paid athletes are using anabolic steroids."

Aside from the steroid crisis in baseball, though, the public's fascination had peaked. The possibilities that baseball's modern day crop of superstars, heroes to millions around the world, had cheated and diluted the sport, would surely be uncovered. The world anticipated.

NOTES

[1]   Doug Krikorian, "Dodgers Glad They Ordered Up a Piazza," *Long Beach Press-Telegram*, May 2, 1993.
[2]   Jeff Miller, "Is Bigger Better?" *Orange County Register*, March 28, 1998.
[3]   Thomas Boswell, "Lifting Raises Standards," *Washington Post*, July 9, 1996.
[4]   Rob Gloster, "Stairs Agrees to Two-year Contract," Associated Press, July 1, 1998.

5   Steve Wilstein, "'Andro' OK in Baseball, But Not Olympics," Associated Press, August 22, 1998.

6   Mike Lefkow, "Life in A," *Contra Costa Times*, June 28, 1998.

7   Tom Verducci, "Totally Juiced," *Sports Illustrated*, June 3, 2002.

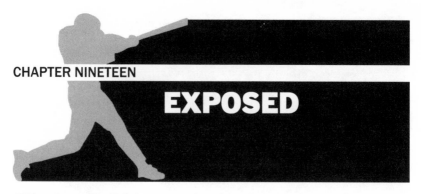

CHAPTER NINETEEN

EXPOSED

"When it was [José's] time to go, they threw him out the door. But they had no reason to and that's why he came out with the book. Because he was open to it [steroids] and spoke out about how he helped other players, they had to make him the guy that's crazy and the outcast. No doubt about it. Because if he's not, and [he's] telling the truth, baseball is fucked."

—Former teammate who preferred anonymity
July 2007

If Canseco had scoffed at McGwire's patriotic, country-adoring stroke in 1998, he certainly didn't convey it. While McGwire electrified the Midwest with unprecedented atomic blasts, up north, in Toronto, the home of Canseco's roof-shaving home run during the 1989 American Championship Series, the thirty-four-year-old Canseco held his own. He had signed a one-year, incentive-laden deal with a reported base salary of $750,000 in February and hoped to resurrect his injury-marred reputation. And he did. Smashing a career-high, forty-six home runs and stealing twenty-nine bases for the Blue Jays in 1998, he flashed his best season since 1988, when he accomplished the groundbreaking feat of hitting forty-two homers and swiping forty bases. The success Canseco had in Toronto helped land him $2.23 million, maximizing the worth of his contract. But that was an elementary amount compared to the $8,928,354 million his once fence-clearing partner McGwire earned in 1998.

Though Canseco had been clearly the more talented, marketable, and electric figure of the two during their prime, McGwire had passed him by. While McGwire rejuvenated baseball and tickled the country, the well-traveled Canseco scheduled court dates and battled for relevancy, pitching his hitter-for-hire services. A decade earlier, the strapping twenty-four-year-old Canseco had boldly grabbed second base and arrogantly lifted it over his head at Milwaukee's County Stadium to confirm his glory as baseball's best specimen. Now McGwire had trumped that feat by flaunting seventy, while saluting Roger Maris in the process. Still, Canseco applauded his former foil. "Mark McGwire to me is the most dominating power hitter baseball has ever seen," Canseco said in September 1998. "Maybe in your lifetime and your children's lifetime."[1] Canseco also raved about McGwire's Herculean build, providing reporters with stimulating thought. "There is, first of all, the man's size," Canseco told Gordon Edes of the *Boston Globe* in 1998. "You don't understand—McGwire is huge. The man has twenty-two-inch forearms. With any other man, those are bodybuilder's arms. They're four times as big as mine." Perhaps Canseco hoped the media would catch on and investigate how McGwire ballooned his physique over the years.

Canseco harbored McGwire's dark secret throughout his career. After leaving Toronto after the 1998 season, Canseco played on three teams in as many years. Despite playing a year and a half in Tampa Bay near his home, he also played briefly with the world champion New York Yankees in 2000. Chronic back problems haunted him and landed him on the disabled list several times, though. By that time his health, allegedly marred by steroids, scared teams away. As one former manager described, "A shadow seemed to follow him wherever he went." In 2001, Canseco, for the first time since he was drafted in 1982, signed a minor league contract with the Anaheim Angels. After batting .231 in thirteen games during spring training, though, thirty-six-year-old Canseco was released for the first time in his seventeen-year career. "This is the first time my ability has ever been questioned," Canseco said after learning of his release in 2001. "It's very awkward. It's beyond belief. I'll probably stay up all night trying to figure it out."[2]

Things became worse when no other teams expressed interest in him, deeming him a bulked up, broken down, one-dimensional player. Humbled and desperate, Canseco latched onto his brother, Ozzie, then with the Newark Bears of the Independent Atlantic League. The previous season Ozzie had clubbed forty-eight homers for the Bears, shattering the Atlantic League record. The reunion would mark the first time he and Ozzie played together since 1990, when they played in Oakland. The reunion didn't last long, however. After batting .284 with seven home runs and twenty-seven RBIs in forty-one games, Canseco was plucked by the Chicago White Sox. The team desperately hoped to fill the void of injured slugger Frank Thomas. Wanting to prove his critics wrong and only fifty-four home runs shy of five hundred, a milestone that had at the time been a ticket into the Hall of

Fame, Canseco returned to the majors. "It's so close I can taste it," Canseco told the *New York Daily News*. Canseco projected he could reach the five-hundred mark in a year and a half. But he also provided punch in the White Sox lineup and meshed well in the clubhouse. "It's a great thing [having Canseco in Chicago] and at the same time, it's kind of sad that a guy who's achieved as much as he has was having to go down to an independent team," teammate Royce Clayton said in 2001. "You look at all the teams in baseball, and they could use a José Canseco."[3]

Canseco muscled closer to five hundred. He averaged a home run every sixteen at-bats for the White Sox. Having already smashed fifteen homers, at an away game against New York on October 3, he faced Mike Mussina. Canseco, needing only thirty-nine more long balls to reach his goal, strolled to the plate, sensing this could be the final series of his checkered career. With healthy designated hitter Frank Thomas scheduled to return to the White Sox the following season, Canseco could be the odd man out. His former club, the Oakland A's, the organization that had drafted him in the fifteenth round as a skinny seventeen-year-old from Miami's Coral Park High in 1982, were rolling into New York the following week to play the Yankees in the American League Division Series.

After Mussina, the same pitcher who had been on the mound when he was dealt to the Texas Rangers in 1992, hurled a pitch in the top of the fourth, Canseco homered no. 462, ranking him twenty-second on the all-time home-run list. Uncertain of his future, Canseco trotted around the bases, savoring each step. "This game has taught me a lot of things and one of them is not to take anything for granted," Canseco told reporters after the game. "Today could be my last at-bat forever. It's a shocking experience no doubt.

"I won't retire. One thing is I'm not a quitter. I never have been and never will be. It's going to take a lot more than that to get me out of the game."

Remaining in the game, though, was out of his control. That trot around the bases in baseball's most marquee stage marked the close of Canseco's colorful career. The following year, in 2002, Canseco inked a minor league deal with the Montreal Expos, but they cut him during the final week of the spring. Though the Expos offered to retain him as an everyday player for their Triple-A club, he declined. In April, Canseco gave it one last shot with the White Sox Triple-A affiliate in Charlotte, North Carolina, and smacked five home runs in eighteen games. Canseco showed he still had pop, but remained in the minor leagues. "The No. 1 thing is that he can still play; this guy has something to offer," White Sox general manager Ken Williams said in May

2002. "And as far as other teams' interest or lack thereof, I can't explain it. I don't understand it."[4]

Canseco couldn't understand it, either. That didn't bode well with the life-steering chip that already rested on his broad shoulders. Although ageless players like Andrés Galarraga, forty-one; Julio Franco, forty-three; and Rickey Henderson, forty-three; had all managed to sell their services to clubs, Canseco, the same age as Barry Bonds at thirty-seven years old, couldn't find an employer. Already feeling that as a Cuban-born superstar dominating an American sport he had been robbed of icon citizenship, the six-time All-Star searched for answers. The most electrifying player in the game in the late 1980s, Canseco was now enduring long bus rides, living out of a suitcase in hotel rooms, and playing at Knights Stadium in Charlotte, facing rejection and pleading for a job.

Those elements seemed all too mysterious for Canseco. Playing in three decades of baseball, he had witnessed the metamorphosis of the sport. He courted steroids in 1985 and soon forged a career-changing romance with the drugs. The affair made him an ambassador for steroids on every team he played. He introduced his fascination to other players. They enjoyed and profited from the benefits, too. Now the sport had betrayed him. Major League Baseball rejected him and he wondered if his association with steroids was the reason why. Peers whispered in his ear. "I've heard from top players in the game, guys making $20 million a year, that I'm being blackballed and conspired against," Canseco said while playing with the Knights. "Every player knows it. The truth will have to come out eventually."[5]

Canseco mentioned that Texas Rangers' Alex Rodriguez and former major league pitcher Alex Fernandez, who had both worked out with Canseco at his Florida home several times in the late 1990s, informed him of the conspiracy. He also confirmed that major league officials told him that teams were collectively plucking him out of the sport. Figuring that teams were essentially banning him from their clubhouses, he wondered if he had been wasting his time trying to climb back into the majors in Charlotte. So, after hitting a lackluster .172, Canseco, thirty-eight home runs shy of five hundred, painfully announced his retirement on Monday, May 13, 2002. In a statement, Canseco claimed he wanted to spend more time with his daughter, Josie. "He still should be proud of himself," said Mike Piazza, after learning of Canseco's retirement. "He really did a lot to further the game and raise the bar for all the players today."[6]

In what ways Canseco furthered the game would be uncovered. Days later, Canseco announced that he and former *Tampa Tribune* sportswriter Bill Chastain would collaborate on a tell-all book unveiling epidemic steroid use in baseball. Uncovering baseball's dark secret, he claimed, would also shed light on why he was exiled from the game. Canseco described, in an interview with FOX Sports radio mogul Jim Rome, that 85 percent of major leaguers were juicing. He claimed his book would be the most shocking in baseball history. "It's (steroids) completely restructured the game as we know it," Canseco told Rome. "That's why guys are hitting fifty or sixty or seventy-five home runs."

His plans to pen his memoir prompted many big leaguers and the media to ridicule and disregard his claims, portraying him as a money-hungry, bitter player who had lost millions during Silicon Valley's dot-com crash. Weeks later, the awareness that steroids had saturated baseball heightened when Ken Caminiti, the National League's Most Valuable Player in 1996, told *Sports Illustrated* that he had used steroids during that season. In the same piece, authored by Tom Verducci, Arizona Diamondback's pitcher Curt Schilling also confirmed the steroid culture in baseball. "I'm not sure how it [steroid use] snuck in so quickly, but it's become a prominent thing very quietly. It's widely known in the game."[7] Three years later, before Congress, Schilling, though, claimed he grossly overstated the problem.

Jason Giambi, who had signed a $120 million, seven-year contract with the New York Yankees on December 13, 2001, scoffed at Caminiti and Canseco's allegations. Six foot three with a beefy physique, Giambi called the claims that steroids were widely used in baseball as "ludicrous." Asked by the *New York Post* if he had ever used illegal steroids, he vehemently denied it.

> I never thought about it. Until I met Mark [McGwire] I never even lifted [weights]. He got me on the program of lifting, and I have the frame at six foot three to carry it off. I got around Mark and hired a trainer. There is something to be said about doing it the right way.[8]

The rumblings directed focus on the legitimacy of thirty-seven-year-old Barry Bonds of the San Francisco Giants, the poster child for increased performance at an age when most players start to decline. "Doctors ought to quit worrying about what ballplayers are taking," Bonds told the Associated Press in 2002, when asked of doctors' concerns over steroid use. Bonds claimed doctors should be concentrating on finding a cure for cancer. "What players take doesn't matter. It's nobody else's business."

The growing concern over the players' health and the game's integrity prompted owners and MLBPA to establish a steroid-testing program in August 2002. Players would be randomly tested for illegal steroids over the next two years (2003–4). The results would be used as an anonymous survey to gauge the scope of the problem. The policy stated that if 2.5 percent or fewer tested positive in consecutive years, mandatory random testing would cease. The Players Association, which had long opposed steroid testing citing privacy concerns for its clients, agreed that implementing testing was a step in the right direction. "We want it," Paul Lo Duca, the Los Angeles Dodger Players Association representative, told the *San Diego Tribune* in August 2002. "It's no big deal to us. It's going to be a pretty strict test, and that's the way it should be."

Though Canseco was a catalyst for creating an awareness of the ongoing steroid crisis, he spent most of the ensuing months battling for his freedom. In November, Canseco and brother, Ozzie, reluctantly pleaded guilty of felony aggravated battery and two counts of misdemeanor battery in a Miami courtroom; they had allegedly broken a man's nose during a tussle at Opium Garden, a Miami Beach nightclub, on Halloween night in 2001. "We basically took a plea bargain," Canseco later told Greta Van Susteren of FOX News Channel.

Though Canseco eluded jail time, Miami-Dade circuit judge Leonard Glick sentenced Canseco to three years of probation and 250 hours of community service. The charges would later haunt him after he violated probation for failing to adhere to the court-ordered provisions. One provision prohibited Canseco from leaving the state for more than thirty days; he had been in California tending to a custody battle for close to forty-five days. He also violated his probation by failing to enroll in anger management classes and failing to make monthly reports to his probation officer. "[Canseco] does not appear to take probation seriously," senior probation officer Ileana Ortiz said in court documents obtained by the *Miami Herald* in 2003.

On Valentine's Day, 2003, Judge Glick issued an arrest warrant on Canseco.[9] Canseco flew back to Florida and arrived in court four days later to surrender. "I understand that I have to take responsibility," Canseco told Glick in the courtroom. "I ask for the mercy and understanding of the court."

"No bond," said Glick, who ordered officers to take Canseco into custody. Canseco, facing fifteen years in prison, handed his wallet and silver necklace to his attorney, Gustavo Lage. Officers handcuffed the former Most Valuable Player and escorted him to the jury box.[10] That Canseco was jailed provided more ammunition for media and players to scorn at him and for him to write a book. Wrote Bay Area columnist Carl Steward:

> Don't hold your breath waiting for it to come out, even if José makes the most of his idle time. While Canseco promised he will name names in this projected tell-all tome, it's highly possible he has not considered

two words that may deter high-profile publishers from moving forward on it—libel and slander.[11]

On March 17, after spending about a month in jail, Canseco was released. Glick soon sentenced him to two years of house arrest, however. But even more trouble found the Canseco family. After police stopped Ozzie's Lincoln Navigator because his tinted windows were too dark, officers discovered a syringe and the illegal steroid Nandrolone in the vehicle. He was also driving with a suspended license. Police arrested Ozzie.

Back at his one-and-a-half-acre guard-gated home in Davie, Florida, serving his house arrest, Canseco profited from his confinement. Launching his website, www.josecanseco.com, he offered his loyal fans an opportunity to come to his home and spend a day with him. For sale on the site, Canseco also peddled several articles of baseball memorabilia he accumulated through the years, including his 1989 Oakland A's World Championship ring. On the online auction site eBay Canseco sold his 1988 Most Valuable Player plaque for $30,000 and his 1986 Rookie of the Year ring for $5,100. "Spend a day with José," as his website described, propositioned bids of $2,500 to spend four hours with Canseco. Doug Ames, his agent, claimed the campaign was geared toward rejuvenating Canseco's battered image.

But the slumber parties at Canseco's home were short-lived. Three months into serving his house arrest, after submitting a court-ordered urine analysis on June 3, Canseco allegedly tested positive for steroids, according to court documents. The probation violation landed him in jail. While Canseco denied he had used steroids during that period, attorney Richard Rosenbaum requested at a July 7 court hearing that the courts hospitalize Canseco, an admitted long-term steroid abuser, for a psychological and physical examination, according to the *Miami Herald*.[12] "It appears that steroids can be as addictive as any other substance out there," Rosenbaum told Judge Glick.

After prosecutors asked why Canseco hadn't sought treatment for his addiction before incarceration, Glick denied Rosenbaum's request and ordered Canseco to remain in custody. He did offer Canseco treatment while incarcerated at Miami's Turner Guilford Knight Correctional Center. What made matters worse was that Ozzie was also incarcerated in the facility. In an interview with Greta Van Susteren of FOX New Channel on July 21, 2003, Canseco reflected on life behind bars.

> The truth will come out. If—if the public and my friends and my family—look, my friends and my family know the truth. I think if the public is a little patient, the truth is definitely going to come out. I have been definitely mistreated.

Canseco's high-profile defense team, Jayne Weintraub and José Quinon, however, soon attacked the reliability of his urine specimen. They argued that Canseco had used steroids for decades and that could have triggered the positive test that violated his probation. The scientific proof of how long steroids could remain in the body now controlled the case's fate. The defense suggested that prosecutors couldn't provide the burden of proof necessary to prove Canseco had used steroids after he was sentenced to probation in November. The strategy worked. On August 25, the state dropped charges on Canseco, admitting it was "progressively unclear" when he had used illegal steroids.[13] After serving over two months in jail, Canseco was released. Asked by Greta Van Susteren what it felt like to be released:

Well, I'll tell you it's—it's—it was a nightmare being in there for two plus months, and I can't believe I'm home. I can't believe I'm here with my family. I was just sitting outside before this call, out there, out there in the grass, actually, with my dogs, just—you know—when you're surrounded by brick walls for two-and-a-half months, just seeing the simple things, you know, grass, the trees, the wind blowing—it's just incredible.[14]

The *San Francisco Chronicle* soon reported that on Wednesday, September 3, 2003, investigators from the Internal Revenue Service, the San Mateo Narcotics Task Force, and the U.S. Food and Drug Administration, raided the Bay Area Laboratory Co-Operative, BALCO. During the search, they seized doping calendars, illegal performance-enhancing drugs, and hundreds of urine samples. Two days later, agents also raided the Burlingame, California, home of Greg Anderson, an associate of BALCO and Bonds's long-time friend and weight trainer. The investigators seized $60,000 in cash, an array of suspected performance-enhancing drugs, and documentation that suggested steroid use of several athletes, including Bonds.[15]

The findings led to several professional athletes, including current and former major leaguers, Jason Giambi, Benito Santiago, Marvin Benard, Bobby Estalella, and Randy Velarde being subpoenaed to testify before a federal grand jury in San Francisco. On December 4, 2003, Bonds told a federal grand jury he used a clear substance and cream given to him by his trainer, Greg Anderson. He also emphasized that he didn't know they were steroids, according to leaked transcripts acquired by the *San Francisco Chronicle*. Jason Giambi also admitted to a federal grand jury on December 11, 2003, that he took steroids obtained from Greg Anderson, according to leaked transcripts acquired by the *Chronicle*.

In November 2003, Major League Baseball announced the results of the random survey, which had been agreed on in the 2002 labor agreement—between 5 and 7 percent of players had tested positive for steroids. Because dozens of players tested positive out of an anonymous 1,438 tests, a testing program carrying disciplinary measures, including unpaid suspensions, would be implemented the following season. If a player tested positive, his name would also be publicly identified. That spurred noticeable changes in the game. In 2004, home-run totals dropped and physiques dwindled. Superstars Jason Giambi and Sammy Sosa arrived to spring training noticeably thinner, and for the first time since 1994, the strike-shortened season, no player reached fifty home runs. Baseball, it seemed, was going through detoxification.

That baseball's doping scandal had dominated newspaper headlines across the country tapped Canseco back into the spotlight. Canseco decided to attend an open tryout for the Los Angeles Dodgers in Vero Beach, Florida, the following March. Many questioned his motives for attending, claiming he would use the opportunity to promote his book, tentatively titled, *Dare to Truth*. Canseco, who had moved to Encino, California, to live closer to Josie year round and explore an acting career after his release, flew back to Florida. When he arrived, he was handed player identification no. 521 to plant on his back. While the Dodgers had informed Canseco in advance that his chances of receiving a contract were bleak, he held onto hope and believed he could return to playing shape in weeks. Playing first base during an intra-squad game, his two-year hiatus from organized baseball showed. Of his eighteen swings in batting practice, the rusty Canseco hit one ball over the fence. Said former A's teammate Doug Jennings, who also attended the tryout:

> He was legitimately trying to get back, I think. He wanted to still get close to 500 [home runs]. He felt like he was cheated away from the Hall of Fame and that's one of the reasons he was on such a major vendetta against Major League Baseball. He got close and did well, but they released him and didn't bring him back. He was always disgruntled with the whole system. He was telling me about his book that was coming out and he was going to expose everybody.

After the tryout, reporters probed him about the details in his rumored steroid-littered memoir, but he answered, "Read the book. "This is probably going to be my last attempt—see you in the movies," confirmed Canseco as he wandered off.

Canseco soon collaborated with former Oakland A's beat writer Steve Kettmann, who covered him in 1997 for the *San Francisco*

Chronicle, to ghostwrite his manuscript. Kettmann knew Canseco through a colleague, Pedro Gomez, the A's beat writer for the *Sacramento Bee* in 1997 and former classmate of Canseco at Miami's Coral Park High.[16] How steroids had infected baseball had always stirred Kettmann. In August 2000, he penned a prophetic piece for the *New York Times*, entitled "Baseball Must Come Clean On Its Darkest Secret." That secret landed Canseco a book advance of $300,000 from controversial publisher Regan Books, a former imprint of Harper-Collins. Canseco also secured an interview upon the book's release with Mike Wallace on CBS's *60 Minutes*. Ironically, *Washington Post* columnist Thomas Boswell first cited Canseco as "the most conspicuous example of a player who made himself great through steroids" on CBS in 1988, a charge Canseco had vehemently denied.

In February 2005, the *New York Daily News* leaked Canseco's explosive allegations in his book, claiming he injected former Bash Brother Mark McGwire with steroids and introduced a handful of players to the drugs. The paper reported that Canseco also acknowledged that he introduced the drug to former teammates Rafael Palmeiro, Juan Gonzalez, and Ivan Rodriguez.

The charges elicited strong reactions around baseball. McGwire, who observers claimed lost more than forty pounds since retirement, was enjoying life away from the public eye on the golf course in Shady Canyon's gated community in Irvine, California. After learning of Canseco's claims, he responded. "Once and for all, I did not use steroids nor any illegal substance," McGwire said in a statement to *60 Minutes*. "The relationship that these allegations portray could not be further from the truth."

Another player, Rafael Palmeiro, who grew up and played baseball with Canseco in the Miami area, now distanced himself from him and adamantly denied his use. "I categorically deny any assertion made by José Canseco that I used steroids," Palmeiro said in a statement. "At no point in my career have I ever used steroids, let alone any substance banned by Major League Baseball."

On Monday, February 14, the two-year anniversary after Judge Glick issued a warrant for his arrest, Canseco's highly anticipated book, *Juiced: Wild Times, Rampant 'Roids, Smash Hits and How Baseball Got Big*, hit the shelves and rocked Major League Baseball. The accusations infuriated Canseco's former teammates and coaches. They ripped his credibility and defended the accused, alleging he squandered a fortune and would go so as far as to manufacture lies to recoup his losses. That didn't sway customers. Amazon.com ranked *Juiced* as the third most popular book on its site.

"I'm so pissed off at him," said Tony La Russa, after learning of

Canseco's claims. "First of all, I think he needs the money. Secondly, I think he's jealous as hell. José had a head start over Mark and screwed it up. The jealousy eats at him."[17]

Others took a different angle to discredit Canseco. Former A's strength and conditioning coach Dave McKay questioned Canseco's mental health and wondered if he had slipped into a trance. McKay said after the release:

> I'm starting to think that maybe José has something wrong with him. He'd tell you a story and you'd know he was making it up, and he'd know it, too. A couple of months later, he'd tell it again and he believed it. You'd tell him it wasn't true. Maybe he believes this now. Maybe he believes he injected Mark McGwire.[18]

The string of denials and character assassination of Canseco was inevitable, said a former teammate, who prefers anonymity. He said baseball had no choice but to smear Canseco.

> When it was his time to go, they threw him out the door. But they had no reason to and that's why he came out with the book. Because he was open to it [steroids] and spoke out about how he helped other players, they had to make him the guy that's crazy and the outcast. No doubt about it. Because if he's not, and [he's] telling the truth, baseball is fucked.

More shocking information labeled McGwire as a steroid user. In March 2005, the *New York Daily News* reported McGwire's name had surfaced during a major federal steroids probe in the early 1990s, citing FBI sources. The investigation, dubbed "Operation Equine," focused on suppliers, preventing agents from targeting McGwire. Two dealers who were nabbed by authorities, however, claimed former steroid dealer Curtis Wenzlaff, a friend of Reggie Jackson's, provided steroids to McGwire and Canseco. One informant alleged Wenzlaff had injected McGwire several times at a Southern California gym, according to the *Daily News*.[19] The groundbreaking report added more unease to baseball's troubled past. Canseco said he had worked out with Wenzlaff, but never obtained steroids from him. McGwire, through his spokesman, Marc Altieri, told the paper he didn't remember Wenzlaff.

Decades of baseball's discreet and neglected past had haunted the sport. The growing crisis raised the eyebrows of U.S. lawmakers in Washington, D.C. They hoped to eradicate steroids from baseball and curb their appeal to overzealous, young athletes by posing its health dangers. The Committee on Government Reform decided to invite a lineup of former and current major league players, including four executives, to attend a congressional hearing on Thursday, March 17, 2005. Mark McGwire, Sammy Sosa, Jason Giambi, Rafael Palmeiro, Frank Thomas, Curt Schilling, and José Canseco were all encouraged to attend the hearing. Also summoned to Capitol Hill were high-ranking baseball executives Sandy Alderson and Rob Manfred, San Diego Padres' general manager Kevin Towers, and Donald Fehr, executive director of Major League Baseball Players Association. A trail of documents tracking baseball's steroid and drug policies since 1970, as well as anonymous test results and penalties since steroid testing began in 2003, were also subpoenaed.

"The committee will conduct a thorough, fair, and responsible investigation. It is important the American people know the facts on baseball's steroid scandal," committee chairman Rep. Tom Davis and Rep. Henry Waxman, the ranking Democrat, confirmed in a statement.

But the House Government Reform Committee faced polite resistance. Though Canseco, Fehr, and Manfred had agreed to attend the hearing, several players respectfully declined. Thomas, who had long been an outspoken proponent of eliminating steroids in baseball, requested to be excused. He claimed that his flight to Washington, D.C., would hinder the recovery of his injured ankle. Palmeiro also asked the committee to be excused, since he claimed the day of the hearing fell on his wife's birthday. Sosa also declined the invitation. Those excuses didn't soften Congress. The committee played hardball with Major League Baseball and fired a head-ducking fastball, demanding their attention. On March 9, the committee flexed their own political muscle and dropped eleven subpoenas on players and executives, including those who had already vowed to attend.

"These people are not above the law," Tom Davis said on NBC's *Meet the Press* on March 13. "They may fly in private planes and make millions of dollars and be on baseball cards, but a subpoena is exactly what it says it is. They have to appear."

The subpoenas infuriated Stanley Brand, a lawyer for Major League Baseball, who accused the committee of misusing its power. He claimed that the steroid probe was beyond the committee's scope of jurisdiction and would interfere with collective bargaining and breach baseball's first amendment privacy rights. Dragging a player from retirement and those playing with their clubs in spring training and suddenly dropping them before Congress's critical eye was unfair, according to Brand. What fueled his frustration was that the two-year-old steroid-testing program had already proved effective and appeared to be pruning steroids from the sport. Since 5 to 7 percent of players tested positive for steroids in 2003, the percentage had trickled down to 2 percent in 2004. Why Congress would criticize an already effective program, according to empirical data, dumbfounded him. "It was already successful and that was my contention," said Brand. "By the time those hearings were held the steroid era was over. The mere threat of survey testing scared most players from doing it."

Additionally, with Giambi's testimony in the ongoing federal investigation of California's Bay Area Laboratory Co-Operative, the hearings could interfere with the case. Brand vowed to fight the subpoenas through federal district court. "It is an excessive and unprecedented misuse of congressional power," he said to reporters during a conference call.

Congress fired back. U.S. lawmakers confirmed they possessed the votes to hold the subpoenaed players and officials in contempt of Congress if they failed to appear. The criminal offense could hand fines up to $1,000 and a maximum one-year sentence for a person. The committee also threatened to revoke baseball's antitrust exception and its tax breaks if they defiantly continued to battle subpoenas.

Brand subdued his position. It was rumored that Major League Baseball and the Players Association began bargaining with the committee behind the scenes, trying to juggle and generate their own line-up card for the hearing. Eliminating crucial subpoenaed players and replacing them with others could prevent a public relation's nightmare for baseball. And with McGwire and Sosa, the two muscle-bound heroes that shouldered baseball back into America's hearts in 1998, scheduled to testify under oath before a body of finger-pointing Congress people, any hint of guilt could smear baseball's heart-pounding resurrection.

San Francisco Chronicle columnist Gwen Knapp confirmed that speculation in a compelling column days before the hearing.

> If McGwire testifies, the magic of 1998 could dissolve. If he says that José Canseco's book is correct, that the two of them used steroids when they played in Oakland, his well-tended reputation will collapse and baseball's image will move another ten steps closer to professional wrestling.

Many sensationalized the hearings as Steroid-Gate and claimed the integrity of America's Pastime was at stake. Fans wondered if the carnival of home runs during the 1990s and 2000s, which awakened fading fan interest, was a chemically fueled hoax. Had performance-enhancing drugs muscled baseball into a billion-dollar empire but ultimately spit on the sport's sacred records? That a central figure of the controversy was missing from the list was baffling. Many wondered why Congress refused to subpoena Barry Bonds. He was baseball's active all-time home-run leader and the most publicized star embedded in the federal investigation. His absence diluted the hearings.

"They [Congress] understood he was never going to come, even if subpoenaed," explained Brand, founder of Brand Law Group in Washington, D.C. "No lawyer—in his right mind—would let him testify at a time when a grand jury [investigation] was hanging over his head."

One significant luminary that decided to show up was Major League Baseball commissioner Bud Selig. Though he had initially offered to send Rob Manfred, one of his five executive vice presidents, to represent him on the panel, he felt compelled to report on the successful strides baseball had made since establishing a testing program. "The players stepped up this past January for an even stricter drug policy beginning this season demonstrating that all of us in baseball are committed to reaching zero tolerance," Selig said in a statement.

The congressional hearings also spurred another unprecedented development: Major League Baseball and the Players Association, widely known for their notoriously fierce quarrels with each other at the collective bargaining table, had suddenly formed a comical, self-serving alliance. That alliance convinced Congress to excuse Giambi from attending the hearing, citing his involvement in the BALCO probe as the reason for his dismissal. Both sides now could mull over the scope of questioning that would be posed to players during the hearing.

The depth of the probes concerned Canseco, who was still on probation in Florida. Just how far Congress would delve into his steroid-littered past could caution him into exercising his Fifth Amendment right. He also wanted to freely discuss his claims that baseball had conspired against him by pruning him out the game and thoroughly expose baseball's rampant steroid use before Congress. But without assurance that his frank statements wouldn't land him back in jail, Canseco requested immunity.

"If they don't give us immunity, we'll take one question at a time and answer those that we can," Canseco's attorney Robert Saunooke told Pat Halpin of FOX News Channel's *Hannity & Colmes* days before the congressional hearings. "We've said already that, you know, José is willing, ready, we cooperated, we want to tell the story, we want people to know about baseball. But if they are going to expose him to possible criminal liability we're not going to answer them."

That was the fate Canseco faced. On the eve of the hearings, Congress denied his request, adding a twist that, Suanooke claimed, questioned the purpose of the hearings. If Congress intended to completely investigate steroid use in baseball, restraining Canseco from fully exposing his experiences would water down the hearings. "They effectively cut the legs off from underneath us," fumed Suanooke.

Still, with the heated reunion of the retired Bash Brothers and a sprinkle of baseball's most prolific players and shrewd executives scheduled to march onto Capitol Hill, a hero-worshipping country focused on Washington, D.C. Amid a dark cloud of hypocrisy, epidemic cheating, head-turning greed, and a rumored cover-up hovering over Major League Baseball, one wondered if baseball possessed the fortitude to survive.

"My interest has been piqued tremendously by the very defensive reaction of Major League Baseball. It's really outrageous," said Christopher Shays, the second-ranking Republican on the committee. "We're not trying to embarrass anyone, unless they embarrass themselves."

NOTES

[1]   Gordon Edes, "His Better Half Canseco Says He Knew McGwire Could Do It," *Boston Globe*, September 10, 1998.

[2]   Cheryl Rosenberg, "Canseco Released as Angels Get Hill," *Orange County Register*, March 29, 2001.

[3]   Jose Miguel Romero and Bob Sherwin, "Canseco Has Had Impact for Chicago," *Seattle Times*, August 11, 2001.

[4]   Stan Olson, "Canseco in Major-League Exile," *Charlotte Observer*, May 12, 2002.

[5]   Dan Le Batard, "Blinded by Hurt and Anger, Canseco Sees Conspiracy," *Miami Herald*, April 28, 2002.

[6]   Nancy Armour, "Canseco Retires," Associated Press, May 14, 2002.

[7]   Tom Verducci, "Totally Juiced," *Sports Illustrated*, June 3, 2002.

[8]   George King and Mike Morrissey, "Yanks, Mets in 'Roid Rage," *New York Post*, May 30, 2002.

[9]   Joan Fleischman, "Warrant Issued for Canseco," *Miami Herald*, February 15, 2003.

[10] Lisa Arthur, "Canseco Is Jailed for Violating Probation," *Miami Herald*, February 19, 2003.

[11] Carl Steward, "As Barry Rides High Jose Hits Bottom," *Daily Review*, February 20, 2003.

[12] Trenton Daniel, "Judge Denies Request, Sends Canseco Back to Jail," *Miami Herald*, July 8, 2003.

[13] Jay Weaver, "Canseco Ends 9 Weeks in Jail But Is Still Under House Arrest," *Miami Herald*, August 26, 2003.

[14] Greta Van Susteren, Interview with Jose Canseco, FOX News Channel, August 25, 2003.

[15] Mark Fainaru-Wada and Lance Williams, "How the Doping Scandal

Unfolded," *San Francisco Chronicle*, December 21, 2003.

16 Interview with Steve Kettman, Amateur Athletic Foundation's SportLetter, April 2005, http://www.la84foundation.org/10ap/ SportsLetter-16-1/SLhome.html#st7.

17 John Shea, "Canseco Swings Away in *Juiced*," *San Francisco Chronicle*, February 7, 2005.

18 Jack Curry, "Canseco Is Only One Doing Bashing Now," *New York Times*, February 13, 2005

19 Michael O'Keeffe, Christian Red, and T. J. Quinn, "McGwire Juiced," *New York Daily News*, March 12, 2005.

CHAPTER TWENTY

A LEGACY SUBPOENAED

"Watching them before Congress took me back to when I was an innocent kid and rooted for the A's. As much as you don't want to believe it, you kind of take a step back and realize they probably were cheating at the time. Not only did they cheat baseball and themselves, they cheated all the innocent little kids like myself. José Canseco and Mark McGwire were my heroes, and even though I'm a grown man, it hurt to watch that."

—Washington Nationals catcher Johnny Estrada
2007

March 17, 2005. As mobs of photographers and reporters crammed into room 2154 inside the Rayburn House Office Building in Washington, D.C., tensions mounted. At 2.375 million square feet, Rayburn boasted the largest dimensions of the three congressional office buildings and seemed the perfect host for two larger-than-life figures. The intrigue traveled beyond Capitol Hill, though. Dozens of Congress people sat on the dias as cameras flickered throughout the room. While some dubbed their motives to launch the congressional probe as pure political grandstanding, others felt they were deeply concerned over a sport they loved.

McGwire marched in first. Surrounded by a parade of attention that he had always shunned when he circled the bases as a player, he sat before the House Oversight and Government Reform Committee. Though he appeared polished and cooperative and even sported a green tie because of St. Patrick's Day, he cringed. After being handed his subpoena two weeks prior, McGwire couldn't understand how his presence could help eradicate steroids from the game. Figuring he would be poked with steroid-laced questions about how those chemicals might have fueled his 583 career home runs, he reluctantly crawled out of retirement. Since he disappeared from the game after the 2001 season, forty-two-year-old McGwire had faded into Orange County's Shady Canyon, a luxurious gated kingdom featuring one of the nation's most exclusive golf courses. It was in Irvine, California, where he had recently purchased two lots on the thousand-acre development to build a custom home. In the sheltered community, he set his sights on his new career as a devoted husband and full-time father.

ESPN.com investigative reporter Wright Thompson wrote a riveting piece titled "Fading Away" in 2006, detailing McGwire's hermit-like exile. He had traveled to Orange County to hunt McGwire down and get the scoop. "I was surprised that he was not only shut off from media; but he was shut off from a lot of people that used to be in his life," Thompson confirmed. During his quest, Thompson dropped by one of McGwire's financial advisers and even left a business card with his secretary. He didn't receive a response. "He doesn't even have a 'no comment' mechanism," said Thompson.

His journey into McGwire's elusiveness helped shape his article. Describing McGwire's sheltered lifestyle behind the guard-gated community of Shady Canyon, Thompson wrote:

> He likes it here on lots 82 and 83 in the Shady Canyon neighborhood, billed as a place for folks with "quiet wealth." Far from the glitz of Beverly Hills and from the O.C.'s ocean-front palaces, it's for people who don't want to be found. A computer system scans license plates for undesirables; security guards stop strangers and, if a home owner doesn't say "yes," send them on their way. From the outside, the houses look like battleships.[1]

Spending time with his second wife, Stephanie, whom he met in St. Louis, and his two toddlers, two-year-old Max and one-year-old Mason, was his priority. Because of his rigorous travel schedule as a major leaguer, McGwire was never able to concentrate year-round on raising his first son, Matthew, who was seventeen years old at the time of the hearing. That pushed him to provide full-time fatherhood to Max and Mason.

McGwire relished retirement. No matter how many offers he received to return to the game, he was stubbornly staying put. Walt Jocketty, the general manager of the St. Louis Cardinals, and manager Tony La Russa asked him if he wanted to return as an honorary coach and tutor up-and-coming players on his terms. McGwire declined. Being away from the boisterous crowds and nagging reporters provided tranquility for him, as did spending obsessive amounts of time on Shady Canyon's golf course. Due to chronic back problems during his final seasons, he wasn't able to play much golf. That changed when he retired. He returned to the sport he cherished as a boy when he caddied for his father, John, at Sierra LaVerne Country Club in Southern California.

His rejuvenated affair with golf elevated his stroke. As an amateur golfer, he even won the PGA Tour's ADT Golf Skills Challenge at Florida's Boca Raton Golf Resort in 2003, edging top-tier golfers Greg Norman, Peter Jacobsen, Nick Faldo, and Paul Azinger. Established golfers marveled at his stroke and felt, in time, he could one day join the PGA Tour. "He has one of the finest golf swings in the game," Peter Jacobsen raved after the competition. "We couldn't find anything wrong with it. Mark has no flaws in his swing."[2]

Besides rekindling his passion for golf, though, McGwire found that his once muscle-packed, 250-pound physique had withered into the lanky frame he carried during the infant stages of his career. In many ways, leaving baseball steered him back to his former self. As reporter T.J. Quinn of the *New York Daily News* wrote in December 2003:

> The best guess is that he has dropped forty pounds since he last swung a bat. The Mark McGwire who once personified baseball hugeness, who strained uniform seams with muscles most people don't even know they have, who introduced the word "andro" to the American public, now just looks like a large, but ultimately human, man.[3]

Not that those muscles could have helped him dodge Congress's arrows. The Congress-issued subpoena had inconvenienced McGwire and dragged him from his post-baseball life. Two months before, McGwire was a can't-miss Hall of Famer. Now, however, his ultimate fate into baseball immortality could be determined by his testimony before Congress. On the golf course, though, accolades from his achievements in baseball still chased McGwire. On April 13, he was scheduled to return to Oakland and be enshrined into the Bay Area Sports Hall of Fame. With a list including tennis icon John McEnroe and mobile quarterback Steve Young, McGwire would be the first member of the late 1980s and early '90s Oakland A's juggernaut to be inducted.

Still, he rarely answered questions about his playing career and distanced himself from baseball. While he earned a lavish lifestyle and gained unrivaled fame from playing, he quietly shoved the sport behind him when he retired. But his past would haunt him.

Fueling his disgust was that his one-time home-run accomplice Canseco authored this fuss. Nervously sipping on bottled water, he waited.

Seconds later, the tension thickened with unease, especially for fans that had revered the once-celebrated duo over the years. Canseco, who had been assigned a room separate from McGwire before the hearing, finally emerged, glaring directly at his seat. Canseco remained an intimidating figure. With tree-trunk arms his sleeves could barely contain, anything less than a beefed-up build for Canseco, playing or retired, was unacceptable for him. After the committee had denied immunity to him, Canseco and his attorney, Robert Saunooke, would nurse each word spoken under oath before Congress.

With only Baltimore Orioles' slugger Sammy Sosa and his attorney lodged between them, for both former superstars, bracing themselves for the dicey moments ahead stirred more discomfort than dodging a sizzling fastball from Nolan Ryan. But sitting before the committee had also kindled a cluster of tangled emotions. This appearance marked the first time since 1997 they had headlined the same lineup, sort to speak. Both, however, flexed different agendas. For McGwire: a rumored past he hoped to escape. For Canseco: a conspiracy he wished to expose.

"Watching them before Congress took me back to when I was an innocent kid and rooted for the A's," recalled Johnny Estrada, a major league catcher who grew up in the Bay Area and idolized the Bash Brothers during the 1980s. "As much as you don't want to believe it, you kind of take a step back and realize they probably were cheating at the time. Not only did they cheat baseball and themselves, they cheated all the innocent little kids like myself. José Canseco and Mark McGwire were my heroes, and even though I'm a grown man, it hurt to watch that." Said A's traveling secretary Mickey Morabito:

> It was painful to watch. And it was sad that they didn't even talk to each other. They were two great teammates; and it was clear that they were never going to be friends or talk to each other again. We had these great years of success and they were both tied at the hip with the "Bash Brothers" thing. Seeing how things were then, and how things are now, bothers me. It's sad.

The mood intensified when committee chairman Tom Davis asked Canseco, "Do you solemnly swear the testimony you're about to give to be the truth, the whole truth, and nothing but the truth?" Canseco, who had lifted up his right arm as he was sworn in, confidently replied, "I do." After sitting down, he grabbed his prepared statement and spoke to the committee.

> My name is José Canseco, and for seventeen years I played professional baseball. . . . Never in my wildest dreams could I have imagined

that my athletic ability and love for America's game would lead me to this place . . .

When I decided to write my life's story I was aware that what I revealed about myself and the game I played for the majority of my life would create a stir in the athletic world. . . . Today, I commit myself to doing everything possible to assist them in conveying to the youth of America the dangers of using steroids will bring . . .

Minutes later, McGwire fastened his eyeglasses, clutched his statement, and, after four years of silence, spoke to the committee.

My name is Mark McGwire, and I played the game of baseball since I was nine years old. I was privileged to be able to play fifteen years in the major leagues; even having the honor of representing my country in the 1984 Olympic baseball team . . .

When McGwire began addressing parents who had lost children victimized by steroid use, he battled for his composure. He paused. Only he knew what inner demons he was wrestling.

There's been a problem with steroid use in baseball. Like any sport, where there's pressure to perform at the highest level, and there has been no testing to control performance-enhancing drugs, problems will develop. It's a problem that needs to be addressed.

McGwire, fighting back tears only he could direct blame on, continued:

What I will not do, however, is participate in naming names and implicating my friends and teammates. I retired from baseball four years ago. I live a quiet life with my wife and children. I have always been a team player. I never been a player who would spread rumors or said things about teammates that could hurt them . . .

Asking me, or any other player, to answer questions about who took steroids in front of television cameras will not solve this problem. If he says no, he simply will not be believed. If he says yes, he risks public scorn and endless government investigations.

Sitting to his left, a fragile Sammy Sosa lingered. Sosa, who months before had been ejected from a game when umpires discovered he was using a corked bat, had taken a public relations beating. That led many to question his power surge. Having spit out three sixty-home-run seasons, he did things the right way, according to Sosa. He tried to convey those feelings to Congress.

Through his prepared statement offered by his attorney, Jim Sharp, he claimed he had never taken "illegal performance enhancing drugs." Aside from his denial, though, his sudden ignorance of the English language troubled some. "Believe me, Sosa knows English," explained a former major league employee. Former Major League Baseball commissioner Fay Vincent, too, noticed that Sosa was out of his element. "Sosa looked very uncomfortable."

In the on-deck circle, Rafael Palmeiro appeared as flawlessly poised as his effortless swing at the plate. Palmeiro, an active player whose twenty-year career exuded a harmonious combination of masterful hitting and an uncanny ability to spray home runs to all fields, had been marred by Canseco's allegations. Hoping to eliminate question marks enveloping his 551 career home runs, he convincingly wagged his index finger toward the committee and pleaded his case. "Let me start by telling you this: I have never used steroids. Period," stressed Palmeiro. "I do not know how to say it any more clearly than that. Never."

By that time, however, many zoomed in on the evolution of his career, one punctuated by Canseco's guidance. Only after Canseco strolled into the Rangers' clubhouse in September 1992 did Palmeiro's career production resemble Willie Mays and Frank Robinson.

The only pitcher on the panel, Curt Schilling, was the next speaker. The one-time outspoken trumpet of how steroids littered the game had since conveniently softened his stance. In 2002, he rambled to *Sports Illustrated* that, "I'll pat guys on the ass, and they'll look at me and go, 'Don't hit me there, man. It hurts.' That's because that's where they shoot the steroid needles."[4] Those frank and revealing remarks convinced Congress to subpoena him. This time, however, he backtracked on his comments he made to the periodical and claimed he had dramatically inflated the crisis. Schilling, who also sprayed venom toward Canseco across the room, admitted:

> I hope the committee recognizes the danger of possibly glorifying the so-called author scheduled to testify today or by indirectly assisting him to sell more books through his claim that what he is doing is somehow good for this country or the game of baseball. . . . The issue was grossly overstated by people, including myself. He's a liar.

The game of baseball was out of its element, it seemed. As compelling as each opening statement appeared, more riveting moments seemed ahead. Feeling like scattered chunks of bread surrounded by a swarm of starving seagulls, Canseco and McGwire threatened to evoke the Fifth Amendment when cornered with a self-incriminating inquiry.

Rep. John Sweeney of New York stimulated the hearings by directing a masterfully packaged question aimed at McGwire. Since McGwire had previously acknowledged that he had used the steroid precursor Androstendione while he was breaking the single-season home-run record in 1998, Sweeney delved into what drove him to use the substance.

"How did you get to that point where that [androstendione] was what you were using to prepare yourself to play?" Sweeney inquired.

The baseball world stopped and listened.

"Well sir, I'm not here to talk about the past," McGwire calmly answered. "I'm here to talk about the positive and not the negative about this issue."

Unsatisfied, Sweeney immediately probed deeper. "Were you ever counseled that designer steroids might have the same impact [as real steroids]?" asked Sweeney.

McGwire stubbornly responded, "I'm not here to talk about the past."

After hearing his hollow response, fans across the nation, especially in St. Louis and the San Francisco Bay area, regions where McGwire thrilled and embraced fans for years, felt saddened, betrayed. He had angrily denied using steroids several times before, but now testifying under oath, he dished out no such denials. As his evasive statements smeared his career, they also diminished his chances of entering Cooperstown. Only months before a reporter had asked McGwire which cap would be engraved on his Hall of Fame plaque. He would be eligible in 2007.

"I don't know. I've heard it's up to Cooperstown now. . . . I'll tell you when the times comes," McGwire told him.[5]

His enshrinement may never come, according to Fay Vincent.

"I think he made a big mistake," said Vincent. "His future is really clouded. I don't know that he'll ever get into the Hall of Fame. He just shot himself in the foot."

Three chairs down, Canseco braced for his own grilling. While he had been the most frank panel member, a contradiction in his book loomed. In his statement before the committee, he adamantly damned steroid use unless prescribed by a doctor. He also discouraged youth from using the drug. But *Juiced*, hailed by many reviewers as his "love affair with the chemicals," revealed a mixed message—his fascination with the muscle-building drugs. That troubled several Congress people.

Rep. Elijah Cummings of Maryland confronted Canseco about his conflicting remarks.

"Help me, Mr. Canseco: You sit here for one moment saying you want to do all these wonderful things to prevent it [steroid use] in the future, but you say the absolute opposite in your book?" Cummings asked.

Canseco calmly leaned toward Saunooke seated on his right, seeking legal advice that could safely shape his answer, and replied, "Steroids are only good for certain individuals—not for everyone."

Moments later, McGwire faced the wrath of Cummings. McGwire, who through his attorney had unleashed a stern denial of any steroid use during his career the day Canseco's book was released, mysteriously had been the only panel member, besides Canseco, to exclude such a denial in his opening statement.

"Would you like to comment on that, Mr. McGwire?" asked Cummings.

McGwire shook his head no, and paused.

"Are you taking the fifth?" asked Cummings, cornering the famed slugger.

McGwire awkwardly leaned into the microphone and mumbled:

"I'm not here to discuss the past—I'm here to be positive about this subject."

Five more times throughout the hearing, a pathetic-looking McGwire refused to delve into his past. Dodging an array of crafty inquiries hurled from Congress, McGwire looked like a boxer dancing around the ring and eluding his opponent, desperately trying to weather the match, round by round, until it ended. It seemed that his records meant nothing. "I wish he would have said something," said George Mitterwald, McGwire's first professional manager in Single-A Modesto. "He was such a good guy, whether he did steroids or not, and I'm sure he did. He was retired, so what difference did it make?"

For once, McGwire couldn't satisfy his loyal fans. Even though he survived the gut-wrenching, two-hour inquiry, uttering his now patented, seven-word response, "I'm not here to discuss the past," his passive display sadly slaughtered his image, according to Steve Wilstein. "It was a pitiful performance and no one could believe him after that," said Wilstein, the Associated Press reporter who discovered the infamous bottle of androstendione in McGwire's locker during his thrilling home-run chase in 1998. "He hurt himself and baseball. He handled that about as badly as [Richard] Nixon handled Watergate. It was like watching an American hero disintegrate before our eyes."

The McGwire on Capitol Hill, though, wasn't the real McGwire, said Mickey Morabito. "Knowing the kind of guy he is and the way he was portrayed that day was sad," said Morabito. "But that's the lasting image people took from that [hearing]. It wasn't him."

At that point, however, McGwire mortgaged his past to desperately return to his future.

After chairman Davis finally dismissed the panel, Canseco and McGwire marched out of Capitol Hill treading on separate paths. For Canseco: exploring an acting career in Southern California, where he hoped to generate more headlines. For McGwire: crawling back to his haven, Shady Canyon. Shouldering an era of weighty dumbbells, mysterious supplements, and revolutionary power before Congress, Canseco and McGwire, the Bash Brothers, will forever be welded as two players who helped inflate baseball, in more ways than one.

"When McGwire, Canseco, and Bo Jackson came into baseball, that was the start of the American League becoming the dominant offensive league," said Merv Rettenmund, the A's former hitting coach from 1989 to 1990. "When those guys started coming in, everyone got bigger. They started it."

With a steroid controversy staining their legacies, McGwire and Canseco headlined the Hall of Fame ballot in 2007. Also featured on the list was Baltimore Orioles' iron man Cal Ripken, Jr., and eight-time batting king Tony Gwynn, a staple for the San Diego Padres. In an era of free agency and players team-hopping in hopes of landing sexy, lucrative contracts, both remarkably played their entire years with one team. That Canseco and McGwire clobbered twice as many home runs (1045) as Ripken and Gwynn (566) didn't sway the Baseball Writers' Association of America. This time, it seemed, heart and hustle overshadowed muscle and power. They voted Ripken and Gwynn into the Hall of Fame.

Most voters, though, shunned McGwire. Hailed as the first Hall of Fame class of the steroid era, he received 128 of the 545 votes— 281 votes short of the 409 needed for enshrinement. Canseco received only six. Perhaps the most piercing quote that best described McGwire's lockout from the Hall of Fame came from Hall of Fame member, baseball writer Hal McCoy of the *Dayton Daily News*. "He doesn't want to talk about the past? Then I don't want to consider his past," said McCoy.

McGwire's next year of eligibility, in 2008, didn't soften most voters' stance. He received fewer votes. And as Canseco continues to fire off more names of players he says doctored their careers and with McGwire's unofficial ban from the Hall of Fame, the Bash Brothers might have helped end the Steroid Era, too.

They were two players whose impacts echoed beyond Oakland.

NOTES
[1] Wright Thompson, "Fading Away," ESPN.com.
[2] Randy Youngman, "McGwire Hit on Golf Course," *Orange County Register*, December 18, 2003.
[3] T.J. Quinn, "McGwire Back in the Swing," *New York Daily News*, December 2003.

4 Tom Verducci, "Totally Juiced," *Sports Illustrated*, June 3, 2002.
5 Joe Ostermeier, "Mac Content," *Belleville News-Democrat*, April 18, 2004.

BIBLIOGRAPHY

Canseco, Jose, *Juiced: Wild Times, Rampant 'Roids, Smash Hits, And How Baseball Got Big.* Regan Books, 2005

Canseco, José, and Dave McKay, *Strength Training for Baseball.* Perigee Books, 1990

Rains, Rob and Mark McGwire, *Home Run Hero.* St. Martin's Press, 1999

INTERVIEWS

Darrel Akerfelds
Sandy Alderson
Jay Alves
Howard Ashlock
Mike Ashman
Leon Baham
Ron Barr
Bill Bathe
Mark Bellhorn
Tim Birtsas
Stanley Brand
Luis Brande
Bruce Buschel
Rick Burleson
David Bush
Greg Cadaret
Tom Carroll
Bob Christofferson
Dave Collins
John Costacos
Rocky Coyle
Ron Cummings

Mike Davis
Rick Davis
Storm Davis
Rod Dedeaux
Jorge Díaz
Glenn Dickey
Andy Dolich
Kirk Dressendorfer
Dennis Eckersley
Roy Eisenhardt
Johnny Estrada
David Fletcher
Susan Fornoff
Steve Friend
Grady Fuson
Bud Geracie
Steve Gokey
Ben Grieve
Brian Guinn
Cynthia Hart
Jack Helber
Dave Henderson

Fred Herman
John Hickey
Rick Honeycutt
Art Howe
Bruce Jenkins
Doug Jennings
Stephen Johnson
Jon Kanter
Dan Kiser
Ron Kroichick
Karl Kuehl
Rene Lachemann
Carney Lansford
Scott Larson
Vance Law
Keith Lieppman
Dick Lobdell
Val Lopez
David Marin
Dennis Mattingly
Bob Mayes
Art Mazmanian
Anna McCarter
Charles McCool
Dave McKay
Joe McIlvaine
Bob Milano
Don Mincher
George Mitterwald
Jackie Moore
Mickey Morabito
Dwayne Murphy
Stan Naccarato
Mack Newton

Steve Ontiveros
Greg Papa
Dave Parker
Camilo Pascual
Amaury Pi-Gonzales
Pamela Pitts
Ted Polakowski
Monte Poole
John Pruett
Merv Rettemund
Randy Robertson
Ted Robinson
Dennis Rogers
David Sharp
Lon Simmons
Phil Smith
Terry Steinbach
Carl Steward
Wright Thompson
José Tolentino
Steven Travers
Ron Vaughn
Fay Vincent
Steve Vucinich
Bob Watson
Dave Weatherman
Bob Welch
Curt Wenzlaff
Darlene Westley
Dick Wiencek
Dave Wilder
Steve Wilstein
Michael Zagaris
Ron Zolo

NEWSPAPERS AND PERIODICALS
Arizona Republic
Associated Press
Boston Globe
Boston Herald
Contra Costa Times
Daily Trojan
Dallas Morning News

Detroit Free Press
Globe And Mail
Huntsville Times
Junior Baseball Magazine
Kansas City Star
Long Beach Press-Telegram
Los Angeles Daily News
Macleans
Miami Herald
Minneapolis-St. Paul Star Tribune
New York Daily News
Oakland Tribune
Orange County Register
Oregonian
People
Sacramento Bee
San Diego Tribune
San Francisco Chronicle
San Jose Mercury News
Santa Rosa Press Democrat
Seattle Times
Sports Illustrated
USA Today
USA Weekend
Washington Post
Wichita Eagle

WEBSITES
http://www.espn.com/
http://www.baseball-reference.com
http://www.baseball-almanac.com/
http://www.baseball-almanac.com/
http://www.retrosheet.org/
http://ccclib.org
http://pressbox.mlb.com
http://www.lexisnexus.com/
http://www.cubanball.com/
http://www.bradmangin.com
http://www.mlb.com

INDEX

THE AUTHOR

Dale Tafoya has interviewed professional athletes, celebrities, and religious leaders for more than a decade. He attended Chabot College in Hayward, California, where he studied mass communications, literature, and journalism. His piece, "A Different Kind of Injection," captured Northen California's Best Sports Feature Story by the Journalism Association of Community Colleges in 2004. His article was later named Honorable Mention in state competitions. In 1997, he began his career in journalism as an intern for San Francisco's KFRC 610 AM, where he assisted radio personalities and interviewed several Oakland A's players. His passion for baseball and fascination with writing helped launch him into the world of publishing. Tafoya lives in the San Francisco Bay Area.